Psychotherapy for Children with Bipolar and Depressive Disorders

Psychotherapy for Children with Bipolar and Depressive Disorders

Mary A. Fristad
Jill S. Goldberg Arnold
Jarrod M. Leffler

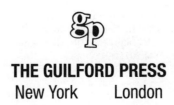

THE GUILFORD PRESS
New York   London

© 2011 The Guilford Press
A Division of Guilford Publications, Inc.
72 Spring Street, New York, NY 10012
www.guilford.com

Printed in the United States of America

This book is printed on acid-free paper.

Last digit is print number: 9 8 7 6 5 4 3 2 1

The authors have checked with sources believed to be reliable in their efforts to provide
information that is complete and generally in accord with the standards of practice that are
accepted at the time of publication. However, in view of the possibility of human error or changes
in behavioral, mental health, or medical sciences, neither the authors, nor the editor and
publisher, nor any other party who has been involved in the preparation or publication of this
work warrants that the information contained herein is in every respect accurate or complete,
and they are not responsible for any errors or omissions or the results obtained from the use of
such information. Readers are encouraged to confirm the information contained in this book
with other sources.

Library of Congress Cataloging-in-Publication Data

Fristad, Mary A.
   Psychotherapy for children with bipolar and depressive disorders / Mary A. Fristad,
Jill S. Goldberg Arnold, Jarrod M. Leffler.
       p. ; cm.
   Includes bibliographical references and index.
   ISBN 978-1-60918-201-4 (pbk.: alk. paper)
   1. Manic-depressive illness in children.   2. Depression in children.
3. Psychotherapy.   I. Goldberg-Arnold, Jill S.   II. Leffler, Jarrod M.   III. Title.
   [DNLM: 1. Bipolar Disorder—therapy.   2. Depressive Disorder—therapy.
3. Child.   4. Psychotherapy—methods.   WM 207]
   RJ506.D4F754 2011
   618.92′8527—dc22
                                                                    2011007928

About the Authors

Mary A. Fristad, PhD, ABPP, is Professor of Psychiatry, Psychology, and Human Nutrition at The Ohio State University. She is also Associate Chair for Academic Affairs in the Department of Psychiatry, as well as Director of Research and Psychological Services in the Division of Child and Adolescent Psychiatry. Dr. Fristad's area of specialty is childhood mood disorders; she is board-certified both in clinical psychology and in clinical child and adolescent psychology. She has published over 150 articles and book chapters addressing the assessment and treatment of childhood-onset depression, suicidality, and bipolar spectrum disorders. She is a coauthor of two books for professionals (*Clinical Manual for Management of Bipolar Disorder in Children and Adolescents* and *Childhood Mental Health Disorders*) and one for families (*Raising a Moody Child*). Dr. Fristad has served on or chaired many National Institute of Mental Health review committees as well as two American Psychological Association (APA) task forces. She has been President of the Executive Board for the Society of Clinical Child and Adolescent Psychology (APA Division 53) and serves on the boards of directors for four web-based education and support groups for children and families with mood disorders. Dr. Fristad has been the principal or coprincipal investigator on over two dozen federal, state, and local grants focused on assessment and treatment of mood disorders in children.

Jill S. Goldberg Arnold, PhD, maintains a private practice in the Boston area, where she specializes in childhood mood disorders. Before moving to the East Coast, she was Clinical Assistant Professor of Psychiatry at The Ohio State University. Dr. Goldberg Arnold has collaborated on both state- and federally funded research projects examining the impact of psychoeducational psychotherapy on families of children with mood disorders. She has multiple publications in the area of childhood mood disorders and, with Mary A. Fristad, coauthored *Raising a Moody Child*.

Jarrod M. Leffler, PhD, ABPP, is Director of Outpatient Group Therapy Programming and Associate Director of the Clinical Child Internship Program at Nationwide Children's Hospital in Columbus, Ohio. He is also Clinical Assistant Professor of Psychiatry at The Ohio State University. Dr. Leffler's research and clinical interests include the assessment, diagnosis, and treatment of bipolar spectrum disorders in youth; group therapy; treatment outcome; service utilization; supervision; and program development, implementation, and evaluation. He has worked on state- and federally funded grants, provided numerous presentations and trainings, and written several articles and book chapters. Dr. Leffler has trained multidisciplinary mental health professionals to implement and evaluate evidence-based treatment and assessment methods, and provides ongoing clinical supervision to trainees and staff. He has also developed a sustainable clinical and financial strategy for providing group therapy in community mental health settings.

Contents

PART III.   Child and Parent Handouts and Group Game Materials

List of Child and Parent Handouts by Chapter

Chapter 7. Teaching Children How to Separate Symptoms from Self and How Treatment Helps Symptoms

Chapter 8. Discussing Medication with Parents

Chapter 9. Discussing Healthy Habits with Children

Chapter 10. Teaching Parents about Systems: Mental Health and School Teams

Chapter 11. The Child's Tool Kit for Coping with Difficult Feelings

Chapter 12. Discussing Negative Family Cycles and Thinking, Feeling, Doing with Parents

Chapter 13. Thinking, Feeling, Doing with Children

Chapter 14. Problem-Solving and Basic Coping Skills for Parents

Chapter 15. Problem-Solving Skills for Children

Chapter 17. The Communication Cycle and Nonverbal Communication Skills for Children

Chapter 18. Communication Skills for Parents

Chapter 19. Verbal Communication Skills for Children

Chapter 22. Wrapping Up with Parents and Children

List of Group Game Materials by MF-PEP Child Session

Session 6

Session 8

PART I

Mood Disorders in Children and How Psychoeducational Psychotherapy Helps

Chapter 1

The Challenge of Treating Children with Mood Disorders

For all of us as therapists, work with children who have with complicated depression or bipolar spectrum disorders (BSD) can be confusing, difficult, and—most of all—humbling. These children push us to be at our very best, and yet very little research has been available until recently to help us determine what "our very best" is. Psychoeducational psychotherapy (PEP) is an evidence-based psychosocial intervention developed by Mary A. Fristad and her colleagues for children ages 8–12 with BSD or depression. The culmination of 25-plus years of clinical experience and research, PEP is an important part of an overall treatment program for these children and their families. This book is a PEP "how-to" guide for clinicians who are looking for a unique and empirically supported way of treating children with BSD or depressive disorders and their families. This book will provide the necessary tools to help such children and families.

What Is PEP?

PEP is the only evidence-based treatment designed for preadolescent children with BSD or complicated depression—the very children clinicians often struggle to treat. PEP combines psychoeducation with elements of family therapy and cognitive-behavioral therapy (CBT). The psychoeducational components give parents and children information about these disorders, as well as how they are diagnosed, treated, and managed. It starts with the basics—offering clear information about the symptoms and diagnosing of mood disorders, along with information about comorbid conditions and other factors that significantly complicate diagnosis. BSD and depression are biological illnesses, but their course is influenced by life stresses, family environment, and daily events. Thus children with these disorders need a wide range of interventions: biological, psychological, educational, and social. Therefore, PEP also provides information about these different types of treatment and gives parents guidelines for establishing a mental health treatment team. Given the challenges inherent in supporting children with mood disorders at school, PEP also provides parents with a better understanding of how school systems work for special-needs children and how to develop and then work effectively with their child's school team.

This psychoeducation is coupled with CBT and other psychotherapeutic exercises practiced during and between PEP sessions. Children learn specific techniques to help them identify and manage difficult moods. Parents, as well as children, learn coping skills such as problem solving, better communication, crisis management, and ways to recognize and prevent or change negative family cycles. In sum, PEP provides information, support, and skills to children, their parents, their siblings, and other caretakers to enable them to manage these lifelong and often debilitating illnesses. Education, support, and new skills lead to better understanding, which in turn leads to better treatment, less family conflict, and ultimately a better outcome. The knowledge that families gain through PEP is only the beginning, and the skills they gain provide a starting point. PEP is designed to help the whole family approach these disorders in a new way—as chronic biological illnesses with a waxing and waning course that typically requires careful medication as well as a problem-solving focus. The skills taught through PEP build resiliency for the whole family.

How This Book Is Organized

Part I of this book offers background information on mood disorders in children, the treatment of these disorders, and practical considerations for implementing PEP. The rest of the present chapter describes the state of our knowledge about psychosocial treatments for children with mood disorders and compares PEP with other such treatments. The chapter concludes with a more detailed overview of PEP. The next three chapters in Part I provide the foundation for incorporating PEP into the treatment of these children and their families. Keep in mind that in order for you to teach families what they need to know about pediatric mood disorders, you will need a strong background in this area. Chapter 2 covers current scientific knowledge about mood disorders in children—the basis of the psychoeducation offered in PEP. Chapter 3 provides more practical details about conducting PEP in either a 20- to 24-week individual-family format (IF-PEP) or an 8-week multifamily group format (MF-PEP). Chapter 4 describes the complexities of diagnosing mood disorders in children.

Part II of this book (Chapters 5–22) provides you with the "nuts-and-bolts" information you need to conduct each PEP session—whether it is with an individual family or with a multifamily group of parents and a group of their children. In IF-PEP, sessions with the child alternate with those for the parents. The chapters in Part II follow the IF-PEP format, with alternating child and parent sessions. In MF-PEP, as explained in more detail in Chapter 3, a group for parents meets separately but (ideally) at the same time as the children's group.

Both formats make use of informational handouts and worksheets, to enable children and parents to practice new skills in session and to reinforce learning through between-session assignments. Part III of this book contains all handouts needed to conduct sessions; these materials may be reproduced and shared with families as needed.

It also includes reproducible materials for group games in MF-PEP. We turn next to an overview of empirically supported psychosocial treatments for mood disorders in children.

Evidence-Based Psychosocial Treatments for Depression in Children

Empirically supported psychosocial treatments are critical approaches for mild to moderate childhood depression, as well as important adjunctive treatments for more severe juvenile depression and BSD. Again, these are biological illnesses that are strongly influenced by psychosocial events (Post & Miklowitz, 2010).

Psychosocial treatments for depression include interventions targeting children at risk for depression (usually in a school-based group format) and therapy for youth diagnosed with depression and their families (in clinic-based group or family formats). The group interventions are based in CBT theory. Most groups include components addressing negative cognitions, negative explanatory style, relaxation, problem solving, coping strategies, positive activity scheduling, communication, and psychoeducation (Asarnow, Scott, & Mintz, 2002; David-Ferdon & Kaslow, 2008; Gillham, Hamilton, et al., 2006; Gillham et al., 2007; Gillham, Reivich, et al., 2006; Pfeffer, Jiang, Kakuma, & Metsch, 2002; Stark, Reynolds, & Kaslow, 1987; Stark et al., 2006; Weisz, Thurber, Sweeney, Proffitt, LeGagnoux, 1997; Yu & Seligman, 2002). The interventions seek to challenge negative cognitions about oneself, situations, other people's intentions, and the future (Abela & Hankin, 2008). Psychoeducational components of group programs teach about identifying feelings and negative thoughts; the relations among thoughts, feelings, and actions; and ways to regulate emotional reactions. These psychoeducational components are closely linked with cognitive strategies.

Studies have found that CBT psychodynamic, and interpersonal approaches to family therapy were effective for children at risk for depression (David-Ferdon & Kaslow, 2008). CBT with families targets many of the same topics covered in group models, with emphases on improving family communication and problem solving and on providing psychoeducation about depression to families (Kovacs et al., 2006; Nelson, Barnard, & Cain, 2003). Psychodynamic psychotherapy focuses on understanding the impact of early experiences on parents and parenting practices, recognizing a child's defensive style, and identifying dysfunctional attachments (Muratori, Picchi, Bruni, Patarnello, & Romagnoli, 2003; Trowell et al., 2007). Tompson et al. (2007) incorporated CBT and interpersonal approaches into a family-based treatment that decreased depressive symptoms and behavior problems. This study did not have a control group, however; thus the efficacy of the combined intervention remains uncertain.

Research on psychotherapeutic strategies for childhood depression supports several group interventions, including school-based CBT programs; a variety of theoretically diverse clinic-based interventions; and individual/family clinic-based interventions from psychodynamic, systems, stress–coping, and CBT perspectives. However, group therapy is not always available. No individual or family-based intervention for childhood depression has the support of a randomized controlled trial (RCT) (David-Ferdon & Kaslow, 2008). Practice parameters for treatment of depression in youth developed by the American Academy of Child and Adolescent Psychiatry (AACAP) state that the minimal standard of care should include "psychoeducation, supportive management, and family and school involvement" (Birmaher, Brent, & the AACAP Work Group on Quality Issues, 2007, p. 1510). PEP combines these elements with the CBT techniques that have proven helpful to groups of children in school-based interventions.

Evidence-Based Psychosocial Treatments for BSD in Children

Several groups of researchers have developed and examined psychosocial treatments for BSD in youth. Two groups have focused their efforts on adolescents. First, David Miklowitz and colleagues have developed an approach called family-focused treatment (FFT); this is described in *Bipolar Disorder: A Family-Focused Treatment Approach* (Miklowitz, 2008). Second, Tina Goldstein and colleagues have adapted dialectical behavior therapy and conducted a pilot trial with adolescents diagnosed with bipolar disorder (BD) (Goldstein, Axelson, Birmaher, & Brent, 2007).[1] Results look promising, but this treatment is still experimental. A third approach, child and family-focused CBT (CFF-CBT), is described in Mani Pavuluri's (2008) book, *What Works for Bipolar Kids: Help and Hope for Parents*; it is a therapeutic program for youth with BSD. Finally, we have developed PEP as described for clinicians in this book and for parents in *Raising a Moody Child: How to Cope with Depression and Bipolar Disorder* (Fristad & Goldberg-Arnold, 2004). All of these treatments are family-based and include four main sets of psychoeducational components: (1) They provide information about the etiology, course, prognosis, and treatments for mood disorders; (2) they emphasize that an affected youth is not at fault for his/her illness; (3) they separate the youth from his/her symptoms/diagnosis and minimize stigma; and (4) they stress the importance of both the patient's and family's responsibilities in managing the illness. In our discussion below of evidence-based treatments for BSD, we focus on those developed for preadolescents: CFF-CBT and PEP.

Child- and Family-Focused CBT

CFF-CBT is designed for for children ages 5–17 and their families (Pavuluri et al., 2004). The 12-session CFF-CBT intervention includes sessions with parents alone, children alone, and parents and children together, and is intended as an adjunctive intervention to medication. The treatment is organized around the acronym RAINBOW: Routine; Affect regulation; I can do it!; No negative thoughts and live in the Now; Be a good friend & Balanced lifestyle for parents; Oh, how can we solve the problem?; and Ways to get support.

---

[1]In this book, "bipolar disorder" (BD) generally refers to bipolar I disorder as defined by the American Psychiatric Association (1994), unless otherwise indicated (see especially the discussions of diagnoses in Chapters 4 and 6). "Bipolar spectrum disorders" (BSD), as the term indicates, refers to the entire range of bipolar disorders.

CFF-CBT uses psychoeducational and skill-building approaches to improve the psychosocial factors that affect the course of illness in children with BSD. These factors include "expressed emotion" (EE); stressful life events; and coping, communication, and problem-solving skills. EE refers to the intensity of critical feedback and emotional involvement of the family in the child's illness (Miklowitz, Goldstein, Nuechterlein, Snyder, & Mintz, 1988). Caregivers in families high in EE tend to direct hostility and negative comments toward, and to become emotionally overinvolved with, the affected children. High EE is associated with poorer outcomes in adults with BD (Butzlaff & Hooley, 1998) and in children with depression (Asarnow, Goldstein, Tompson, & Guthrie, 1993). Stressful life events can have a larger impact on affectively dysregulated children. Skills in coping, communication, and problem solving help decrease EE, improve family communication, improve social interactions, and reduce stress. Through psychoeducation and CBT strategies, families learn about the illness and ways to address symptoms. Therapists also offer to educate school personnel and conduct a session with siblings of affected children, focused on helping the sibling understand BSD and develop coping skills.

Psychoeducational Psychotherapy

PEP was tested in children ages 8–12 with mood disorders and their families. However, we have used these techniques clinically with children both younger and older than this age range. As noted earlier, PEP can be delivered in an individual-family format (IF-PEP) or a multifamily group format (MF-PEP). MF-PEP consists of eight weekly 90-minute sessions in which a parents' group and a separate children's group meet (ideally, at the same time). IF-PEP typically consists of 20–24 weekly 50-minute sessions, alternating between parent sessions and child sessions. Like FFT and CFF-CBT, PEP focuses on educating families about the children's illness and its treatment; decreasing EE; and improving symptom management, problem solving, and communication skills. PEP also provides parents with education about how to be effective and active members of a child's treatment team. Coping strategies for issues common to mood disorders—including emotion regulation, problem solving, and communication—are important foci of PEP. Family patterns are explored, along with ways to reduce negative cycles. PEP with individual families includes session time focused on helping children develop healthy eating, sleeping, and exercising habits, in addition to a sibling session when relevant.

Unlike FFT and CFF-CBT, PEP is designed for children with any mood disorder, including depressive disorders (i.e., major depressive disorder [MDD], dysthymic disorder [DD], and depressive disorder not otherwise specified) as well as BSD. This is important, because longitudinal studies suggest that one-quarter to one-half of children with prepubertal-onset depression will eventually develop BPD (Geller, Zimerman, Williams, Bolhofner, & Craney, 2001; Geller, Fox & Clark, 1994; Strober & Carlson, 1982); Therefore, learning about the warning signs of BSD, as well as about treating and coping with these disorders, may decrease delay in getting effective treatment for these children. IF-PEP and MF-PEP have both elicited clear consumer satisfaction from children and parents (Davidson & Fristad, 2008; Fristad, 2006; Goldberg Arnold, Fristad, & Gavazzi, 1999).

Efficacy of MF-PEP

The efficacy of MF-PEP has been demonstrated through a small RCT ($N = 35$) (Fristad, Gavazzi, & Soldano, 1998; Fristad, Goldberg Arnold, & Gavazzi, 2002, 2003; Goldberg Arnold et al., 1999), as well as through a larger RCT of 165 children ages 8–12 diagnosed with depressive disorders or BSD (Fristad, Verducci, Walters, & Young, 2009; Mendenhall, Fristad, & Early, 2009). In the latter study, MF-PEP plus treatment as usual (TAU) ($n = 78$) was compared to a wait-list condition ($n = 87$). Assessments occurred at baseline and at 6, 12, and 18 months. Intervention occurred between baseline and 6 months for the immediate-treatment group and between 12 and 18 months for the wait-list group. PEP was associated with lower Mood Severity Index (MSI) scores (the MSI combines scores from the Young Mania Rating Scale and the Children's Depression Rating Scale—Revised). The wait-list group showed a similar decrease in MSI scores 1 year later after treatment. In conclusion, MF-PEP is associated with improved outcome for children ages 8–12 with major mood disorders.

Given the documented efficacy of PEP, potential mediators of treatment outcome were investigated by Mendenhall et al. (2009). Participation in MF-PEP significantly improved quality of services utilized, which was mediated by parents' beliefs about treatment. Participation in MF-PEP also significantly decreased the severity of children's mood symptoms, which was mediated by quality of services utilized. As intended, MF-PEP appears to help parents become better consumers of the mental health system, leading them to access higher-quality services, which in turn lead to subsequent improvement in children's symptom severity.

Efficacy of IF-PEP

To meet the needs of varying clinical practice settings, an individualized version of MF-PEP (IF-PEP) was developed and tested. The original version of IF-PEP consisted of 16 sessions lasting 50 minutes each. Fifteen sessions dealt with specific issues associated with mood disorders (the same topics as in MF-PEP), while one flexible ("in-the-bank") session could be scheduled as needed for families to deal with crises and/or review previous material.

The efficacy of IF-PEP was tested in a small RCT of 20 children with BSD and their parents (Fristad, 2006). Children's mood improved immediately following treatment, with gains continuing 12 months after treatment. There was a trend toward improved family climate and treatment utilization, but a larger sample size would have been needed to find significance. Consumer evaluations from parents and children were positive.

Following completion of this study, we conducted a review of our treatment program. This review led to an increase in the number of IF-PEP sessions from 16 to 24, thereby matching the amount of therapist–family "face time" for IF-PEP with that for MF-PEP. The expanded IF-PEP includes 20 (vs. 15) content-specific sessions and 4 (vs. 1) flexible ("in-the-bank") sessions, to be used as needed to reinforce learning or manage crises. This is the version of IF-PEP described in detail in Part II of this book. Parent information on mental health services and school services, originally covered in one IF-PEP session, is now covered in two separate sessions; also added is a second child session on developing healthy habits (i.e., sleep, exercise, and eating). A new parent session has been added for meeting with the child's school team; in another new session, siblings meet with the therapist. This expanded version of IF-PEP has been demonstrated to be associated with reduced mood symptoms and improved family climate in children with BD (Leffler, Fristad, & Klaus, 2010), and the session format is generally acceptable to families (Davidson & Fristad, 2008).

Overview of PEP Sessions and Interventions

A fundamental principle of PEP is reflected in its nonblaming motto: "It's not your fault, but it's your challenge!" In PEP, mood disorders are conceptualized as "no-fault" brain disorders with a biological foundation. Acknowledgment that the *cause* of mood disorders is often biological can decrease the blame and guilt parents feel for their children's problems. At the same time, psychosocial influences greatly affect the *course* of illness, which is part of the reason why an intervention like PEP is so important for overall recovery.

PEP not only educates parents and children about mood disorders and treatment, but also gives them tools for managing symptoms, for establishing a treatment team, and for effectively participating on the team. In both formats of PEP, child sessions and parent sessions follow the same general sequence; the topics build on each other as the program progresses. The early sessions are primarily (but not exclusively) psychoeducational, and they provide a foundation for the skills emphasis of later sessions. Take-home projects are assigned at the ends of both parent and child sessions to reinforce learning. Although some projects are primarily for either the parents or the child, several are family projects that require collaboration. These help to shift family interactions in a more positive direction.

The topics of IF-PEP sessions appear in Table 1.1 in their suggested order. The table also lists the corresponding chapter in Part II that covers each session's conduct and content. With one session per week, on average, child sessions alternate with parent sessions over the course of 20–24 weeks. As noted earlier, each session runs 45–50 minutes. There are important parent check-ins at the start and at the end of each child session, but the therapist and child spent most session time alone. The child does not attend parent sessions. IF-PEP offers more sessions and covers some topics not covered (or not covered as thoroughly) in MF-PEP. These include developing healthier habits, a meeting with the child's school team, and a session with siblings.

The topics of MF-PEP sessions appear in Table 1.2 in their suggested sequence along with the corresponding chapters in Part II. Over the course of 8 weeks, a group of children and a separate group of their parents meet (again, ideally at the same time) once a week. Sessions run for 90 minutes each. Parent session content in MF-PEP is generally similar to that in the corresponding IF-PEP sessions. Each children's MF-PEP session, however, includes a period of group games and activities not included in IF-PEP. These games and activities are explained further in Chapter 3.

In both formats of PEP, parents and children learn in their first two sessions about mood disorders, symptoms, and treatments, including medications (see Chapters 5–8).

TABLE 1.1. IF-PEP Session Order and Content

Week	Attendees Session no.	Session topic	Chapter
1	Child[a] Session 1	Mood disorders and symptoms	5
2	Parents Session 1	Mood disorders and symptoms	6
3	Child Session 2	Treatment, including medications	7
4	Parents Session 2	Treatment, including medications	8
5	Child Session 3	Healthy Habits	9
6	Parents Session 3	Mental health services/school services	10
7	Child Session 4	Building a coping Tool Kit	11
8	Parents Session 4	Negative family cycles and Thinking, Feeling, Doing	12
9	Child Session 5	Thinking, Feeling, Doing	13
10	Parents Session 5	Problem solving	14
11	Child Session 6	Problem solving	15
12	Parents Session 6	Revisiting mental health/school issues and services	10
13	Child Session 7	Healthy habits	9
14	Parents Session 7	School issues (meeting with school personnel)	16
15	Child Session 8	Nonverbal communication skills	17
16	Parents Session 8	Improving communication	18
17	Child Session 9	Verbal communication skills	19
18	Parents Session 9	Symptom management	20
19	Siblings	Sibling session	21
20	Child and parents Session 10	Wrap-up/graduation	22
	As needed[b]	In the bank	
	As needed	In the bank	
	As needed	In the bank	
	As needed	In the bank	

[a]Parents attend the beginning and ending of every child session.
[b]Therapists should use their discretion to determine when to hold an "in-the-bank" session, what its content will be, and who will participate. If a previous session's content is repeated, the handouts and projects for that topic should be used.

TABLE 1.2. MF-PEP Session Order and Content

Week	Attendees Session no.	Session topic	Chapter
1	Children[a] Session 1	Feelings and mood symptoms/patterns	5
1	Parents Session 1	Mood disorders and symptoms	6
2	Children Session 2	Treatment, including medications	7
2	Parents Session 2	Treatment, including medications	8
3	Child Session 3	Building a coping Tool Kit	11
3	Parents Session 3	Mental health and school systems	10
4	Children Session 4	Thinking, Feeling, Doing	13
4	Parents Session 4	Negative family cycles	12
5	Children Session 5	Problem solving	15
5	Parents Session 5	Problem solving	14
6	Children Session 6	Nonverbal communication skills	17
6	Parents Session 6	Improving communication	18
7	Children Session 7	Verbal communication skills	19
7	Parents Session 7	Symptom management	20
8	Children and parents Session 8	Wrap-up/graduation	22

[a]Parents and children begin and end every session together.

For children, this is a basic introduction allowing them to understand more about their own specific disorders and symptoms, and helping them to distinguish symptoms from core features of personality. An exercise we call "Naming the Enemy" (see Chapter 7) is an example of what White and Epston (1990, p. 38) have referred to as "externalizing the symptom." This builds on the PEP motto, which is introduced in the first child session: "It's not your fault, but it's your challenge!" Parents receive more in-depth information in their sessions, including discussion of the etiology and course of these illnesses and the role of medication (Chapters 6, 8). Starting in their first and second sessions, parents also learn to chart their child's mood and, if relevant, medication regimen. The Mood Record or Mood–Medication Log is then briefly reviewed at the start of every child session, when parents check in with the therapist. These charts are crucial tools for tracking symptoms and evaluating what does and doesn't work to manage them. Families also collaboratively develop what we call a "Fix-It List" of realistic goals for the time they are in PEP.

Psychoeducation for parents in IF-PEP includes an overview of the types of mental health treatment, the range of professionals who may be on the child's treatment team, and the role of parents as team members (see Chapter 10). It also offers parents information on how school systems allocate services for special-needs children, the range of educational professionals who may be on the child's school team, and ways to build a coalition with the school (Chapters 10 and 16). In MF-PEP, mental health and school teams are discussed in one session.

The first child sessions also begin to teach emotion regulation and coping skills, including CBT. Developmental psychology suggests most children cannot distinguish thoughts, feelings, and actions until they possess metacognitive skills, which typically develop at about age 11 (Grave & Blissett, 2004). However, Vygotsky (1978) argued that a child can learn new skills by "scaffolding," a process by which a parent or therapist teaches the skill, provides input to help the child complete the task, and models or demonstrates the solution (Vygotsky, 1978). Children's understanding can be supported and raised through this social interaction; hence the term "scaffolding." In this way, the connections among thoughts, feelings, and behaviors can be taught to children who have not yet developed solid metacognitive skills (Fristad, Davidson, & Leffler, 2007).

PEP scaffolds cognitive content by teaching basic skills individually during early sessions, continually reinforcing them, and then connecting and building on them during later sessions. Starting with the first session (Chapter 5), children practice identifying their feelings, considering what events triggered those feelings, and rating the feelings' strength. These skills are particularly useful for mood-disordered children, given their emotion-processing deficits (see Chapter 2). Every subsequent child session begins with this brief three-step feelings exercise. As the program progresses, children become better able to recognize their emotions, to determine what triggers them, and to rate their feelings' strength; these are prerequisites for learning when and what kind of emotion regulation skill to use. The first emotion regulation skill, which we call "Belly Breathing," is taught at the end of the first child session. Deep breathing is probably the most universal calming and stress-relieving technique; it can be used any time, anywhere, and by anyone. Two other breathing techniques, "Bubble Breathing" and "Balloon Breathing," are introduced in subsequent sessions, and a breathing technique is practiced at the end of every session. We chose these names for the techniques because using imagery to which children can relate increases the likelihood that they will use the techniques, and therefore increases the likelihood of their success. We refer to them as the "three B's" in PEP. Practice of each breathing technique is assigned as a take-home project.

Better symptom management is a key purpose of two IF-PEP child sessions on developing healthy habits (Chapter 9). Sleep is often problematic for children with mood disorders, and pharmacological treatments for BD in particular are often associated with weight gain. Thus attention to eating and exercise becomes an important part of comprehensive care. Exercise also functions to alleviate depressive symptoms, and so increasing exercise can reduce a child's core symptoms. Children pick the area of greatest concern to them to work on first (selecting from among sleep, eating, and exercise). They revisit healthy habits later in treatment. For children in MF-PEP, there is not a specific session focused on healthy habits, but related concepts are interwoven throughout the various sessions.

The session on building what we call a "Tool Kit" for coping (Chapter 11) builds on a child's previously learned skills. By this point, children should have some ability to identify feelings, including mood symptoms ("mad, sad, bad" feelings) and what events tend to trigger them. Children are next taught to recognize the physical sensations that can signal difficult emotions and to consider how they act in response. Children may not have a choice about how they feel ("It's not your fault ... "), but they do have a choice about how they respond—with either hurtful or helpful actions (" ... but it's your challenge!"). With help from the therapist and family, the child begins to develop a Tool Kit of helpful activities for responding to difficult emotions. Four categories of activity tools are discussed in this session: Creative, Active, Rest and relaxation, and Social (CARS). The breathing techniques taught early in the program can become some of the child's tools in the R category. Children go home after this session with the assignment of putting together a Tool Kit for taking charge of difficult feelings. This kit can be used across settings—at home, in school, or with peers.

The next child session, on what we call "Thinking, Feeling, Doing" (Chapter 13) connects thoughts to feelings and actions. It introduces a child to the idea that hurtful thoughts or actions increase hurtful feelings, and that these all lead to more problems. Changing hurtful thoughts and actions to more helpful ones can alter mood states. The exercise and worksheet on Thinking, Feeling, Doing helps the child see the relationships among a trigger situation and hurtful thoughts, emotions, and actions. Developing and using more helpful thoughts and actions can result in less difficult feelings.

Parents also learn the CBT-based linkage among thoughts, feelings, and actions as a way to begin changing negative family cycles (Chapter 12). With this parent session, the focus shifts from providing information to improving the internal workings of the family. As noted earlier, multiple studies have shown that high EE in families (patterns of critical comments, hostility, and emotional overinvolvement) predicts poorer outcome, and that EE can be changed (see Chapter 2 for a review of research). Joan Asarnow and her colleagues have focused on EE and childhood depression; they have shown that EE rates are higher in families of depressed children than in families of nondepressed children, and that high EE is associated with a more insidious onset of depression (Asarnow et al., 1993).

Helping parents understand negative family cycles is a first step to changing them, reducing EE, and improving family functioning. When parents' efforts fail to help their child feel better, they usually respond with frustration and anger, and may withdraw until guilt fuels further attempts to change the way the child feels. Empathy is crucial in conducting this parent session and in helping parents recognize how this or a similar negative cycle may play out in the family; at the same time, parents are taught that responding differently to the child can improve family interactions. To help parents catch negative interactions as they happen, they are asked to complete the same Thinking, Feeling, Doing exercise given to the child.

The next parent and child sessions (Chapters 14 and 15) each teach basic problem solving. The parent session also covers key coping skills and includes important dos and don'ts for responding to a moody child. The goal for both parents and children is to view mood symptoms and challenging behaviors as problems to be solved by using the basic steps of problem solving. Children learn five steps: "Stop" (take a moment to calm down); "Think" (define the problem and brainstorm strategies); "Plan" (select and plan a strategy to use); "Do" (carry out the strategy); and "Check" (evaluate the outcome and decide on future action). For parents, problem solving is taught as an approach to symptom management and family conflicts. The importance of adequate problem definition is emphasized, and parents learn one additional step (deciding who needs to know about the problem). Parents are also taught to examine pros and cons as a way to pick which possible solution to try.

The parent session (Chapter 10) covering the school system and the child's school team is a useful foundation; however, many parents still struggle with how to work with their child's school. Therefore, in IF-PEP (but not MF-PEP), a meeting is scheduled for the parents, the therapist, and personnel at the child's school to discuss the child's particular school issues (Chapter 16). This is not a typical parent session, and it does not follow the usual session format. The therapist's goal for the meeting is to improve communication between the parents and the school staff. The therapist also assists in the development or enhancement of school services or accommodations. The meeting is typically scheduled after the parents have been taught problem-solving skills; these skills are helpful for planning, as well as during the meeting itself. In preparation, the therapist should help parents define the child's school problems and plan an agenda for the meeting. The parents typically arrange this meeting with school personnel.

Attention next shifts to communication skills and patterns. For children, there are two separate sessions, one for nonverbal communication (Chapter 17) and one for verbal communication (Chapter 19). Research suggests that children with mood disorders have difficulty reading nonverbal cues in others (see Chapter 2 for a summary). Therefore, children first learn about the communication cycle—sending, receiving, responding, and understanding the response. They then learn about the types of nonverbal communication (facial expression, gestures, posture, tone of voice, and personal space). Role play is used to help children practice sending and reading the emotional messages in nonverbal cues. The child session on verbal communication emphasizes ways to stop hurtful words and phrases and to replace them with more helpful expressions, including "I" statements. Parents receive one session on communication (Chapter 18), with an emphasis on making family interactions less stressful. Less daily stress and less EE help to reduce the frequency or severity of the child's symptoms and can significantly improve both child and family functioning. Parents are first counseled on general communication traps to avoid, as well as traps specific to mood disorders. They are then coached on how to communicate effectively with moody children. Next, family members are given the assignment to catch themselves using old, hurtful words, and to develop and use more helpful phrases as replacements.

The final parent-only session (Chapter 20) reinforces the skills learned in previous sessions and helps parents plan for the future regarding suicidal, manic, or other dangerous mood-related behavior. Being a "good enough" parent does not automatically equip one with the skills needed for these situations. This session emphasizes the importance of maintaining a Mood Record or Mood–Medication Log for catching symptoms early to prevent crises, and reviews strategies for managing manic and depressive symptoms. Other issues covered include the need for a safety plan and guidelines for creating one; ways of responding to a child's suicide threats; and times when hospitalization may be needed. Techniques for parent stress management are reviewed.

Not all children with mood disorders have siblings, but when they do, the siblings can struggle under a heavy emotional burden. Sibling issues are an important part of managing a child's mood disorder within a family. When such issues are relevant, a session in IF-PEP is devoted to a meeting of therapist and siblings without the mood-disordered child (Chapter 21). The session allows siblings to speak freely, to voice their own concerns and issues, and to receive age-appropriate information about mood disorders. The therapist then helps siblings raise their issues with parents and facilitates family problem solving in regard to these. There is no sibling session in MF-PEP, but sibling issues are frequently discussed in both the parent and child group sessions.

The final session (Chapter 22) is devoted to a review of material learned over the course of treatment. Warning signs of relapse are reviewed, and transition plans are confirmed. In MF-PEP, a graduation ceremony is held. In some cases, after the end of IF-PEP, families will continue with the therapist for maintenance treatment; in such cases, goals are set and treatment continues.

As noted earlier, IF-PEP provides for four "in-the-bank" sessions to be used as needed at any time during the program. For example, some parents enter the program without a mental health team or school team in place and need additional help to establish them. The child or parents may need an additional session to consolidate such skills as problem solving, changing negative family cycles, making use of the coping Tool Kit, or crisis management.

In the next chapter, we review what current scientific research tells us about childhood mood disorders and their treatment. The information given to parents and children about mood disorders in PEP is based on this research. As also discussed in Chapter 2, many of the skills taught to children in PEP are designed to address cognitive deficits found in youth with mood disorders.

Current Scientific Knowledge about Childhood Mood Disorders

In this chapter, we provide an overview of the current scientific knowledge about the biological (and, to a lesser extent, the psychosocial) underpinnings of childhood mood disorders, as well as evidence-based biological treatments. Awareness of the causes of these disorders is an important component of treatment. You will not need to be an expert on these details to be an excellent PEP therapist, but having a general sense of the "hows" and "whys" of mood disorders will help you convey the complexity of the disorders to your families in treatment. It will also help families appreciate why a biopsychosocial approach to treatment makes so much sense.

Why Mood Disorders Occur

As yet there is no definitive understanding of what causes mood disorders; however, research indicates that genetics plays an important role. Differences in brain structure and cognitive abilities have also been found in those with mood disorders. In this section, we summarize key findings in these areas.

Genetics

Substantial evidence points to a significant genetic role in the development of mood disorders in general and BSD in particular. For example, identical twins are concordant for BD between 40% and 70% of the time; for fraternal twins, the concordance is less than half that rate. Children with a positive family history of BD in first-degree relatives have a 10–20% risk of developing BD, compared to 1% in children without a family history (Craddock & Jones, 1999). In addition, risk seems to be additive or multiplicative, given that when there is a history of BD in first-degree relatives on one side of the family and a history of depression or BD on the other side, the lifetime risk of developing depression or BD rises to 70% (Birmaher et al., 2009). This is probably due to the complicated and multicausal basis of inherited vulnerability combined with environmental influence.

For example, single-nucleotide polymorphisms (SNPs) commonly result from a single-nucleotide variation in DNA that leads to the substitution of a single amino acid in a protein, which is made up of hundreds or thousands of amino acids. It is becoming increasingly likely that many SNPs act as vulnerability or protective factors in the risk for mood disorders, as well as other psychiatric illnesses (Post, 2009). Although, our knowledge about the genetics of mood disorders has grown exponentially over the past decade, we are still a long way from translating it into treatment. Here we briefly review some promising advances in research. For further details, please see Post (2009).

The focus of much research has been genetic vulnerability to stress. For example, brain-derived neurotrophic factor (BDNF) is a substance necessary for neuronal growth and survival and for new synaptic connections critical for long-term learning and memory (Post, 2009). Stress can lead to decreases in BDNF, and BDNF has been shown to be decreased during episodes of depression and mania; greater decreases are associated with more severe episodes (Post, 2007a, 2007b). A significant genetic vulnerability that has been identified involves a single amino acid substitution that has been associated with less efficient functioning of BDNF in cells (the Val66Met allele). This finding has been replicated multiple times in adults with BD. Interestingly, adults who do not have BD but who have this same genetic variation have smaller hippocampal and frontal lobe volumes, as well as minor declarative memory deficits (i.e., problems with memory for specific information, such as lists of words).

The more efficient BDNF allele (the Val66Val allele) has also been associated with BD in general and with the early-onset and rapid-cycling variants of BD in particular, as summarized by Post (2009). The reason for this finding is not entirely clear, but it may be related to findings of increased creativity associated with BD. It is also possible that rapid, pressured speech and expansive thinking are symptoms associated with this variation (Post, 2009).

A clear example of gene–environment interaction has been noted in the area of unipolar depression. There is a common genetic variation in the serotonin transporter (where selective serotonin reuptake inhibitors [SSRIs] act), with a short form and a long form. The short form is less efficient than the long form. Without environmental stress, individuals with both forms have the same risk for depression. With a history of early adversity combined with the presence of current adult stressors, however, individuals with the short form are at twice the risk for the onset of a depressive episode (Caspi et al., 2003; Kaufman et al., 2006). It is likely that many SNPs have a small individual impact on clinical outcome. When they co-occur in the presence of adverse environmental factors, they are likely to play a more significant role in the onset and course of psychiatric illness (Post, 2009).

Neuroanatomical and Cognitive Differences

Although we cannot yet use brain imaging to diagnose mood disorders, researchers have found specific differences in the brains of people with and without mood disorders. For the most part, these brain differences are more pronounced than the differences among individuals with specific mood disorders (Serene, Ashtari, Szeszko, & Kumra, 20007). In the first parent session of PEP, a handout is reviewed that outlines documented brain differences (see Part III, Handout 16). Connections in the brain, and the ways messages are sent between brain structures, differ between children with mood disorders and children with typically developing brains. Once parents understand this, they may find it easier to shift from a child-blaming perspective to a coping perspective. In addition, the basic science findings reviewed with parents support the interventions included in PEP. The therapeutic exercises used throughout PEP are designed to remediate some of the cognitive deficits that correspond to the structural brain deficits associated with having a mood disorder. Below, we describe first the evidence for differences in brain structure and next the differences in cognitive functioning between those with and without mood disorders.

It is important to note that most of the available research has been conducted with adolescents (13–18 years old) rather than with all youth (<18 years old). We still have much to learn about younger developing brains.

TABLE 2.1. Brain Regions and Their Functions

- *Amygdala*—produces fear, rage, and other emotional reactions in response to stimuli in the environment; closely connected with sensory organs; also stores emotional memory

- *Association cortex*—part of the "higher-thinking" brain dedicated to processing certain types of stimuli (e.g., fear-provoking)

- *Dorsal anterior cingulate cortex (dACC)*—monitors interference between top-down reappraisals that neutralize emotions and bottom-up evaluations of emotion-provoking stimuli

- *Limbic system*—a set of structures that serve as basic processors of emotion; includes the amygdala, hippocampus, hypothalamus, and pituitary glands

- *Prefrontal cortex (PFC)*—a combination of smaller regions responsible for a variety of cognitive processes; includes the ability to generate and maintain alternative ways of thinking about emotional stimuli

- *Dorsolateral PFC (DLPFC)*—involved in attention shifting, working memory, response inhibition, and regulation of emotional responses in a context-dependent manner

- *Ventrolateral PFC (VLPFC)*—controls reactions in the peripheral nervous system, endocrine system, and motor system; in other words, controls how the rest of the body reacts to varying stimuli

- *Junction of the DLPFC and VLPFC*—provides information about anticipated and past reward and punishment to guide behavior, and is involved in modulating emotions

- *Medial PFC*—involved in the subjective experience of, and physiological reactions to, internal emotional responses to external stimuli; also involved in inhibiting self-perspective to allow a person to take another's perspective

Neuroanatomical Foundations for Deficits in BD

Recent advances in brain imaging techniques have been used to investigate the anatomical differences associated with skill deficits. Table 2.1 includes a basic explanation of the functions of various brain structures and systems implicated in BD. Below are brain regions associated with deficits in BD.

ASSOCIATION CORTEX

A recent study on facial emotion recognition found that adolescents with BD had less connectivity between the *amygdala* and the temporal lobe *association cortex*, which are involved in processing facial expressions and social stimuli (Rich et al., 2008). In other words, fewer neurons connect the brain structures involved in perception and processing of emotional signals.

PREFRONTAL CORTEX

One function of the *prefrontal cortex* (PFC) is to control emotional responses by decreasing activation of *limbic system* structures (e.g., the amygdala and pituitary gland; see below). In people with BD, the amygdala is more activated and the PFC is less activated in response to emotional stimuli. This indicates that automatic, emotion-focused responses are more highly activated than rational, modulating responses to these stimuli (Green, Cahill, & Malhi, 2007).

Executive functioning deficits appear linked to the ventrolateral PFC (VLPFC), which also has hierarchical control over affect regulation and the integration of affective and cognitive control systems. The VLPFC is less activated in people with BD during emotionally charged situations (Green et al., 2007). An associated area, the dorsal anterior cingulate cortex (dACC), tends to be smaller in people with BD (Green et al., 2007). Together, a less activated VLPFC and a smaller dACC allow the emotion circuitry to be more responsive in people with BD. Thus their physiological reaction to stress is more intense, making ordinary situations feel more like emergencies. Lithium treatment increases the concentration of *N*-acetylaspartate, an indicator of neuronal health, in the VLPFC in adolescents and adults (Marsh, Gerber, & Peterson, 2008). Improving functioning in the VLPFC may be one mechanism by which lithium improves symptoms in people with BD.

The junction of the dorsolateral PFC (DLPFC) and VLPFC is also less activated in people with BD than in nondisordered controls. Thus emotions are not sufficiently modulated, making it more difficult for those with BD to focus on the facts of a problem and think about it rationally. This dysfunction leads to difficulty understanding and appropriately reacting to emotionally laden material in the environment, because youth with BD have difficulty distancing themselves enough from the emotion of a situation to think about it clearly. Likewise, decreased activation in the medial PFC is related to difficulties understanding the perspectives of others and taking them into consideration when making choices about behavior. These problems with executive functioning add to difficulty in inhibiting immediate responses.

LIMBIC SYSTEM

Overall, research suggests that BD is associated with dysregulation in the anterior limbic network, which includes regions of the PFC, several subcortical structures (e.g., thalamus, striatum, amygdala), and the midline cerebellum; all these structures are active in emotion regulation and specific cognitive processes (Adler, DelBello, & Strakowski, 2006). The anterior limbic network perceives and processes emotional stimuli and regulates responses to those stimuli. This dysfunction appears to worsen across time with repeated episodes (Adler et al., 2006). Findings suggest that the emotion-focused parts of the network are more active and the thinking-focused parts of the network are less active in those with BD than in nondisordered controls.

Neuroanatomical Foundations for Deficits in Depression

Less research has been conducted on neuroanatomical bases of depressive spectrum disorders than on BD in youth. Most of these studies are cross-sectional, which does not allow for control of individual differences (Serene et al., 2007).

AMYGDALA

Youth with MDD have lower amygdala volumes; however, the implications for this are not clear from the research to date (Rosso et al., 2005). Lower amygdala volumes may be associated with poor responses to social and emotional situations and to the decreased intensity of emotional reactions noted in MDD (i.e., anhedonia and flat affect).

ANTERIOR CINGULATE CORTEX

Likewise, the ACC has been found to have lower glutamate levels in youth with MDD than in healthy controls (Rosenberg et al., 2005). This may indicate less activity in the ACC, which would lead to increased emotional reactivity to stimuli (Magistretti, Pellerin, Rothman, & Shulman, 1999). Thought-driven reappraisals of the stimuli are suppressed, thus allowing feelings to overwhelm thinking about a situation.

PREFRONTAL CORTEX

The PFC also appears to be different in youth with MDD than in healthy youth. Depressed youth with familial MDD (those who have both MDD and a family history of MDD) have a smaller proportion of frontal lobe volume compared to cerebral volume than healthy controls do (Steingard et al., 1996). Youth with nonfamilial MDD (those who have MDD but no family history of MDD) have a higher PFC volume than healthy controls do (Nolan et al., 2002). These volume differences may indicate dysfunctional development in both groups (Serene et al., 2007).

Cognitive Deficits in BD

Recent research on neurological correlates of pediatric BD provides biological evidence for several of the skill deficits noted in youth with this disorder. Table 2.2 lists impairments found in executive functioning and other cognitive areas. There are significant difficulties in many areas of attention, learning, memory, and other important cognitive skills, as discussed in more detail below.

IQ AND LEARNING DISORDERS

One study (Mayes & Calhoun, 2007) investigated cognitive ability and learning disorders in children with various psychiatric diagnoses. This study found that children with BD had significantly lower IQ scores (mean [*SD*] = 93 [17]; 22% with IQ < 80) than children with attention-deficit/hyperactivity disorder (ADHD) or anxiety/depression (the researchers combined these groups), but not lower than those with disruptive behavior disorders. The IQ scores of children with BD in this sample were not significantly different from those of children with autism, spina bifida, or traumatic brain injury.

Mayes and Calhoun (2007) also found that a majority (79%) of their sample of children with BD had a learning disorder. Disorders of written expression were the most common (74%), but substantial percentages of the children with BD also had reading disorders (28%), mathematics disorders (32%), and significant spelling problems (24%). These global ability measures indicate that children with BD are likely to have difficulty in school. Additional studies have examined specific skills and abilities.

TABLE 2.2. Cognitive Impairments in BD

Impairments in executive functioning
    Sustained attention
    Selective attention
    Inhibitory control
    Cognitive flexibility
    Processing speed
    Working memory

Impairments in other skills
    Verbal fluency
    Verbal learning
    Verbal memory
    Visual–spatial memory
    Problem solving
    Perspective taking

EXECUTIVE FUNCTIONING

A major deficit area shown in people with BD is in "executive functioning," an umbrella term for the planning and self-control processes of the brain, includes the abilities to inhibit impulses, plan, shift attention from one task to another, initiate tasks, use working memory, and maintain goal-directed effort; it also includes metacognition and perspective taking (Riggs, Jahromi, Razza, Dillworth-Bart, & Mueller, 2006). Executive functioning and some of the same neural pathways also appear to be impaired in children with ADHD (Pavuluri & Sweeney, 2008). Although common executive functioning measures assess different aspects of such functioning, the overall picture is one in which children with BD have difficulty stopping their automatic reactions, changing strategies to fit new reward and punishment contingencies, planning globally to facilitate completing a task, and holding several pieces of information in mind at the same time. Each of these abilities is essential not only to academic success, but also to social and interpersonal functioning.

THEORY OF MIND

"Theory of mind" refers to the ability to infer what others are thinking and feeling from their nonverbal and verbal communication. Deficits in this area directly influence social functioning. Schenkel, Marlow-O'Connor, Moss, Sweeney, and Pavuluri (2008) found that children with BD had more difficulty than healthy controls with inferring the true intentions behind subtle actions. Many studies have examined facial emotion processing, and though some find few or no deficits in BD, others have found specific problem areas (see Getz, Shear, & Strakowski, 2003, and Green et al., 2007, for reviews). Youth with BD misinterpret neutral faces as more threatening than control children do (Marsh et al., 2008). They also misinterpret happy, sad, and fearful facial expressions in adults and children; in particular, extremely happy and sad faces are interpreted as only moderately to mildly happy or sad (Pavuluri & Sweeney, 2008).

Cognitive Deficits in Depression

Learning disabilities have been shown to be more common in children hospitalized with major depressive disorder than in the general population (Fristad, Topolosky, Weller, & Weller, 1992). Similarly, children with learning disabilities have, on average, higher scores on depression measures than same-aged peers without learning disabilities (Maag & Reid, 2006). In addition, school performance often deteriorates in children who are depressed; clinical referrals are often initiated by school personnel concerned about a child's decline in academic and social functioning.

Behavioral Manifestations of Deficits in Mood Disorders

Children with mood disorders exhibit numerous difficulties resulting from the brain dysfunctions summarized above. When confronted with an emotionally intense situation, such a child is likely to focus on the emotions rather than the task at hand, possibly misinterpreting the type or intensity of the other person's emotion and making impulsive decisions about how to respond. These neurological findings help explain the "rages" often described by parents of youth with BD in particular, and suggest why consequences do not seem to curb the out-of-control behavior. Increasing awareness of the links among thoughts, feelings, and actions (see Chapter 13) helps children gain control over previously dyscontrolled behavior.

Children with mood disorders will usually benefit from taking a moment to stop and calm down before taking action. This is why PEP teaches these children calming breathing techniques (Chapter 5), and why the first problem-solving step the children learn is "Stop," so they can use these and other Tool Kit strategies to decrease emotional intensity (see Chapters 11 and 15). Teaching these children to generate several possible actions increases their ability to inhibit an impulsive hurtful response. This is the "Think" step of problem solving, as described in Chapter 15.

These children will usually also benefit from coaching in the interpretation of their own and others' emotions, using both nonverbal and verbal cues. Each PEP session begins with having children identify and rate the strength of their feelings and link those feelings to events that have occurred in their lives. The PEP sessions covered in Chapters 17 and 19 provide coaching in sending and receiving nonverbal and verbal communication. Children with BD show compromises in their thinking and feeling circuitry and in the connections between the two (Pavuluri & Sweeney, 2008); thus scaffolding of cognitive concepts, culminating in the Thinking, Feeling, Doing exercise, helps children unite these disparate cognitive processes (see Chapter 13).

Although our knowledge is still in its infancy, research over the past decade has given us a much better understanding of the role of genetics in mood disorders as well as differences in brain structure and cognitive abilities. Knowledge about these differences can only serve to encourage research on interventions for mood disorders—psychopharmacological, nutritional, and psychosocial.

Psychosocial Influences on Course of Illness

The general consensus is that the *causes* of mood disorders are fundamentally biological; however, the *course* of a mood disorder (including onset, duration, offset, and recurrence) is greatly affected by psychosocial events. For instance, Post and Miklowitz (2010) provide a thorough review of the role of stress in the onset, course, and progression of BD and its comorbidities. They review the evidence for how environmental stressors interact with BDNF and other biological factors to affect (1) vulnerability to onset; (2) onset of manic and depressive episodes; (3) onset of, and relapse into, substance abuse; and (4) relapse into manic or depressive episodes. Given the importance of stress in affecting course of illness, teaching children and their parents stress management and other coping skills becomes paramount in the overall treatment of childhood mood disorders (Fristad, 2010).

Abuse History

One stressor that has received considerable attention is physical or sexual abuse. Adults with BD who experienced abuse as children are more likely to have an earlier age of BD onset (Post & Miklowitz, 2010). Multiple pathways may be involved with this link. Children with mood disorders often have parents with mood disorders, as previously noted. If those parents were not well treated, they are at risk for using maladaptive parenting strategies, including physical abuse as punishment. If the parents are hypersexual during manic episodes, they are at greater risk of sexually abusing their children. Conversely, children with mood disorders can be highly demanding and place particular stress on their parents' coping capacity. Thus children at risk for mood disorders are also at elevated risk for abuse.

Blaming and Parental Guilt

In addition to the difficulty of managing symptoms, parents often find it stressful to work with treatment providers who maintain a blaming attitude toward them or who lack fundamental knowledge about childhood mood disorders (Mackinaw-Koons & Fristad, 2004). In fact, this study also documented that providers sometimes know less about symptoms and treatment for depression and BSD than the parents do. In a national online survey, parents named the following as top contributors to their stress levels: isolation, financial strain, guilt, blame, physical illness, worry about the future, care for their high-needs children, advocating for their children at school, and exhaustion (Hellander, Sisson, & Fristad, 2003).

Family Climate and Family Functioning

High degrees of conflict, hostility, intrusive relationships, and lack of warmth are associated with poor outcomes in persons of all ages with mood disorders (see review by Miklowitz & Goldstein, 2010). Conversely, a loving, warm, stable, supportive, and non-blaming family can serve as a protective factor in a child's recovery. Negative family environments can lead to negative child outcomes, including a slower course of recovery, more frequent relapses (Asarnow et al., 1993), and higher rates of child diagnosis (Schwartz, Dorer, Beardslee, Lavori, & Keller, 1990).

It is developmentally normative for children to be dependent on their families. In general, the younger a child, the greater the dependence. Children rely on their parents to provide structure, safety, guidance, and comfort. This has two treatment implications: (1) The younger the child, the greater the influence of family climate on how the mood disorder evolves over time; and (2) interventions must occur at the family level for maximum recovery. In reviewing the treatment literature, Lofthouse and Fristad (2004) identified the following as the bases for effectively improving family climate and child outcomes: information sharing with family members, and parent and child skill development that incorporates training in problem solving and communication. PEP includes all of these components.

Next, we turn to what we know about medications, nutritional interventions, and healthy habits.

Current Knowledge about Medications for Mood Disorders

The decision to give medication to a child with a mood disorder raises complicated issues. It is particularly important for clinicians to understand these issues, so that they can guide parents through this very difficult set of decisions. (See Chapter 8 for the PEP session on helping parents understand medications for children and evaluate the pros and cons of embarking on medication trials.) One of the biggest challenges for clinicians, particularly prescribing clinicians, is that although they are constantly learning about which medications work, there is still much they do not know.

Medication can be especially helpful in moderate to severe depression and in BD. Medication can reduce acute distress from severe symptoms and stabilize mood, thus enabling children to benefit from psychosocial interventions such as coping, problem solving, and communication. Medications can also reduce risk for future episodes or decrease their intensity and the associated impairment. However, medication does not solve every problem or completely alleviate mood symptoms in most youth (Kowatch et al., 2005). Most medications will also produce side effects ranging in severity from mildly annoying (e.g., increased thirst/urination, increased skin sensitivity) to moderate (e.g., excessive weight gain, impaired sleep) to life-threatening (e.g., Stevens–Johnson syndrome, liver damage).

In addition, most research on the effectiveness of medication for mood disorders has been conducted with adults. We cannot assume that children and adolescents will obtain the same results as adults from medication. This lesson became obvious when research revealed that several antidepressants found to be efficacious in adults did not improve children's mood (Birmaher et al., 2007), and that some antidepressants were related to increased suicidal ideation (Bridge et al., 2007). Many clinical trials testing the efficacy of psychotropic medications in children are underway, but current knowledge remains limited. The information about medications provided to families in PEP is not meant to dictate what should be prescribed for a particular child. It is meant to educate parents on how to be active participants in medication management, how to understand the target symptoms for which medications are prescribed, and how to manage side effects. Knowing what to expect from the medication and keeping careful Mood–Medication Logs can help parents use appointments with their children's prescribers more effectively. The goal is to empower, not overwhelm, children and parents.

Here we review what we do know about medication, so that in your clinical work you will be equipped to help parents make educated decisions. For more detailed information, a good resource is the *Clinical Manual for Management of Bipolar Disorder in Children and Adolescents* (Kowatch, Fristad, Findling, & Post, 2009).

Antidepressant Medications

PEP provides general information about the medications frequently prescribed for the treatment of mood disorders in children. Only fluoxetine (Prozac) is approved by the U.S. Food and Drug Administration (FDA) for treatment of child and adolescent depression (U.S. FDA, 2004), but several other SSRIs and other classes of antidepressants are prescribed for child and adolescent depression, based on the research support for effectiveness in adults (Birmaher et al., 2007). All antidepressants prescribed in the United States must carry warnings that they may increase suicidal ideation or behavior in persons up to age 25 (U.S. FDA, 2004). It may be helpful to explain to parents that the risk of suicide can increase when youth start to have more energy but still have low mood. In fact, many of the antidepressants take a few weeks to make a significant impact on mood, although physical symptoms (e.g., energy level, appetite, sleep) respond more quickly (Kramer, 2004). A child who has had suicidal ideation but has been too fatigued and lethargic to act on it may now have the energy to act while still in a dysphoric mood or feeling hopeless. Members of the treatment team need to carefully monitor children's suicidality, especially in the first 2 months of treatment (Birmaher et al., 2007). Likewise, parents benefit from learning that asking their children about suicidal ideation will not inspire it. Studies have shown that inquiring about suicidal ideation does not increase the risk of its occurring (Gould et al., 2005; Herjanic, Hudson, & Kotloff, 1976).

Mood-Stabilizing Medications

For children and adolescents with classic manic symptoms (i.e., episodes of persistently and unusually elevated mood for a period of 1 week or more), mood-stabilizing medication is usually a primary treatment strategy (Kowatch, 2009a; Kowatch et al., 2005). Lithium is FDA-approved for use in children age 12 or older for acute mania and maintenance therapy. Valproate (Depakote) has some support for its use in children and adolescents, as well as adults (Kowatch, Strawn, & DelBello, 2010), although side effects are common and there is particular concern about development of polycystic ovarian syndrome in females. Carbamazepine (Tegretol, etc.) is not recommended as a first-line agent, and it has multiple drug–drug interaction problems that interfere with its use (Kowatch et al., 2010).

Atypical antipsychotics have received much attention in recent years (Kowatch, 2009b). A handful of clinical trials have led to U.S. FDA approval of risperidone (Risperdal), aripiprazole (Abilify), olanzapine (Zyprexa), ziprasidone (Geodon), and quetiapine (Seroquel) in the treatment of manic symptoms in children ages 10–17 (Kowatch et al., 2010). However, all the atypical antipsychotics carry with them varying degrees of risk for a wide variety of significant side effects, including drug-induced parkinsonism, akathisia, tardive dyskinesia, neuroleptic malignant syndrome, excessive weight gain, hyperlipidemia, increased prolactin levels, and cardiac QTc changes.

Other medications include lamotrigine (Lamictal), which has promising open-label results but no RCT data; gabapentin (Neurontin), which may be beneficial in treating comorbid anxiety but does not have evidence for antimanic properties; topiramate (Topamax), which has inconclusive results from an adolescent study discontinued when adult studies had negative findings; and oxcarbazepine (Trileptal), which has one negative RCT (Kowatch et al., 2010).

One goal of PEP is to help parents understand that the trial-and-error nature of the medication process is due to our still-developing knowledge about mood medications, and not an indication of incompetence on the part of their prescribing doctor. This understanding often helps parents to be more patient and to cooperate more effectively with the physician as medication trials are conducted.

Other Psychotropic Medications

Other psychotropic medications are also discussed with parents. Antihypertensives (e.g., clonidine [Catapres], guanfacine [Tenex]) are typically used to decrease agitation or assist with sleep (Campbell & Cueva, 1995; Ming, Gordon, Kang, & Wagner, 2008; Schnoes, Kuhn, Workman, & Ellis, 2006). However, there is some possibility that Tenex can precipitate hypomanic and manic symptoms, according to a small anecdotal study by Horrigan and Barnhill (1999).

Medications for ADHD, including stimulants (e.g., lisdexamfetamine [Vyvanse], methylphenidate [Ritalin, Concerta], dexmethylphenidate [Focalin], amphetamine plus dextroamphetamine [Adderall]) and one nonstimulant (i.e. atomoxetine [Strattera]), are sometimes prescribed for children with mood disorders who also have ADHD symptoms (Pliszka & the AACAP Work Group on Quality Issues, 2007). As previously discussed, mood disorders are often comorbid with behavior and anxiety disorders; thus parents can benefit from knowledge about medications to treat these other conditions.

In sum, medication has the potential to provide some relief for children with mood disorders, but no study has demonstrated robust response to medication. In addition, side effects are problematic for many children who take psychotropic medication. It is important for families to understand that medication can play a role in recovery, but that child- and family-based strategies are critical for a good outcome.

Current Knowledge about Nutritional Interventions

Nutritional deficiencies have been tied to a variety of notable psychological problems, and nutritional supplements have recently been linked to a wide range of health improvements, ranging from neuronal development to decreased depression (Hibbeln, 1998; Noaghiul & Hibbeln, 2003). Early clinical trials in adults and children show promise for nutritional supplements in the treatment of mood disorders. Multinutrient supplements and omega-3 fatty acids have been examined.

EMPowerplus (EMP+) is a multinutrient supplement containing 14 vitamins, 16 minerals, 3 amino acids, and 3 antioxidants. It has been shown to reduce manic symptoms in adults with BSD in open-label trials (Kaplan, Crawford, Gardner, & Farrelly, 2002;

Kaplan et al., 2001; Simmons, 2003). In open-label trials, participants know they are taking the active agent, as do the researchers assessing them; thus results can be related to the participants' and researchers' expectations. Double-blind placebo-controlled trials, where neither the participants nor the researchers know which participants are taking the active agent and which are taking a placebo, address this limitation. Double-blind placebo-controlled trials are underway with EMP+ in adults and children. In a double-blind placebo-controlled trial of another vitamin–mineral supplement, children ages 6–12 who took the supplement had fewer antisocial behaviors (e.g., threats/fighting, vandalism, being disrespectful, disorderly conduct, assault/battery, defiance) than those on the placebo. A series of case studies showed significant decreases in mood and behavior problems in children taking EMP+ (Frazier, Fristad, & Arnold, 2010; Kaplan et al., 2002; Kaplan, Fisher, Crawford, Field, & Kolb, 2004; Popper, 2001). Several of these studies have had participants who were previously on psychotropic medications remain stable on EMP+ alone (Frazier et al., 2009; Kaplan et al., 2004; Simmons, 2003). One open-label pilot study of 10 children with severe mood dysregulation demonstrated tolerability and safety of EMP+ as well as decreased depressive and manic symptoms over an 8-week trial (Frazier, Fristad, & Arnold, 2010). Side effects of EMP+ include nausea and other minor gastrointestinal problems, but EMP+ is generally well tolerated by participants. Overall, the EMP+ results are promising for reduction of manic symptoms in children with BD, but additional studies are needed.

Omega-3 fatty acids are one of two series of essential fatty acids, the other being omega-6. Although these two series can substitute for one another, omega-3 appears to be more important for neuronal function (Hibbeln, Ferguson, & Blasbalg, 2006). The critical omega-3 fatty acids are long-chain, 20-carbon eicosapentaenoic acid (EPA) and 22-carbon docosahexaenoic acid (DHA) (Owen, Rees, & Parker, 2008). These fatty acids support neuron communication in the brain (Owen et al., 2008). Decreased rates of depression and BD have been noted in populations with high seafood consumption, the main dietary source of omega-3 fatty acids (Hibbeln, 1998; Noaghiul & Hibbeln, 2003). Research reviews have found inconsistent evidence for the effectiveness of omega-3 supplements in reducing symptoms of depression, BSD, and ADHD in adults and children (Parker et al., 2006; Schachter et al., 2005). Symptom improvement was noted in several compelling double-blind placebo-controlled studies, but other studies show no effect for omega-3 supplementation (Parker et al., 2006). This may be due to lack of consistency in the EPA-DHA ratio, as well as in the dose of omega-3 fatty acids used in the studies. One recent double-blind placebo-controlled study of 28 children ages 6–12 with MDD found significant effects of omega-3 supplementation on depressive symptoms, with many children meeting remission criteria by the end of 16 weeks of treatment (Nemets, Nemets, Apter, Bracha, & Belmaker, 2006). Side effects of omega-3 fatty acids are generally minor and include a fishy aftertaste and some gastrointestinal problems, but omega-3 supplements are generally well tolerated (Parker et al., 2006). Omega-3 fatty acid supplements also tend to be less expensive than many psychotropic medications. At this time, appropriate doses of omega-3 fatty acids and the optimal ratio of EPA to DHA are not well established.

Current Research Supporting Healthy Habits

As part of PEP, significant emphasis is placed on maintaining healthy habits—in particular, good sleep hygiene (i.e., regular habits that allow for sufficient sleep), regular exercise, and healthy eating habits. (See Chapter 9 for the PEP sessions on developing healthy habits.) Our premise is that healthy habits support mood stability and help to alleviate the impact of medication side effects. In short, building healthy habits around sleep, eating, and exercise amounts to "free" medicine. Here we review the science behind this premise.

Sleep

Sleep disturbance is common in persons of any age with a mood disorder. Depressed children can take longer to fall asleep, and their REM sleep patterns differ from those of nondepressed children (Emslie, Rush, Weinberg, Rintelmann, & Roffwarg, 1990). Youth with BSD also have many sleep problems, most typically delayed sleep onset due to evening mood elevation, followed by difficulty awakening or morning hypersomnia (Staton, 2008). Over half of children with BSD report decreased need for sleep (Lofthouse et al., 2008). Other commonly reported sleep problems include waking in the middle of the night and waking too early. Some of these sleep problems are related to comorbid diagnoses (e.g., separation anxiety, generalized anxiety, enuresis, and fear of the dark) (Lofthouse et al., 2008).

Sleep deprivation or reduction can trigger mania or hypomania in persons with BD (Plante & Winkelman, 2008). Not surprisingly, improved sleep is associated with increased cooperation and decreased irritability for adults with BD (Barbini, Bertelli, Colombo, & Smeraldi, 1996). Some evidence suggests that taking melatonin may lengthen sleep duration and improve manic symptoms (Bersani & Garavini, 2000). Similarly, enforcing darkness for 14 hours has been demonstrated to help adults who are experiencing a manic episode (Wehr et al., 1998). It is speculated that regulated light–dark cycles may have a therapeutic effect on manic episodes, because persons with BD might otherwise literally keep the lights on all night long, prolonging such episodes (Barbini et al., 2005). Together, these findings suggest that good sleep hygiene may be a powerful intervention in achieving and maintaining mood stability in persons with BD.

Exercise

Exercise is important for children with mood disorders, for several reasons. First, children and adults who engage in more physical activity have fewer depressive symptoms, suggesting that exercise may be preventative. Second, physical activity can provide relief from dysphoric mood states, suggesting exercise as a symptom management strategy. Third, weight gain is common among children and adolescents with mood disorders because of the appetite changes associated with mood. Fourth, many of the medications prescribed for mood disorders can also cause increased appetite, leading to weight gain; thus exercise can be a key component of side effect management as well as symptom management. Finally, given the well-established health benefits of exercise, children with mood disorders can benefit overall from regular exercise.

Several epidemiological studies have found exercise to be associated with fewer depressive and other psychiatric symptoms. Adults who engage in regular physical activity or exercise have fewer depressive symptoms (Stathopoulou, Powers, Berry, Smits, & Otto, 2006). In a study of 16,000 respondents age 15 years or older from the European Union, those who were more physically active had better mental health, regardless of their age, gender, marital status, gross household income, or educational status (Abu-Omar, Rütten, & Lehtinen, 2004). British youth ages 11–14 who engaged in 1 hour of physical activity daily were somewhat less likely to have self-reported emotional problems (Wiles et al., 2008). In a large community sample of German 14- to 24-year-olds, those who engaged in nonregular or regular physical activity were less likely to have dysthymia immediately or at a 4-year follow-up than those who engaged in no activity (Ströhle et al., 2007). In a group of 70 Welsh children ages 9–11, a child's amount of physical activity (defined as low, moderate, or high, based on a week's pedometer readings) was significantly related to anxiety, depression, and self-esteem: Anxiety and depression decreased and self-esteem increased as physical activity increased (Parfitt & Eston, 2005). In a community sample of 1,500 youth ages 10–17, 30% of those with five or more major depressive symptoms and functional impairment used the Internet for at least 3 hours a day, compared to 12% of youth with no depressive symptoms (Reeves, Postolache, & Snitker, 2008). Sedentary activities such as watching TV, Internet activity, and playing video games are often appealing to children; however, these activities are often conducted in social isolation. Engaging in physical activities with other children gives the benefit of social reinforcement from enjoying time with peers in addition to the physical activity (Reeves et al., 2008). The link between physical activity and depression is probably bidirectional: Increases in depression lead to decreases in physical activity, and decreases in physical activity lead to increases in depression. This link has been demonstrated with adolescents and adults who have mood disorders (e.g., Harris, Kronkite, & Moos, 2006). Though research has not been conducted with children, it is plausible that they are likely to get the same benefit from increasing physical activity.

As previously mentioned, weight gain is associated both with mood symptoms and with the medications used to treat mood disorders. When depressed, children may experience increased appetite along with decreased energy or psychomotor retardation. This increased caloric intake and decreased activity level can lead to weight gain. Many antipsychotic and mood-stabilizing medications are also associated with weight gain (Kowatch et al., 2009). In fact, development of metabolic syndrome is a very real concern for youth taking these medications (Correll & Carlson, 2006; Kowatch et al., 2005). Exercise can decrease the likelihood of this side effect.

In addition, lack of sleep—a common problem in childhood mood disorders, as described above—can lead to increased hunger (Reeves et al., 2008). The connection of sleep insufficiency and carbohydrate craving with depressed mood may be linked with serotonin, a major neurotransmitter whose deficit is implicated in depression (Reeves et al., 2008). The link between being overweight and being depressed may be bidirectional as well: Being overweight may lead people to feel down or depressed, and being depressed and seeing themselves negatively may cause them to eat more and become overweight.

Finally, children in general benefit from engaging in physical activity. The Centers for Disease Control and Prevention (CDC, 2008) emphasize the importance of exercise to decrease risk of cardiovascular disease, Type 2 diabetes, and some cancers. Exercise strengthens bones and muscles, improves the ability to engage in daily activities, and increases longevity.

Eating

A healthy diet is likewise beneficial for all children, but can be especially important for children with mood disorders. Increases and decreases in appetite are common mood symptoms, and increases (sometimes decreases) in appetite often occur as a side effect of medications for mood disorders as well as comorbid disorders. This puts children with mood disorders at particularly high risk for obesity and sometimes inadequate nutrition. Childhood obesity in general has become a major concern. Data from the National Health and Nutrition Evaluation Survey (NHANES) indicate that 16.3% of youth ages 2–19 are obese (defined as at or above the 95th percentile on the CDC growth charts), and that 31.9% are overweight (defined as at or above the 85th percentile on these charts) (Ogden, Carroll, & Flegal, 2008).

Summary

Research on the assessment and treatment of childhood mood disorders is rapidly growing. There are several promising avenues of treatment, including psychopharmacological, and nutritional interventions (as reviewed in this chapter) and psychosocial treatments (as reviewed in Chapter 1); however, much more research is needed for all these interventions. Staying abreast of research findings will aid clinicians in individualizing treatment for children with these chronic and often severe disorders. In the next chapter, we turn to the practical details of how to set up and deliver PEP to individual families or to multifamily groups.

Chapter 3

Implementing Psychoeducational Psychotherapy

In Chapters 1 and 2, we have reviewed in general terms what PEP is, for whom it is intended, and what we know about mood disorders in children. In this chapter, we turn to how to deliver PEP. We review therapist qualifications for conducting PEP; characteristics of those families and children who are likely to benefit; setting considerations; session structure for conducting both IF-PEP and MF-PEP; and general issues relevant to conducting PEP in either the individual or the multifamily format.

Therapist Qualifications and Preparation

If you are a therapist interested in conducting PEP, you should have the following skill sets: (1) a basic understanding of mood disorders in children and their evidence-based treatment; (2) a working knowledge of children's development and family functioning; (3) experience with CBT and family-based interventions; and (4) familiarity with different classes of medication, the medications in those classes, and current issues regarding medication in general. You should also familiarize yourself with the components of PEP as described in this book. Finally, if you are planning to conduct MF-PEP, you should have some knowledge of group therapy. This manual is intended to serve as a useful supplement to your existing knowledge base, and it describes in detail how to conduct the specific PEP treatment components.

As a therapist for children with complex disorders, you will also need to be knowledgeable about your local community, state, and online resources. This is especially the case in delivering PEP, which educates parents about mental health and educational services. You should know about, and consider joining, your local National Alliance on Mental Illness (NAMI) and/or Mental Health America (MHA) chapter. Mental health resources vary from state to state and from community to community. Each state government has a department that addresses mental health needs; make sure you know the relevant department and agencies for your state. If you are not a psychiatrist and don't know local psychiatrists, make some contacts. If therapy does not seem to be providing enough support, think about what other resources a family could access to provide more intensive services. Case management? Wrap-around services? To pursue such questions, you will need to know what is available in your clients' community, as well as how to access those services. PEP also gives parents information on school systems and how they allocate services to special-needs children; IF-PEP devotes a parent session to a meeting with the child's school team. Therefore, you should know your local school districts, understand how they work, and be familiar with their special education resources.

Countering Stigma

Society's views of heart disease, cancer, and multiple sclerosis, among other physical ailments, are very different from mood disorders and other psychiatric illnesses. Interestingly, these physical disease states were once also stigmatized; therefore, societal change is possible. In the meantime, the stigma surrounding mental illness can affect individuals deeply, and social isolation is one of its most profound sequelae. Throughout each PEP session, you will need to help families think creatively about how to lessen their own isolation. The easiest route to an understanding community is through the Internet. There is power in numbers when it comes to fighting stigma. Know how to access online support groups and other resources, so you can tell families how to do so. (See the Appendix for a listing of resources.)

In addition, prepare to be a voice for lessening stigma in your community. When opportunities arise, raise awareness. By attending school meetings and educating school districts, you can take a step toward fighting stigma. Educate those around you; every little bit helps. If you are comfortable with public speaking, give a talk at your local library or place of worship. Many religious organizations are great at providing support for families experiencing physical illnesses, but do not know how to support families struggling with mental illnesses. If you are affiliated with a church, synagogue, temple, or mosque, work with clergy on how to make families dealing with mental illness feel comfortable reaching out to the clergy, and make sure clergy members have some idea of how to support families.

Families often feel particularly stigmatized by their children's schools. In addition to social struggles and feeling ostracized by the parents of peers, parents can feel judged by school personnel. By encouraging families to share PEP materials as well as other sources about mood disorders with school personnel, you can help to change perspectives. And by helping to educate the school staff about mood disorders, you have the opportunity to reduce stigma in the school setting.

Finally, never underestimate the value to a child and family of a clinician who cares and "gets it"—who understands the unique and painful struggles they are experiencing and who can, within the framework of PEP, give them the tools they need to move forward constructively in their family life.

Children and Families Who May Benefit

IF-PEP and MF-PEP can be delivered to a broad array of children and families. Both formats were tested with children ages 8–12, and the children's exercises are particularly appropriate for that developmental age group. However, we have used PEP materials with both younger and older children. Younger children may need more coaching through the various exercises; in particular, they may not fully grasp the cognitive aspects of the Thinking, Feeling, Doing exercise, and so may need more scaffolding. Older children will have additional issues related to adolescence, but the general concepts of the therapeutic exercises will still hold. You may decide to replace the handout graphics to make them more appealing to teenage clients.

Families new to treatment often benefit most from PEP, but we have worked with many families who were "therapy-wise" yet still found the PEP materials to be helpful. This is especially true in MF-PEP, where a significant benefit cited by many families was meeting others struggling with similar issues.

On the basis of our research, we can say that children diagnosed with any mood disorder, either bipolar or depressive, benefit from PEP. However, you do not need to be certain about a child's precise diagnosis to recommend a family for PEP. In fact, participating in PEP may help family members learn to become better informants and so lead to a clearer diagnostic picture. A suspected diagnosis is certainly enough.

> Carol, a licensed social worker at a large multidisciplinary clinic, had been working with 9-year-old Todd's family for about 3 months. Todd had been diagnosed with ADHD due to his considerable distractibility both at home and at school, as well as his almost constant high energy and talkativeness. He had begun seeing one of the psychiatrists in the clinic, who had started Todd on a stimulant for ADHD. Initially, the medication seemed to help, especially at school. However, Todd's parents had described some irritability and explosiveness prior to medication, and these symptoms worsened with the medication. As a result, the medication was stopped and now Carol was grappling with whether Todd had a mood disorder. When she learned that PEP was being offered by one of her colleagues at their associated clinic across town, she immediately thought of Todd and his family.

Families such as Todd's have a great deal to gain from PEP. The more they understand what to look for, the better able they will be to provide information that will help to hone the diagnostic process. Following PEP, such families will be better equipped to participate actively with mental health professionals in managing ther children's symptoms.

Individual-Family or Multifamily Format: Staffing and Setting Considerations

Although the majority of our research has focused on MF-PEP, the same therapeutic topics and skills are covered in IF-PEP, along with expanded coverage of some topics. IF-PEP with individual families is a practical delivery model for clinicians in private practice.

One therapist can conduct both parent and child sessions, which are held on alternate weeks. Scheduling is flexible, and there are no unusual space requirements.

MF-PEP ideally requires sufficient space for running a child group and a parent group simultaneously, along with a staff of three therapists (one for the parent group, two for the child group). If space or staffing do not allow for simultaneous sessions, parent and child groups can meet on different days, either within the same week or on alternate weeks. A center or clinic may be the most realistic setting for running the multifamily format.

General Therapeutic Issues

The following general therapeutic issues are relevant to both IF-PEP and MF-PEP.

Children's Behavioral Management System

Whether you are implementing IF-PEP or MF-PEP, plan to establish a few basic rules in the first child session, and keep these rules posted at subsequent sessions. Describe the reward system to be used, as well as the general structure for each session. Point systems are ideal in the 8–12 age group. Points can be awarded for on-task behavior, participation, demonstration of breathing techniques to parents, teaching the session's content to parents, and so on. You can involve children in the reinforcement system; for example, have them put tokens in a cup or mark points on a sheet of paper. In addition, we have found it helpful for MF-PEP child therapists to come to each session equipped with a cache of candy (e.g., Starbursts) to give out as immediate reinforcers for positive behavior during sessions.

Sessions can feel long to children, especially younger children. Giving tokens or points at planned intervals to earn prizes at the end of treatment can help to encourage attention and concentration. Intervals will vary according to the children's age and degree of impairment: but every 10 minutes will work for many, every 5 minutes may work better for others. Prizes should be interesting but inexpensive. Party supply stores and dollar stores are good places to look. Be sure that prizes are age-appropriate and that different interests are represented (e.g., trading cards, pencils/erasers, key chains, stress balls, puzzles, stickers).

Other Tips for Motivating Children

Children may say, via their words or actions, "I don't want to put the time in." This provides you the opportunity to discuss how putting time and effort into PEP can ultimately save the children time for things they would prefer to do, and enable them to do these things successfully. Children may also be concerned about missing out on other after-school activities. In IF-PEP, you can work to schedule appointment times flexibly, to meet all family members' needs as well as possible. In MF-PEP, emphasizing its short-term nature (8 weeks) is probably most useful.

Confidentiality

As in any therapy, the topic of confidentiality should be explained in the first session—to parents and children together, as well as separately. Children need to know what you will, and will not, tell their parents. In IF-PEP, you and the parents will meet in one session with school personnel, and parents may have particular concerns about what the school will learn about their child. In MF-PEP, the importance of group members' maintaining confidentiality for each other warrants review.

Take-Home Projects and Use of Handouts

Homework assignments are given after every session in both PEP formats. We refer to these as "take-home projects"; "homework" is typically an unpopular word for children. Projects are designed to reinforce skills presented during sessions. Some are for parents to do on their own; some are for parents and children to do together as family projects; and some are for children to do on their own or with some parent support. Handouts are used in the session, as well as distributed for completion as take-home projects. Each session begins with a review of the previous session's assigned projects.

Handouts for each session are listed by title and number at the beginning of each chapter in Part II. The handouts themselves can be found in Part III of this book and may be copied and shared with families. Parents and children should be encouraged to keep all handouts together in a binder and bring them to each session. Some therapists and families may prefer to have a comprehensive workbook for parents and/or children that contain all the handouts (these workbooks are available at *www.moodychildtherapy.com*).

Conducting IF-PEP

IF-PEP can be individually tailored and it is particularly flexible in terms of meeting the needs of a wide variety of families. Unlike MF-PEP, it can be implemented at any time, allowing families to begin treatment when their motivation to do so is high. As described in Chapter 1, IF-PEP parent and child sessions are held on alternate weeks for a total of 20 content-specific sessions and 4 open "in-the-bank" sessions. Each session lasts 45–50 minutes. The in-the-bank sessions are intended to be used flexibly, to address crises or to allow additional time to consolidate a skill before moving on to a new topic. Therapists are encouraged to use these in-the-bank sessions as needed, while ensuring that the family completes the "standard" content before terminating treatment.

Expanded Coverage Unique to IF-PEP

With more sessions than MF-PEP, IF-PEP allows more thorough coverage of several therapeutic topics. Specifically, it provides for two child sessions devoted to developing healthy habits—sleep, eating, and exercise (see Chapter 9)—plus a session for siblings (see Chapter 21). Also unique to IF-PEP, as noted earlier, is a parent session in which the parents and therapist meet with staff from the child's school (see Chapter 16).

Session Sequence and Staying on Track

In both PEP formats, the session topics build upon each other sequentially. For children in particular, each session teaches skills that serve as building blocks for subsequent sessions, as described in Chapter 1. Skills are reinforced by handouts and between-session assignments. When you are working with individual families, we encourage you to apply this treatment manual with "flexibility within fidelity" (Kendall & Beidas, 2007). If an issue scheduled later in the treatment protocol is particularly challenging for a family (e.g., functioning in the school setting), it can be moved up in the schedule. Approaching session order flexibly and addressing a troublesome topic early may prevent it from becoming a crisis. Also, some families may begin therapy with an extensive preexisting knowledge base (e.g., if another sibling has already been treated for a mood disorder). Such families may not need as much time to review the basics, and in these cases, session content can be combined. In other cases, certain topics will be not relevant for families, and the sessions on these topics can be completely skipped (e.g., the sibling session for an only-child family) or greatly streamlined. If a child has intact sleep hygiene, eats a well-balanced diet, and gets plenty of exercise, then devoting two sessions to healthy habits is not necessary. A brief review of why these three healthy habits are good for mental health should suffice, and this can be accomplished during the Tool Kit session. A child with mild depression who is not on medication will not need a parent or child session devoted exclusively to learning about medication; a brief mention of medication as a future option, if the situation calls for it, will be adequate. Similarly, teaching about symptoms may go more quickly if the child has mild depression; in such a case, the separate parent and child sessions on teaching about symptoms may be combined. Furthermore, there may be practical limitations to the number of sessions a family is able to attend: The family's mental health benefits may be limited; a long travel time to and from appointments may make attending 20–24 sessions impossible; or parents' work schedules may not be flexible enough to allow for all sessions.

Although modifications in session order are allowable, many families come to PEP in crisis, and it is tempting for clinicians to try to put out every fire as it arises. It is useful to keep in mind that the tools gained while progressing through PEP are designed to keep fires from erupting in the future. Incorporating parents' concerns into the Lesson of the Day (see below) will allow you to meet their needs while covering the therapy content. At times, it may help to direct the conversation gently back to session content, with a reminder that the skills the parents are learning will help them solve future problems and avoid future crises. So, while recognizing that families may come with different priorities, you also need to make sure that each family ultimately benefits from all the PEP content.

> Ricky (age 9) and his parents, Jim and Rhonda, came to the first child session of PEP looking tense and apprehensive. After brief introductions, Rhonda said, "We need help with Ricky at school." Ricky immediately shouted, "I hate school! Why do you make me go?" Rhonda launched into a description of their typical morning, which included outbursts and tears on Ricky's part, and yelling and cajoling on his parents' part. The afternoons seemed to consist of explosions and arguments about homework, which rarely got completed. Given that this was meant to be the first child ses-

sion, Sandra, their therapist, stopped Rhonda and suggested that they dedicate the first parent session to school-related issues. Rhonda relaxed at this suggestion, which allowed the session in progress to proceed as planned. At the next parent session, Sandra delivered the content of the session on working with school systems (normally Session 6; see Chapter 10) to Jim and Rhonda . After reviewing Ricky's current school situation, Sandra discussed various interventions they might wish to consider, as well as how to approach the school to get modifications. She suggested that Jim and Rhonda schedule a meeting with school personnel (normally Session 14; see Chapter 16) as soon as possible, and she would participate via a conference call. She also mentioned that since school issues were so dominant, Jim and Rhonda could use an in-the-bank session to address the issue further. Sandra also talked to Jim and Rhonda about how some of the other concepts they would learn in PEP could help alleviate problems that were aggravating the school issue. Sandra thus brought the session topics back on track to maintain fidelity to the model, while being flexible about the timing of delivery.

By making a plan to address working with the school system early in treatment, Sandra was able to assist this family out of crisis mode. This can be done effectively within the IF-PEP model.

IF-PEP Session Format

Child and parent sessions in IF-PEP follow similar but slightly different formats. Both formats are outlined in Table 3.1 and discussed below, starting with child sessions. Time allotments shown in the table are estimates; vary these as needed to address each specific session's content with parents and children. The chapters in Part II of this book follow the formats shown on Table 3.1, with the exception of the sessions with school professionals (Session 14; see Chapter 16) and with siblings (Session 19; see Chapter 21).

Child Session Format

BEGINNING THE SESSION (10 MINUTES)

Parent–Child Check-In and Review of Mood Record/Mood–Medication Log. Parents are invited to join the beginning of each child session, and the therapist briefly checks on how the parents and child have been doing since the last session. After the first child session, this check-in is facilitated by a review of the Mood Record or Mood–Medication Log that parents are taught to keep in their first or second session, respectively.

Review of Take-Home Projects. Take-home projects from the previous child session are reviewed while the parents are still in the room. As noted earlier, we refer to these assignments as "projects" rather than "homework." The projects are designed to reinforce skills presented during sessions. Some projects are for parents and children to do together, and some are for children to do independently or with some support from parents. (Parent-only take-home projects are reviewed in the parent sessions.) Following this review, parents typically leave the room, rejoining the session at its end. However, depending on the child's

TABLE 3.1. Standard Session Formats for IF-PEP

Child sessions

Beginning the session (10 minutes)
    Parent–child check-in, review of Mood Record or Mood–
        Medication Log, and review of previous take-home projects
    Identification and rating of feelings (child only)
Lesson of the Day (25 minutes)
    Session topic
    Practice and assignment of new take-home project
Breathing Exercise (5 minutes)
Session review with parents (10 minutes)
    Child "teaches" parents the Lesson of the Day
    Review of new take-home project

Parent sessions

Beginning the session (10 minutes)
    Check-in (see above)
    Review of previous parent take-home projects
Lesson of the Day (30 minutes)
    Session topic
Assignment of new and ongoing take-home projects (10 minutes)

age and developmental level, some child-focused sessions (e.g., the session on healthy habits) may work better as conjoint sessions, with parents sitting in for the entire session.

Child Identification and Rating of Feelings. Starting with the first session, children learn to identify how they are currently feeling, to consider why they feel that way, and to rate the intensity of their strongest emotion. This exercise is repeated in all subsequent child sessions; it is a building block for learning the connections between situational triggers and feelings, and among feelings, thoughts, and actions.

LESSON OF THE DAY (25 MINUTES)

The main content of each topic-specific session is presented to children as the "Lesson of the Day" and is taught through various exercises and handouts. The child's take-home project is practiced and assigned during this part of the session.

BREATHING EXERCISE (5 MINUTES)

The child-only portion of the session concludes with the practice of a breathing technique. Three breathing techniques are taught to the child, one each in the first three child sessions: Belly Breathing, Balloon Breathing, and Bubble Breathing. Practice of each breathing technique is assigned as a take-home projects.

SESSION REVIEW WITH PARENTS (10 MINUTES)

Parents rejoin their child at the end of the session, and the child then "teaches" the Lesson of the Day to the parents. This allows parents to stay abreast of their child's treatment, consolidates the session content in the child's mind, and allows the therapist to check on the child's comprehension of the session content.

Parent Session Format

Parents' sessions follow a format similar to that of the child sessions. Each session begins with an approximate 10-minute check-in, review of the Mood Record or Mood–Medication Log, and review of any parent-only take-home projects assigned in the previous session. The Lesson of the Day is then presented to parents (approximately 30 minutes), and the session ends with assignment of ongoing and/or new parent-only take-home projects (approximately 10 minutes). The format is also outlined in Table 3.1.

Conducting MF-PEP

MF-PEP offers the same basic therapeutic content as IF-PEP in a time-efficient group format. A group of children and a group of their parents meet once a week over 8 weeks; ideally, the two groups meet simultaneously. MF-PEP differs from IF-PEP in offering a shorter treatment course with fewer sessions (a total of 16 MF-PEP sessions, compared to 20+ IF-PEP sessions). MF-PEP sessions are also longer (90 minutes each), and child sessions include an opportunity for *in vivo* social skills training via a group games section unique to the group format. Staffing requirements are also different: One therapist is needed for the parent group, and two therapists for the children's group. The latter is usually staffed with a lead therapist and a cotherapist (often a trainee), who assists with behavior management. As mentioned earlier, if space or staffing does not allow for simultaneous group sessions, parent and child sessions can alternate weekly or twice weekly.

In the MF-PEP format, there is limited flexibility to change the order of topics. When parents come to a session in crisis, incorporate their concern into the lesson of the day if possible. You can briefly and privately touch base with parents, as needed, at the beginning or end of the session to make any additional referrals.

Group Composition

Six to eight children are ideal for the children's group. A group with more children has the potential to become chaotic; fewer children result in a very small group for adequate discussion if one or two are missing on any particular week. Having six to eight children also typically results in adequate reimbursement for multiple therapists.

For the parent group, plan on two parents per child attending, on average (12–16 adults). Whenever possible, both parents should be encouraged to attend, as well as all other primary caregivers (e.g., stepparents). Family members determine among themselves who will attend the group. The only restriction, requested by parents in previous groups, is that older siblings not be invited to attend the parent group, as parents wish to speak candidly about their children. Families should contract to do the entire course of PEP, so that they can learn all the content covered sequentially during the scheduled sessions.

When you are organizing an MF-PEP group, take into consideration the overall group composition. As a general rule of thumb, you will want to be mindful about inviting a family to participate that is an outlier on some relevant demographic or clinical parameter, such as being the only high- or low-income family, the only family of a girl with a mood disorder if all other participating children are boys, or the only family with a severely manic child in a group of moderately depressed children. Careful thought and discussion with referring colleagues may be helpful in determining whether inclusion in the group would be beneficial to the family, as well as to others in the group.

In many settings, families new to treatment will primarily be referred to MF-PEP. These families often find the organized materials presented in MF-PEP to be highly beneficial. However, if your parent group includes participants at later stages of coping with childhood mood disorders, these "veteran" families frequently contribute in a very important way to the group. The support a parent receives from a therapist can pale in comparison to that received from another parent who has experienced and survived a similar stressor. In our experience, parents who are experienced at managing the ups and downs of their children's mood disorders are pleased to share their knowledge, and often join MF-PEP to provide their children with the opportunity to meet others struggling with similar issues.

Staffing Requirements

Again, one therapist is needed for the parent group, and two therapists for the child group. One child therapist should be experienced and be prepared to deliver session content; as noted earlier, the other therapist can be a trainee, primarily in charge of managing children's behavior and assisting the group leader. This cotherapist provides reinforcement, sits strategically in the group to support children who need assistance to behave appropriately, escorts children for bathroom breaks or time outs as needed, and assists with any crises (e.g., a child who becomes agitated and needs to leave the room to calm down). All three therapists should plan on meeting before and after the group sessions. This allows for coordination of therapeutic efforts between the child and parent therapists; the child therapists can give feedback on the child's functioning to the parent therapist, and vice versa. Prior to sessions, the child therapists will also need to prepare the room and set out materials.

Session Scheduling

Sessions are probably best scheduled midweek (Tuesday, Wednesday, or Thursday), in the late afternoon/early evening (e.g., 5:00 to 6:30 P.M.). Midweek scheduling takes into consideration the extra fatigue many children experience on Monday after returning to school from a weekend, as well as the fact that many families have competing weekend activities on Friday, Saturday, or Sunday. Late-afternoon/early-evening scheduling allows parents to attend after work, but allows sessions to be completed before children (and parents) become too hungry. It is advisable to have water and snacks (e.g., cheese crackers or pretzels) for the children and water and/or coffee for the parents.

Space Requirements

Ideally, MF-PEP is conducted with parent and child groups running simultaneously, as noted above. This requires the availability of two group rooms. Since sessions begin and end with a brief joint group meeting, one of the rooms must be large enough to include all parents and children.

The children's room should be equipped with a whiteboard, SMART Board, and/or easel for writing. It will ideally also have a large table that the children and therapists can sit around during the first portion of their group session. The room must be large enough (and free of breakable objects) to accommodate group activities, and there must be floor space for breathing exercises toward the end of each session.

Advantages of MF-PEP

Groups give parents an opportunity to hear multiple perspectives; families have the opportunity to learn from each other as well as from the PEP therapist. Many families are extremely appreciative of the social support gained from meeting others who struggle as they do.

> When the Brown family came to group, the parents, Barbara and Dave, really thought that their situation could not be worse. Christopher had been hospitalized several times, and it was proving difficult to find medications that made an appreciable difference. He was spending most of his school time in the quiet room supervised by an adult after his frequent disruptions in class; he was doing no schoolwork. At home, Christopher's aggression seemed intolerable to his parents, who were very worried about the impact on their two younger children. They were losing hope. As Barbara and Dave listened carefully to the stories of other families, however, they began to realize that theirs was not the only family dealing with such challenges. They listened to Jan and Bob talk about how bad their situation had been a year ago. Their daughter, Myra, had been hospitalized twice last year. Her rages had led to aggression on a daily basis; Jan described having bruises up and down her arms. Myra seemed driven at times—angrily insisting on following her ideas immediately, even if they were unrealistic. At other times, she became distraught and hopeless. She often refused to go to school, and when she was at school, she spent most of her time in the nurse's office. After several medication changes, the aggression had largely stopped. Myra still had significant ups and downs in her moods, but compared to last year, the family's situation had improved significantly. Myra was readily going to school daily and participating in class much more consistently. Jan and Bob's experience with Myra began to give the Browns hope.

Children with mood disorders are often socially isolated. In MF-PEP, children often meet peers for the first time who experience the same struggles and challenges, and they can derive considerable comfort from this. The children's common experiences lead to acceptance in addition to peer support. The group format also provides the children with opportunities to practice newly acquired social skills that are more difficult to practice in an individual setting.

MF-PEP Session Format

MF-PEP Children's Group Session Format

The standard format for children's group sessions in MF-PEP is outlined in Table 3.2 and briefly discussed below. Like the child sessions in IF-PEP, sessions begin and end with parents and children joining each other in whatever room is large enough to accommodate all participants. MF-PEP makes use of the same handouts and take-home projects as IF-PEP, and also uses materials for group games and activities, described below and later in this chapter. Again, the time allotments shown in Table 3.2 and presented below are estimates only.

BEGINNING THE SESSION

Parent–Child Check-In and Review of Take-Home Projects (10 Minutes). Children's group sessions begin with a conjoint check-in with parents. Take-home projects from the previous child session are also reviewed.

Sharing Feelings and News of the Week (10 Minutes). After the child and parent groups separate, children begin their session with "Sharing Feelings" and telling their "News of the Week" to the other child group members and therapists. Sharing Feelings is the group version of identifying and rating feelings. The Feelings Chart and Strength of Feelings thermometer (see Handouts 1 and 2) are good resources to use in early sessions; children quickly acclimate to this process and usually don't need visual prompts after several weeks in the group, particularly as the group leaders can serve as role models in sharing this information. For News of the Week, children are asked to report on one or two important events that have happened in their lives since the group last met.

LESSON OF THE DAY (40 MINUTES)

The main portion of each children's group session is working on the Lesson of the Day. The same content is covered as in the corresponding IF-PEP session, with exercises adapted for a group. The lead therapist asks the group questions and uses a whiteboard, SMART Board, or easel to write down children's contributions to the lesson. Working as a group has multiple advantages: It allows children to take leadership roles, provides role models for children who might otherwise be too insecure or shy to contribute, and offers social support. These children all have struggles in common. The lesson ends with preparation, practice, and assignment of the children's take-home project.

TABLE 3.2. Standard Session Formats for MF-PEP

<u>Children's group sessions</u>

Beginning the session
    Parent–child check-in and review of previous take-home projects
       (10 minutes)
    Sharing Feelings and News of the Week (children and therapists only)
       (10 minutes)
Lesson of the Day (40 minutes)
    Session topic and exercises
    Assignment of take-home project
Group games and activities (15 minutes)
Breathing exercise (5 minutes)
Session review with parents (10 minutes)
    One or more selected children teach parents the Lesson of the Day
    Review of new take-home project

<u>Parents' group sessions</u>

Beginning the session (see above, 10 minutes)
    Parent–child check-in and review of previous session's take-home projects
    Review of any parent-only take-home projects (parents only, 10 minutes)
Lesson of the Day (60 minutes)
    Session topic
    Assignment of new and ongoing parent-only take-home projects
Parent–child check-out (10 minutes)
    One or more selected children teach parents the Lesson of the Day
    Review of any new family take-home project

GROUP GAMES AND ACTIVITIES (15 MINUTES)

Children next engage in *in vivo* social skills training via directed group games and activities. This portion of the session is unique to MF-PEP. Its rationale lies in the realities of working with children in general, and children with mood disorders in particular. As noted earlier, MF-PEP is typically run in the late afternoon/early evening; by that time, children are often tired, hungry, and cranky, and need a physical outlet for their bottled-up physical energy. Frequently group members have comorbid ADHD, and the effects of any stimulant medications are likely to be waning, decreasing these children's ability to concentrate and increasing their activity level and irritability. It's unrealistic to expect group members to remain focused on therapeutic material while sitting around a table for 90 minutes at this point in the day, even if the therapeutic exercises are presented in a fun way. Session-specific instructions for these activities are given later in this chapter; reproducible supporting materials are described there and are provided in Part III of this book.

BREATHING EXERCISE (5 MINUTES)

As in IF-PEP, children end the child-only portion of the session by practicing a breathing technique (Belly Breathing, Balloon Breathing, or Bubble Breathing). Following the physical activity, this exercise helps the children calm down and get ready to rejoin their parents.

SESSION REVIEW WITH PARENTS (10 MINUTES)

Parents join their children at the end of the session. Three child volunteers are selected to "teach" parents the Lesson of the Day, and describe the take-home project, and demonstrate the breathing exercise.

Parents' Group Session Format

The session format for the parent group is also outlined in Table 3.2. Each session begins and ends with an approximate 10-minute check-in with the children, as described above. These combined check-ins allow for families to connect as a unit. The previous session's parent-only take-home project is then reviewed in the parent-only group.

The bulk of each parent session is spent discussing the topic of the day, plus reviewing any parent-only projects to be completed prior to the next session. Material is presented in a more didactic format than in IF-PEP. Parents may feel less confronted or blamed, since information is addressed to all the parents. The session closes with parents and children coming together (in whatever room can accommodate all the participants), at which time one child each (1) teaches parents their Lesson of the Day, (2) reviews the family project to be completed before the next session, and (3) demonstrates the breathing technique of the day.

Most of this book focuses on how to deliver IF-PEP, although the session content in Part II is relatively easy to transfer to the group format. The games and activities in MF-PEP children's groups, however, are unique to that format. The balance of this chapter describes the specifics of these activities for therapists who will run the children's groups in MF-PEP.

Children's Games and Activities in MF-PEP

We have developed a set of physical activities and games related to session-specific MF-PEP topics. As noted above, these allow children a physical outlet and a structure for interaction during the last part of each group session. Think of this time as *in vivo* social skills training: You can frequently refer back to that session's Lesson of the Day (or past lessons) if conflict arises (e.g., checking in on a group member's current feelings, using a tool from a child's Tool Kit to calm down). Feel free to develop your own exercises and to fit these activities into the time and space you have available and the needs of your group members. For example, if your group includes multiple members who have reading difficulties, you may wish to delete the activities that involve reading. This part of the session is supposed to maximize enjoyment, not frustration, for the children.

The "Where" of Games

If you have access to both a child group room and a large playroom or gym, you can escort the children after the Lesson of the Day to the playroom or gym to play games. If you have just a child group room, you may wish to move the table and chairs to one side of the room to give you more floor space. Examples of small-space and large-space activities are provided for many of the games described below.

The "When" of Games

Some groups are very chatty and use up all their time on the Lesson of the Day. Other groups plow through material quickly, use the activities described below, and still have time before the session is over to engage in "free-choice" games. Examples of additional group games that may be played, depending on the available physical space, include kickball, Monkey in the Middle, Steal the Bacon, charades, and Simon Says. Group members may also play a card game (e.g., Go Fish, Uno, Memory, Spoons) or a board game (e.g., Sorry!, the Ungame) together. You and your cotherapists should encourage activities that foster group cohesion and improve relationships. The key is to be flexible; for every group you run, this latter portion of each group session may flow differently.

Game Materials

Some of the games and activities use unique materials (in addition to common items, such as a ball, playing cards, paper, and crayons or other writing implements). For example, the Medication Match game described for Session 2 requires cards created in advance, which list diagnoses, symptoms, and medications. Samples of these cards and of other unique group game materials can be found among the Game Reproducibles at the end of Part III. Descriptions of specific MF-PEP games and activities are given next.

Getting to Know Each Other Better (Session 1; See Chapter 5)

An important goal of the first session is to build rapport within the group. Getting to Know Each Other Better is a physical activity that continues to work toward that goal by helping group members learn more about one another and see characteristics they have in common. This is a very simple exercise requiring only one resource, a ball. Depending on the size of the space, a playground ball, basketball, tennis ball, plastic golf ball, or ball of yarn can be used. Using a ball of yarn has the added benefit of producing a visual representation of the links between group members and leaders.

For the activity, all of the group members (including the group leaders) stand in a circle, with space between them appropriate for the ball being used; obviously, more space should be left if children are bouncing a playground ball than if they are tossing a plastic golf ball. Next, a group leader explains that the person holding the ball will share something about him-/herself that the person has not already told the group. That person passes the ball to the next person. If a ball of yarn is used, each person holds onto the string, and a web is created among all of the group members. As the group leaders, you and your therapist begin by sharing something about yourselves, passing the ball to each other, and then passing it to a child group member. Encourage full participation so that everyone gets a chance to share and learn about each other. The ball can be passed until time runs out or until the ball of yarn (if one is used) reaches its end.

Medication Match (Session 2; See Chapter 7)

Medication Match expands on the medication information learned in the second session and requires some preparation ahead of time to create cards used in the game. This exercise will be most meaningful if the cards reflect the medications actually being used by the group members; therefore, you will need to collect that information from parents at the first group session.

Depending on the size of the group, two to four sets of cards are needed—one set for each team of two to four children. Each set of cards should be on a different color of paper, but should have the same information, in three categories: diagnoses (e.g., Depression, Bipolar Disorder, ADHD, Anxiety); medications (e.g., Risperdal, Abilify, Lithium, Zoloft, Prozac, Concerta, Strattera, Ritalin, Depakote); and symptoms (e.g., sad, really irritable, grouchy, angry, worried, nothing is fun, worried, no energy, scared, too excited, thinking too fast, talking too fast, can't pay attention, can't concentrate, hyperactive, etc.). Include about 15 cards per set, although the number can be adjusted to fit the developmental and intellectual levels of the group members. If laminated or printed on card stock, these cards can be used repeatedly for multiple groups. Game Reproducible 1, in Part III, includes sample cards that can be copied onto colored paper and cut for use.

Before the game starts, the sets of cards should be mixed together, and you group leaders (the children can help) should spread the cards randomly around the room. Next, divide the group into teams of two to four children, and assign each team a color of cards to collect. Teams have to walk or run around to pick up the scattered cards; this is the physical part of the activity. Teams can consist of children with similar abilities, to let them work at the same pace while you group leaders help lower-functioning groups. Alternatively, teams can consist of children with different abilities, so that the more advanced children can help others on their team. Teams may also reflect groups of children who take similar medications or have similar diagnoses, as they will be familiar with those symptoms and medications. On the other hand, teams of children with different diagnoses will allow each child to make a unique contribution. Use your best judgment in creating groups.

Explain the game to the group members as follows:

1. Team members need to pick up all the cards in their assigned color.
2. When they have all their cards, they find a space to work and sort the cards into the three categories: diagnoses, symptoms, and medications. For younger or lower-functioning groups, you can preselect each team's work space and mark it with a sheet of paper listing the categories.
3. Next, for each diagnosis, the team members match the medications and symptoms. This step is where children are most likely to need help from you. Two therapists for two to four teams should allow time for each group to receive some

assistance. When the team is finished matching the cards, they give their card sets to you and your cotherapists.

Body Tracing (Session 3; See Chapter 11)

To build on the physical awareness of feelings that children discuss in the third session, ask them to trace their bodies. For this activity, the necessary supplies are one large piece of paper per child (longer than the child is tall), and several sets of black, red, green, and blue markers or crayons. Children work in pairs at first. One partner lies down on the paper, and the other partner traces around him/her with a black marker. Then partners switch places. Keep in mind that some children may be sensitive about being touched, due to abuse history or other experiences; tell the children to lie with their feet together, so that the partner doing the tracing does not need to trace between the other partner's legs. Tracing can also be several inches from the body, so that the children don't actually touch each other. Next, children take the outlines of their own bodies and mark the places where they feel mad (in red), sad (in blue), and bad (in green) feelings. They should have several ideas from the worksheet they completed during the session (e.g., fists when angry, stomachache when sad, furrowed eyebrows when feeling bad). You and your cotherapists can circulate around the room to offer ideas and encouragement. Children can take their tracings home and discuss them with their parents. Their parents may learn some nonverbal signals of their children's moods.

Expanding on Thinking, Feeling, Doing (Session 4; See Chapter 13)

The fourth session's activity follows the discussion of relationships among thoughts, feelings, and actions when a trigger occurs. For this activity, the children will need to *think* and *feel* so that they can then *do* a fun activity. The word "Feeling" in this game refers to its tactile sense. It's important to explain to the children that this is not the same "feeling" (i.e., emotion) talked about during the Lesson of the Day.

Supplies needed for this activity include Thinking, Feeling, Doing Activity Cards, a bag, playground equipment, and/or writing implements and ordinary playing cards. The Activity Cards can be made by reproducing and cutting up Game Reproducible 2, which lists activities appropriate for large and small spaces. You can laminate or copy the cards onto card stock for repeated use. An example of an activity in a small space is "Use a skinny marker to connect the dots in the PEP Connect the Dots game." If you have a large space, a possible activity is "Using a cone, whiffle ball, and bat, set up a batting-T and hit the whiffle ball into the large end of another cone." Game Reproducible 2 has more activity ideas. Other ideas can be substituted, given the characteristics of the therapy space and the equipment available to you.

Each child receives a card with an activity on it. In order to complete the activity, the child will need to *think* about what materials are needed, *feel* in a bag for the right supplies, and then *do* the activity as listed on the card. The key supplies needed for each activity should be in a large bag, and children must locate supplies for their activity by touch alone. Other supplies can be available from you and your cotherapist. When you are working with a group in a small space, a grocery bag can be used to hide writing implements. In order to "Use a pencil to complete one of the PEP Mazes leading from 'My Symptoms' to 'Me.'" a child will have to reach into the bag and feel the difference among the skinny marker, the highlighter, and the pencil. After the child finds the pencil, he/she can ask one of you for a version of the PEP Maze to complete (see Game Reproducibles 9–11). PEP Connect the Dots or one of the PEP Word Search games (see Game Reproducibles 3–6) can also be handed to the child once the skinny marker or highlighter is located, as specified in the Activity Cards on Game Reproducible 2. Game Reproducibles 7 and 8 are Color by Number pictures. The Activity Cards can be gathered and redistributed if time allows. Answer keys for PEP Connect the Dots, the PEP Word Searches, and the PEP Mazes are provided on Game Reproducibles 12–18. When the children are working in a large space, searching the room for other items needed to complete the task can be part of the game.

Problem-Solving Task (Session 5; See Chapter 15)

Children learn and discuss the steps of problem solving during the fifth session. The physical game at the end of the session presents them with a problem to solve. The only material needed is one sheet of paper for each two-member team. The pairs of children line up along one wall of the room, and each pair is given a sheet of paper. Their goal is to get across the room and back within the following rules:

1. Both members of each team have to cross the room.
2. Feet and shoes cannot touch the floor directly.
3. The only equipment they can use is the piece of paper.

Encourage the group members to see which team can get across the room and back the fastest. As the activity begins, members usually ask for clarification of the rules, such as "Do we have to go at the same time?" or "Can we tear the paper?" You can reply, "Whatever will get you both across the room the quickest while following the rules." Monitor the game for safety concerns (e.g., one member trying to carry another), and intervene to prevent any potential injuries; judge when the task has been completed. Possible solutions include these:

1. Tearing the sheet of paper in fourths, and have each team member use a piece under each foot to traverse the floor. This can be accomplished by sliding on the paper or picking the pieces up and using them like steppingstones to advance.
2. Tearing the sheet in half, and having each player advance by scooting his/her feet on the half sheet.
3. Having both players stand on the same sheet of paper and try to advance by scooting their feet.

As one team begins to move successfully, other teams usually begin to imitate the successful idea. Once all teams have completed the task, process with the members what skills they needed to complete the activity. Inquire about how problem solving can help not only with difficulties related to their mood, but also with other daily problems.

Follow-the-Leader Charades and Letter Scramble (Session 6; See Chapter 17)

In the sixth session, children have worked on nonverbal communication skills. They will need to use these skills for this session's physical activity. Group members are divided into teams of two or three. Each team receives two cards: one for Follow-the-Leader Charades and one for the Letter Scramble game. Game Reproducibles 19 and 20 can be copied and cut up to create these cards. The Follow-the-Leader Charades card has instructions for an activity. One team member reads the card to him-/herself and must then get his/her partner(s) to carry out the activity without using words; the reader can model the desired action (charades). For instance, one card reads, "Without talking, get a peer to play underhand catch with you." The only feedback the reader can give his/her partners is a nod for "yes" or a head shake for "no," depending on how close the partners are to accomplishing the task.

Each Letter Scramble card lists six activities to complete, but the words in the directions are scrambled. The team has to unscramble the words to complete the activities. All teams get the same card. (Letter Scramble may be omitted if group members' average reading level is relatively low.)

As an alternative activity, some groups express the desire to keep doing charades as they did during their Lesson of the Day. If that happens, go with it—it's hard to object to the desire to practice new skills!

Game of the Children's Choice (Session 7; See Chapter 19)

In the seventh session, verbal communication has been discussed. Using their new communication skills, children are asked to select collectively what group game to play, based on available resources. (See "The 'When' of Games," above, for such games. Again, you and your cotherapist should encourage activities that foster group cohesion and improve relationships.)

PEP Review Game (Session 8; Chapter 22)

The majority of the final session with children is spent reviewing topics discussed in MF-PEP. This can be done in the form of a game that spans most of the session, not just the final 15 minutes. The review is set up like a game show or trivia game, and the children are asked questions about information in four categories: (1) Symptoms/Medications; (2) Thinking, Feeling, Doing; (3) Anger Management/Coping; and (4) Problem Solving/Communication. Questions within each category are worth 100, 200, 300, 400, or 500 points, with higher point values for harder questions. There are also several "bonus questions," for which there is an immediate reward if answered correctly. Children take turns until all of the questions have been asked. Whoever has the most points after the last question is asked wins the game.

Game Reproducible 21 lists suggested review questions by category and point value. Questions are provided at three difficulty levels (i.e., easy, medium, hard). Therapists can choose the appropriate level of difficulty for each group member. Answers to closed-ended questions are provided in **boldface.** In addition to the list of questions, supplies needed for the review game include a poster (or blackboard) showing the four question categories and choice of point values, immediate rewards to be given for correctly answered bonus questions, paper and pencil to keep track of points, and sticky notes to cover the point values that have been asked. It can be helpful for one of you therapists to read the questions and the other to keep track of points.

You may establish the rules of play as you see fit, but suggested procedures are as follows:

1. The child whose turn it is selects a category and point value (e.g., Symptoms/Medications for 200 points).
2. The therapist who is serving as "master of ceremonies" covers that point value on the poster board with a sticky note, or otherwise indicates that it has been chosen.
3. The therapist asks the child the question.
4. If the child answers correctly without assistance, he/she is awarded the points; if the child is unsure of the answer, he/she can ask another group member, and if that member gets it right they each earn half of the points; if the child answers incorrectly, the therapist tells the group the correct answer, and play moves on to the next member.
5. If the question is answered correctly and there is a bonus associated with it, the therapist asks the bonus question; if the child gets it right, he/she gets an immediate reward; if the child gets it wrong, play moves on to the next player (no points are lost or gained). Bonus questions are listed below the category questions on the PEP Review Game reproducible (Game Reproducible 21).
6. If there is no bonus question, play moves on to the next player.

Summary

This chapter provides the overarching framework to conduct IF-PEP and MF-PEP and also describes how to implement games for the child MF-PEP groups. Subsequent chapters describe in greater detail content of the specific PEP child and parent sessions.

Chapter 4

The Complexities of Establishing a Mood Disorder Diagnosis

A definitive diagnosis is not necessary for a referral to PEP, but clinicians running PEP need to have a clear understanding of what depressive spectrum disorders and BSD are and of how they differ from, but often co-occur with, other disorders. Differentiating BD from ADHD is a particularly important diagnostic task. A key to careful assessment of pediatric mood disorders is encouraging parents to keep records that help to identify moods and co-occurring symptoms. In their first PEP session, parents are taught to keep a Mood Record on their child (see Chapter 6). The more parents know about mood symptoms, the better observers they become. Both parents and clinicians need to understand that diagnosing a mood disorder is a process that takes time and a carefully obtained history. Because depressive spectrum disorders are no longer considered controversial in child assessment, we offer some brief comments about diagnosing depression, but we focus in most of this chapter on the diagnosis of BSD in children.

Assuming that a child's moods appear to be a problem, there are two initial assessment questions to consider: (1) What are these mood states? (2) How significant is the mood problem?

Defining Mood States

Depressive spectrum disorders are characterized by dysphoric, anxious, and/or irritable moods. BSD are characterized by moods changing from too high (mania or hypomania) to too low (depression). Specific mood states range from euphoria and rage (mania) to sadness and irritability (depression). Many researchers consider euphoria to be the hallmark of BD (e.g., Geller et al., 2002). Euphoria in children may be seen as excessive silliness or giddiness that is inappropriate to a child's situation. For example, an 8-year-old acting giggly and silly while playing dress-up with a close friend is behaving appropriately in the situation, whereas an 11-year-old giggling uncontrollably during math class is not.

TABLE 4.1. Comparison of Symptoms for Depression and Mania

Symptoms	Major depression	Mania
Mood state	Sad/irritable/angry	Elevated/expansive/angry
Interest	Loss of interest	Excessive interest in many activities or topics
Sleep	Too much sleep or difficulty sleeping with fatigue	Reduced sleep without fatigue
Appetite	Increased or decreased	—
Thoughts	Morbid or suicidal	Grandiose, rapid
Concentration	Impaired	Impaired
Activity level	Restless or lethargic	Increased
Self-appraisal	Worthless/guilty	Inflated/grandiose
Behavior	Withdrawn/isolated	Reckless or foolish

Note. From Fristad and Goldberg Arnold (2004). Copyright 2004 by The Guilford Press. Reprinted by permission.

Although mania can be the more dramatic phase of BD, depression is often longer-lasting and, over time, more debilitating. It is important for both parents and clinicians to understand how the two phases differ, as recognizing mood states often helps to guide psychopharmacological intervention.

A euphoric mood and a dysphoric mood may occur simultaneously or alternate rapidly during a particular time period. This is described as a "mixed" state.

Symptoms that accompany dysphoric and euphoric mood states, and that constitute depressive spectrum disorders and BSD, are summarized in Table 4.1.

Determining the Significance of the Mood Problem

After you determine which mood states are occurring, the next task is to establish how significant the mood problem is. We use four metrics to determine this: Frequency, Intensity, Duration, and Impairment (FIDI). FIDI can be rated in different settings and used initially to assess the problem, then subsequently to evaluate treatment response.

- *Frequency* describes how often the mood states occur. Periods of excessive silliness that occur once a month probably do not significantly interfere with a child's functioning. However, periods of excessive silliness that occur most days in a week are more likely to cause problems.

- *Intensity* refers to the severity of mood symptoms when they occur. Being somewhat giddy may not cause problems. However, when silliness moves into euphoria and the behavior seems bizarre to anyone who observes it, then the symptom is more severe and the intensity of the mood state is more significant. Similarly, if a child is a little bit sad after school in response to an argument with a friend, a parent may be sympathetic but not overly worried. However, if a child comes home miserably sad and distraught without a notable stressor, this is more concerning.

- *Duration* refers to how long a mood state lasts when it occurs. Giggling and being silly for short periods (10–15 minutes) throughout the day may be noticeable but may not cause significant problems. Excessive silliness that continues for 4 or more hours during a given day (not necessarily all at once) and continues for several days in a row is likely to be disruptive to the whole family and to be problematic.

- *Impairment* refers to the degree to which a child's mood states cause problems for the child and those around him/her. A child who gets a little weepy before bedtime but is able to get a reasonable amount of sleep, and whose crying doesn't interfere with the rest of the household's sleep routine, has relatively low impairment caused by sadness. On the other hand, a child who becomes weepy and distraught during the school day, is unable to complete work, and causes a distraction for other children has relatively high impairment due to sadness. Irritability after school can be a nuisance, or it can result in disruption to the household and an inability to function socially and within the family. A high energy level with an elevated mood may not be disruptive during weekend play time, but may cause considerable impairment during the school day.

It is important to explore all possibilities before assuming that a child or teen's symptoms can be explained by a mood disorder. Be a good detective. As children grow older, consider the possibility that recreational drugs and/or alcohol are contributing to the symptoms observed. Environmental stressors should also be considered. If issues occur primarily at school, the possibility of learning disabilities or other school-related issues, such as bullying, should be explored. Finally, it is important to rule out any physical causes. Mood symptoms can be signs of diabetes; thyroid disease; anemia and other nutritional deficits (e.g., low vitamin D); side effects from medications; and many other physical illnesses (e.g., mononucleosis).

Defining Childhood Mood Disorders

One of the best ways to understand mood disorders, and to help parents understand them, is to look at graphs of mood patterns. Figure 4.1 shows a variety of patterns, including those of several BSD and depressive spectrum disorders. Panel A depicts normal fluctuations in mood. Panel B shows dysthymic disorder (DD; a mild to moderate depressive disorder, which lasts at least 1 year in a child or adolescent). Panel C illustrates Major Depressive Disorder (MDD; more severe depression lasting at least 2 weeks). Panel D shows Bipolar Disorder I (BD-I; manic episodes lasting at least 1 week, alternating with periods of depression lasting 2 weeks or more). (In most of the book, BD-I is referred to simply as BD.) Panel E shows Bipolar Disorder II (BD-II; hypomanic episodes lasting at least 4 days, alternating with periods of depression lasting 2 weeks or more). Panel F illustrates cyclothymic disorder (hypomania alternating with periods of mild depression for at least 1 year). The fourth edition of the *Diagnostic and Statistical Manual of Mental Disorders* (DSM-IV) was published by the American Psychiatric Association in 1994. Our knowledge of early-onset BSD has developed considerably since then. Changes to BSD diagnoses have been suggested for DSM-5—most notably, that 2 days might be consid-

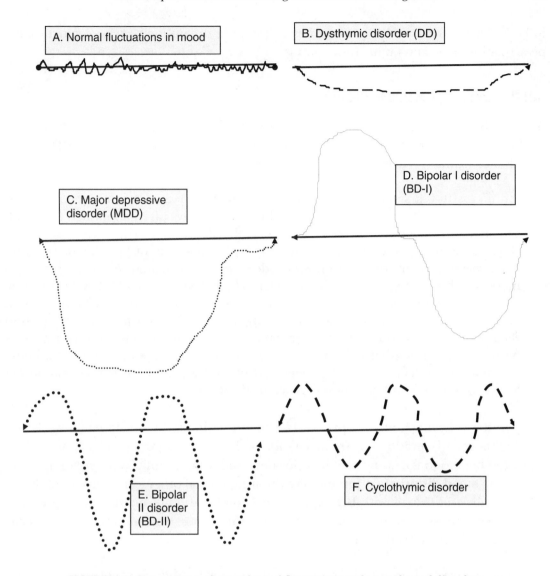

FIGURE 4.1. The patterns of normal mood fluctuations and several mood disorders.

ered a sufficient duration for a hypomanic episode. However, at this writing, final decisions on criteria alterations have not been made. Since BD-II and cyclothymic disorder in children have not been well studied, we concentrate below on BD-I and on a residual BSD category.

Disorders Involving Depression in Children?

Depressive spectrum disorders include MDD, DD, and depressive disorder not otherwise specified. Depression is also a highly impairing component of BD and other BSD. Although BD can occur with only a manic episode, depressive episodes are the more common and ultimately the longer-lasting phases of BD. The depressive symptoms tend to be harder to treat, and over time they cause more disruption to school functioning, peer relationships, and family functioning.

BD: Occurrence of Mania in Children

BD (i.e., BD-I as defined above), also called manic–depression, is diagnosed when an individual has experienced mania. Even if depression has not yet occurred, BD is diagnosed once mania has occurred.

> Jennifer is 10 years old and in fourth grade. She has always been a high-energy kid with lots of interests and ideas. Her teachers have always raved about her. Although she has always made friends easily, it has been harder for her to develop close friendships as she has gotten older; her intensity has made some of her friends shy away from spending more time with her outside of school. During the spring, Jennifer's mood has begun to get overly happy. Her energy level has made it stressful to be in the house with her. She becomes intensely excited about a project, starts it, then gets distracted and leaves it; there are multiple piles of unfinished projects around the house. She has also begun talking loud, fast, and almost constantly. Her parents have been enforcing her normal bedtime, but it has been taking her up to 2 hours to actually fall asleep, and she has been getting up about an hour earlier than usual. She goes full steam all day and never seems tired.

> Jennifer is having a manic episode. Her mood is elevated most days in a week (*frequency*); the mood elevation is extreme (*intensity*); this has been going on for a week (*duration*); and her mood is causing problems for her and for her family (*impairment*). In addition to the mood disturbance, Jennifer is exhibiting several other symptoms of mania.

Typically, individuals with BD experience a combination of mania and depression. Sometimes depression and mania occur at separate times, and sometimes they occur simultaneously in a mixed episode.

> Mike, who is 10, lives with his mother and his baby brother. His mother's boyfriend lived with the family until 6 months ago. Mike has always struggled at school and has typically been very oppositional at home. He is frequently irritable, especially after school, and his irritability has been getting increasingly intense in recent weeks. For instance, he has been lashing out at his baby brother, with whom he previously had been very patient and kind. Due to support from a resource room teacher, Mike brings home very little homework. When he does have a little bit of homework, he flies into a rage when his mother asks him to complete it. Also, Mike has been having periods when he seems excessively agitated. He is unable to settle down during these periods, and it is a struggle for him to stay seated. Mike's sleeping has become erratic; some nights he sleeps only 5 hours but is full of charged up energy the next day. Mike can be very giddy and laugh too hard at things that are not funny, and then begin crying about how much he hates his life. When he cries, he sometimes talks about how nobody loves him and how he makes everyone go away. During these crying spells, Mike talks about his father and his mother's boyfriend. Crying can turn into screaming, yelling, and throwing things in an instant.

Bipolar Disorder Not Otherwise Specified

Bipolar disorder not otherwise specified (BD-NOS) is a category for individuals whose bipolar symptoms negatively affect their functioning, but do not fit the descriptions and criteria established in DSM-IV. Here are some examples:

> Krista is 9 and has been easily irritated for as long as her parents can remember. Last year, Krista became extremely sad and tearful, lost interest in all of her favorite activities, developed psychomotor agitation, had trouble sleeping, lost her appetite, and told her mother that she wished she were dead. This depressive episode lasted for about 6 weeks. Currently Krista is back to being easily irritated, but about once a week she gets very silly and extremely energized, to the point that it seems strange to family members. At these times she seems just on the edge of losing control. During these energetic phases, Krista thinks of projects that she insists she needs to do right away; she talks incessantly; she describes grandiose plans that a 9-year-old could never carry out; and her thoughts jump around as if they were racing. These episodes last from a few hours to an entire day. After these episodes, everyone in the household is exhausted, and the house is a huge mess. Krista has the requisite number of symptoms for a manic episode, but the duration does not reach either the week-long threshold required to diagnose BD-I or the 4-day threshold required to diagnose BD-II; thus she has been diagnosed with BD-NOS.

> Eleven-year-old Trevor was adopted at birth and is an only child. He was never an easy child, but this past year has brought increasing challenges for Trevor and his parents. It seems as if he is irritable much of the time and is bothered by everything anyone else does. He has withdrawn significantly from the kids in the neighborhood and tends to spend a lot of time in his room reading. At other times, his activity level increases, and he gets interested in big projects, overestimates his abilities, and oversteps boundaries. Recently he decided to start a dog-walking business and asked his mother to print 1,000 large colored signs for him on the computer to post around the city. During these high-activity times, which last 1 or 2 days, he gets extremely irritable if he doesn't think his parents are supporting him. Trevor does not have a

TABLE 4.2. COBY and LAMS Criteria for BD-NOS

A. Elated mood + *or* irritable mood + three or more of the following:
- Inflated self-esteem/grandiosity
- Decreased need for sleep
- More talkative/pressured speech
- Flight of ideas/racing thoughts
- Distractibility
- Increase in goal-directed activity/psychomotor agitation
- Poor judgment/involvement in risky behaviors

B. Demonstrated change (increased or decreased) in functioning

C. Duration: ≥4 hours within a 24-hour period

D. Frequency: Four or more episodes of ≥4 hours' duration

Note. Based on Birmaher et al. (2010).

sufficient number or duration of symptoms to be diagnosed with hypomania, but he certainly has some hypomanic symptoms that are causing interference, making BD-NOS an appropriate diagnosis.

Two ongoing large-scale studies funded by the National Institute of Mental Health— the Course and Outcome of Bipolar Youth (COBY; Birmaher et al., 2006) and the Longitudinal Assessment of Manic Symptoms (LAMS; Findling et al., 2010)—have used the same set of operationalized criteria for BD-NOS, which are summarized in Table 4.2. Using these criteria may help you in your diagnostic work.

Developmental Considerations

The descriptions of mood symptoms provided in DSM-IV were based on adult manifestations of mood disorders. It can be harder to recognize the patterns in children. Part of the challenge in diagnosing children is their significant developmental differences, making it more difficult to figure out what is normal and what is not. A 4-year-old claiming that he is Superman and refusing to answer to a name other than "Superman" may be behaving within normal limits. The same behavior by a 10-year-old who really seems to believe that he has superhero powers may reflect grandiosity. The younger the child, the wider the range of developmentally appropriate behavior. This makes diagnosing young children particularly difficult.

Co-Occurring Disorders: Defining Symptom "Piles"

Children typically come to us with long histories of difficulties and often with other psychiatric disorders. One of our jobs, as clinicians is to help parents and others on the treatment team sort these problems into categories, or "piles," and make a plan to deal effectively with each one.

Life has been a challenge for Bobby since he was a baby. He has never slept well and from infancy has seemed to be in perpetual motion. Bobby loved preschool, but would become distraught when he had to separate from his mother. Separation complicated bedtime as well. Out of sheer exhaustion, his parents began allowing him to fall asleep with them. Bobby was diagnosed with BD a year ago, when he was 7. At the time, his energy level had ramped up considerably. He spent most of the day in what the family came to call "hyperspeed." He jumped from activity to activity, intensely interested in each one, describing grandiose ideas about how important these projects were and how they would ultimately help people. When Bobby talked about them, he talked quickly and loudly, and it was very difficult to interrupt him. If he couldn't do the activity he was interested in, he would become extremely angry and rage for up to 1½ hours. Following rages, he would cry and tell his mother that he wished he had never been born. Since his diagnosis with BD, Bobby has been taking a mood-stabilizing medication. At age 8, some of his mood symptoms have improved, but he continues to have multiple problems. Currently he falls asleep in his own room, but insists that his mother stay on the second floor until he is asleep. He still wakes in the middle of the night and gets in bed with his mother. Bobby's teachers have repeatedly raised concerns about his attention and his activity level. At home, Bobby throws a fit whenever he doesn't get his own way. These problems often overwhelm his parents and confuse his treatment team.

So what are Bobby's "piles"? His problems can be sorted into the four groupings shown in Figure 4.2. First, Bobby has a mood disorder, and its symptoms constitute one pile. He experiences periods of excessively high mood, extreme irritability, and extreme sadness. Accompanying these changes in mood state are grandiosity, periods of high energy, and racing thoughts. In addition to the mood pile, he has always been easily distracted and impulsive. These issues are particularly notable at school and indicate ADHD. Thus they are grouped under ADHD in Figure 4.2. In addition, Bobby worries a lot and experiences considerable separation anxiety at a level that is inappropriate for his age. These issues make up an anxiety pile. Finally, there is Bobby's disruptive behavior pile: He tends to be oppositional and to defy parental requests.

Children with mood disorders often have comorbid disorders. These can be grouped into several categories: behavior disorders, anxiety disorders, eating disorders, developmental disorders, elimination disorders, and psychotic symptoms. Below, we briefly review how these tend to interact with mood disorders and how differential diagnoses can be made.

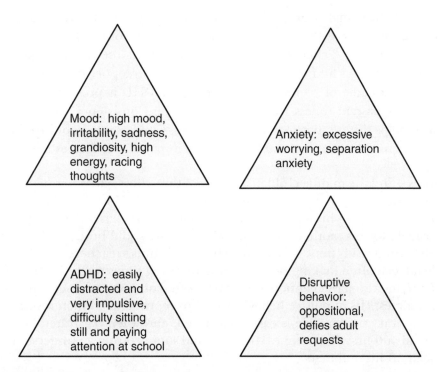

FIGURE 4.2. Bobby's symptom "piles."

Behavior Disorders

One or more behavior disorders occur in many children with depression and probably most children with BSD. These include ADHD, as well as two disruptive behavior disorders: oppositional defiant disorder (ODD) and conduct disorder (CD). Based on a recently completed treatment study by the Ohio State University Mood Disorders Program, the rate of ADHD in children diagnosed with depression was 88%, whereas the rate in BSD was 90% (Fristad et al., 2009). Similarly, rates for ODD were 86% for children with depression and 90% for children with BSD. Rates for CD were 22% for children with depression and 30% for children with BSD.

Children with mood disorders often have difficulties with impulse control and with maintaining attention and concentration. Making a differential diagnosis can be challenging, partly because mood symptoms can mimic ADHD. To complicate things further, some research suggests that stimulant medication can worsen manic symptoms (DelBello et al., 2001), while other research suggests that it does not worsen or trigger manic symptoms (Pagano, Demeter, Faber, Calabrese, & Findling, 2008; Carlson, 2009). This makes it particularly important to differentiate between ADHD and BSD. Although it is common for children with BSD to have ADHD, the reverse is not true: Children with ADHD do not have a high rate of BSD. Thus identifying symptoms that are specific to BSD can significantly aid the diagnostic process.

ADHD versus Mania

Look first for the cardinal symptoms of mania—expansive or elevated mood and grandiosity. It is important to differentiate impulsivity, or behavior resulting from poor judgment, from grandiosity. A child with ADHD runs into the street because he/she did not look before running. A child with mania runs into the street because the child believes he/she can win a game of "chicken" with the cars. ADHD is present by age 7, and its symptoms are consistent unless treatment is in place. Consistency, or the lack of consistency, also helps differentiate the two conditions. Consistently impulsive/hyperactive behavior is a sign of ADHD; noticeable change in impulsivity indicates mania.

> Dennis is 9 and the middle child in a family of three boys. He is frequently in conflict with his older brother, due to his impulsive behavior and his high activity level. Getting Dennis through his morning and evening routines has always been an exhausting struggle for his mother, who notes that his 7-year-old brother is more independent in getting ready for school than Dennis is. Dennis's teachers complain that he is highly fidgety, often making noises during teaching times when the rest of the class is quiet. They also have mentioned that he is often off task and does things to irritate his classmates. His impulsive behaviors lead to reprimands, which result in remorse and temporary sadness. He is easily frustrated, and when frustrated he is prone to emotional outbursts. Sometimes structure and support from an understanding adult can head off his outbursts.

> Joanna is 10 and the elder of two children in her family. She has always been a high-energy child, in contrast to her 7-year-old brother, whom her mother describes as "mellow" and "cautious." Joanna has trouble staying on task and can be disruptive

at both home and school due to her high activity level. Recently her energy level has revved up even more. She tends to be intrusive in peer groups: She tries to direct peer activities overzealously and with exaggerated emotion, and she seems to grossly overestimate the importance of her ideas as well as the importance of her role in the group. Peers have been shying away from Joanna as these behaviors have been increasing. When the other children laugh, she laughs longer and louder, and sometimes is overly silly when the other children are not laughing. Her ideas about projects she can do with her classmates have been getting bigger and grander, so that her peers are reluctant to go along with her even when her enthusiasm typically would have convinced them to do so.

Dennis's high energy and impulsivity are significant, but indicate ADHD with no current hallmark symptoms of mania. Joanna, on the other hand, is struggling with expansive mood, grandiosity, and elevated mood, as well as with attentional impairment and overactivity.

The impulsivity of ADHD also applies to emotional reactions. Children with ADHD can be emotionally labile. They can have low frustration tolerance and be prone to severe tantrums when they do not get their way. Thus it is important to determine whether a child's rages occur only in the context of being thwarted or when others' expectations are beyond their perceived capability. This requires a careful environmental analysis. For example, if a child gets frustrated on a daily basis at home, but only when reminded to do chores he/she has forgotten about or when doing homework, these symptoms are impairing but confined in scope.

In some cases, mania and ADHD co-occur. Sometimes high energy, rapid "meltdowns" following minor provocations, and poor concentration can reflect severe ADHD. In other cases, what appears to be co-occurring ADHD turns out to be symptoms of mania. Regardless, the first step is to determine whether the child is experiencing mania. If so, pharmacological treatment for the mania may be necessary. Once the child's mood is effectively treated, it will be easier to determine whether ADHD is co-occurring. It is important to stabilize mood prior to treating ADHD.

ODD versus Mania

The most difficult issue related to co-occurring ODD is helping family members figure out when a child "can't" comply and when a child "won't" comply. This becomes a very important and often ongoing differential diagnosis issue: Are the behavioral issues that crop up a result of a child's being oppositional and defiant, or are they a result of mood symptoms?

During a typical week, 10-year-old Melanie tends to want her way and insists on immediate gratification. However, she had been doing relatively well—keeping her behavior together at school and generally responding to firm redirection at home. But at a recent therapy appointment, Melanie's parents came in looking very stressed. Melanie loudly insisted that her time to meet alone with the therapist needed to come first, before her parents' turn. During her time alone with the therapist, she was domineering and difficult to redirect. When her time was up and she was asked to switch with her parents, she began arguing and ultimately had to be carried out of the office by her father. Her parents described a very difficult couple of weeks at home and some challenges at school. Melanie had been railing against the word "no" and had become both verbally and physically aggressive at times. The parents' behavioral strategies were not working, and they were exhausted.

After spending time with Melanie and listening to her family, their therapist was able to help them see that Melanie's mood was destabilized. Although her behaviors were similar to ODD, Melanie was demonstrating an underlying level of agitation and elevated mood that persisted throughout the day; sometimes she was able to continue meeting expectations, and sometimes her mood was getting the best of her. After a slight increase in one of her medications and a shift in the timing of another of her medications, Melanie's mood improved somewhat, and her behavior improved considerably. She was no longer having behavioral challenges at school, and at home she was becoming more responsive to limit setting and consequences for inappropriate behavior.

At her most recent visit to her therapist, Melanie began to throw a fit about giving her parents time alone with the therapist. The therapist reminded her that her behavior was going to determine whether she could pick where the family would have dinner after the appointment. With that reminder, Melanie was able to contain her behavior and act appropriately until the end of the session.

In the first paragraph of the vignette above, Melanie provides a great example of a child who "can't" comply because the behavior is driven by an underlying mood episode. In the third paragraph above, she provides an example of a child who "won't" comply because she wants what she wants when she wants it. Helping parents to separate behavioral problems from mood episodes is a critical part of separating mood disorders from co-occurring disorders. Oppositional behavior is particularly challenging to manage and can be hard to pick out from the irritability related to a mood episode. Many children experience both "can't" and "won't" behaviors, just as Melanie does.

The behavior problems of substance use and abuse are relatively rare in preadolescent children with mood disorders. However, if you are seeing adolescents with mood disorders, substance use and abuse are much more common. Teens sometimes resort to self-medication with alcohol and other drugs in an attempt to get relief from untreated or partially treated mood symptoms or from other co-occurring disorders.

Tic disorders, including Tourette syndrome, are sometimes included with behavior disorders; many now argue that they are better classified with anxiety disorders or as neurological disorders. In some cases, children with tics can learn to suppress them or to engage in activities that prevent tics (e.g., chewing gum, holding something in one hand). For other children, medications such as clonidine (Catapres) can be used to reduce or eliminate tic activity. The same atypical antipsychotic medications that are often prescribed to stabilize mood (see Chapter 2) are also helpful to reduce tics. Some medications, stimulants in particular, can cause or increase tic activity.

Anxiety Disorders

Anxiety disorders include separation anxiety disorder, generalized anxiety disorder, specific phobias, social phobia, panic disorder, acute stress disorder, and posttraumatic stress disorders. Anxiety symptoms need to be carefully included in treatment planning for a child with a mood disorder. Anxiety symptoms can be addressed with therapy and/ or with medication. CBT has been shown to be helpful for treating anxiety. Antidepressant medications are frequently used for anxiety as well as depression. However, while a child's mood is labile, it can be very difficult to treat anxiety effectively in therapy. Also, the medications that are typically used to treat anxiety can trigger manic symptoms. Therefore, manic moods need to be well stabilized first; then the plan to manage anxiety can include CBT alone or combined with very cautious use of medications. In some cases, mood destabilization in a child with BSD brings with it a substantial increase in anxiety that resolves when the child's mood is stabilized. This increase in anxiety during a mood episode serves to remind us how uncomfortable it must be for the child experiencing the mood symptoms, as well as for those living with the child.

Obsessive–Compulsive Disorder

Although obsessive–compulsive disorder (OCD) is usually classified with the anxiety disorders, it has some distinctive features that set it apart, in terms of its apparent overlap with bipolar symptoms as well as its treatment. A child with OCD who is thwarted in completing his/her compulsions will often respond with intense rage; this can appear, on the surface, like the rages seen in a manic episode. The key to determining whether the rage is due to mania or to OCD is identifying its antecedent as well as its co-occurring features. For example, a child who rages while also not needing much sleep for days on end is more likely to have BSD; the child who rages when a ritual is interrupted is more likely to have OCD. Also, CBT for OCD is highly specific, and focuses on principles of exposure and response prevention.

Eating Disorders

Many issues related to eating affect children with mood disorders. Changes in appetite can be a symptom of depression. Emotional eating is a common feature of depression. Children who overeat in the context of their depression will typically gain weight, but generally do not meet criteria for an eating disorder.

Many medications prescribed for children with mood disorders can cause increases in appetite and thus weight gain. In some cases, medications can cause reductions in appetite and thus weight loss (see Chapters 2 and 8 for more detailed information about various medications and their side effects).

Anorexia nervosa is a serious eating disorder that is diagnosed when significant weight loss (i.e., weighing <85% of expected body weight) accompanies preoccupation with body image. Children with anorexia nervosa see themselves as overweight despite being within normal weight limits or underweight. This is different from children who do not eat simply because their appetite is gone due to a medical condition or medication side effect, or because they are depressed. Anorexia nervosa can be life-threatening and requires specialized treatment, often in a residential setting.

Bulimia nervosa is also associated with preoccupation about body image, but involves consuming large amounts of food in one sitting (e.g., an entire package of crackers or cookies) and then finding ways to rid the body of the calories (e.g., vomiting, laxative misuse, excessive exercise). This is distinct from the bingeing or foraging for excessive amounts of food that can be a side effect of some medications for BD, particularly the atypical antipsychotics.

Childhood obesity is rapidly becoming an epidemic in Western society. Overeating, underactivity, and poor eating habits can all lead to obesity. Children with mood disorders are particularly at risk for becoming overweight or obese. Many experience sleep impairment, have excessive fatigue, and have little interest in physical activity. Eating as a way to soothe difficult emotions (such as those associated with depression and anxiety) can also contribute to the problem. In addition, many medications prescribed to manage mood symptoms slow metabolism and/or increase appetite. In Chapter 9, we review ways to incorporate healthy habits (good eating habits, sleep hygiene, and exercise) into treatment for children with mood disorders.

Developmental Disorders

The term "developmental disorders" refers to problems in cognitive development, such as intellectual deficiency, and in social development, such as autism and spectrum disorders (also known as pervasive developmental disorders). Also in this category of co-occurring disorders are specific learning disorders (i.e., reading, writing, and math), speech and language impairments, deficits in motor development, and nonverbal learning disorders. Managing developmental disorders while also managing a mood disorder can get very complex, depending on the severity of the problems. As with any problem, identifying and defining the problem is the first step in developing plans to address it. A complete cognitive or neuropsychological battery is recommended, preferably when the child's mood is stable.

Elimination Disorders

Encopresis and enuresis are frequent co-occurring problems for children with mood disorders. Depending on the frequency and type of elimination problem, the level of interference varies. Nighttime enuresis can be frustrating for families, but can be managed so that the child experiences minimal interference in his/her daily life. Daytime enuresis for school-age children can be extremely distressing. Some medications, lithium in particular, can cause an increase in bladder activity and thus an increase in enuresis. This may be noted either when a child starts the medication or when a dose change is initiated. Encopresis can be even more taxing on families, and requires attention to diet, exercise, and parent–child communication. Both enuresis and encopresis can significantly aggravate social problems, so the sooner they are treated, the better.

Psychotic Symptoms

During mood episodes, especially severe episodes, it is not uncommon for children to experience psychotic symptoms. *This is almost never schizophrenia.* Barbara Geller and her colleagues found that 60% of children with BD experienced hallucinations (Geller et al.,

2000). Children with severe episodes of depression may also experience hallucinations, including hearing voices, seeing things, and sometimes smelling or feeling things. Delusions may also occur; for example, children with BD may believe that they are receiving special messages or have special powers, or may have other unusual thoughts or ideas. All these symptoms occur when mood symptoms are severe. Importantly, they go away when a mood disorder is treated.

Assessment Procedures: The Lifeline and Genogram

Unfortunately, there is no easy screening measure, instrument, or test that can make a definitive diagnosis of a childhood mood disorder. There is absolutely no substitute for a careful clinical assessment that documents the onset, offset, and duration of symptoms, as well as how symptoms occur in the context of the child's developmental, social, school, medical, and family history.

We recommend organizing an intake evaluation via two principal devices: a "lifeline" and a "genogram." A lifeline can guide the collection and integration of the child's developmental, social, school, and medical history, as well as information on the child's current family situation. Box 4.1 lists the content to summarize in a lifeline.

A three-generation family genogram can be used to summarize familial transmission of mood, anxiety, substance use, developmental, and psychotic disorders. Figure 4.3 shows the graphic conventions for recording information on a genogram. Below, we summarize the information to collect and make some suggestions for interview questions.

Document the People

Start with the child's nuclear family: Draw symbols for the parents (and stepparents if relevant), the child, and siblings. Work backward to draw symbols for the child's paternal grandparents, aunts, and uncles, then for the maternal grandparents, aunts, and uncles. If the child is adopted, record the current nuclear family, and also record anything that is known about the birth family.

Document Each Parent's Psychosocial History

The following questions can help obtain a "nutshell" version of each parent's developmental history and will provide insight into what they both naturally bring to their own parenting:

> "What was growing up like for you?"
> "How did you get along with your parents/siblings?"
> "Were there any problems with drinking or drugs or family fights?"
> "How far did you get in school?"
> "When did you meet your spouse/your partner/the child's other parent [as appropriate]?"

BOX 4.1. Contents of a Lifeline

Pregnancy and early development

- Mother's physical and emotional health during pregnancy
- Mother's use of tobacco, alcohol, illicit drugs, and prescription drugs during pregnancy
- Labor and delivery complications
- Developmental milestones
- Temperament

Child care

- What child care arrangements has the child had throughout his/her life?
- How has the child functioned in those settings?
- If there were problems, what was the apparent quality of the child care setting?

Home environment

- Who lives in the home?
- How does the child get along with those persons?
- If any immediate family members live outside the home (e.g., a parent), how much contact does the child have with that person or persons and what is the quality of the relationship?

School history

- Starting with preschool, how has the child done in each placement (behaviorally and academically)?
- If there were problems, what was the apparent quality of the educational setting/teacher?
- Have any grades been repeated?
- Have there been specialized school services (e.g., a 504 plan, an individualized education program [IEP])?
- Has the child changed schools?

Stressful life events

- Document family moves, abuse, separations, divorces, deaths, domestic violence, and so on.

Physical health

- Document any physical health concerns and their treatment, including allergy and asthma treatment

Mental health

- Document prior treatment history, including medication and psychotherapy

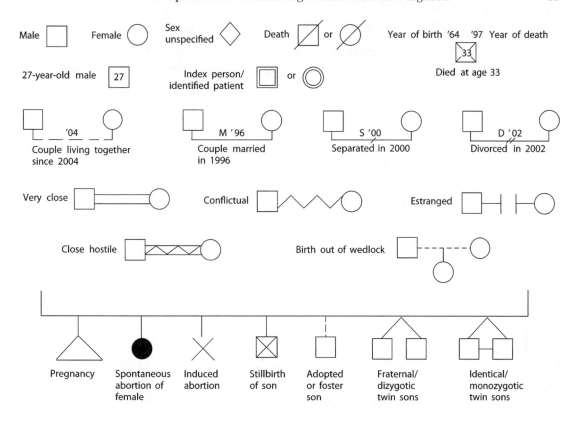

FIGURE 4.3. Graphic conventions for recording a genogram. From Zuckerman (2010). Copyright 2010 by Edward L. Zuckerman. Reprinted with permission from The Guilford Press.

Document Family History

Rather than asking about diagnoses per se, it is useful to ask about problematic behavior in general categories of disorders. This avoids the problem of underreporting (i.e., if family members were not given a diagnosis for an existing condition, or if the informant simply isn't aware of any diagnosis), as well as that of inaccurate reporting (e.g., if someone was diagnosed with schizophrenia, but your review of symptoms appears more consistent with recurrent depression with psychotic features). Have each informant look at the genogram while reporting; the visual representation can help remind him/her of all the persons to report about. The following general questions can get at suspected family history (follow-up questions can be added to clarify the information received):

"Has anyone in your family ever been in treatment or been hospitalized for mental/emotional/behavioral problems?"
    If yes: "Who and for what reasons?"

"Did anyone in your family ever attempt to kill themselves?"
    If yes: "Did that person complete suicide?"

"Did anyone in your extended family ever have problems with...."
    "Periods of time when they were really down in the dumps, sad or depressed?"

"Being unable to continue with their usual responsibilities?"

"Periods of time when they seemed to be "too high," or got into trouble for spending way too much money or doing outrageous things?"

If yes: "Was this the result of using drugs or alcohol, or for some other reason?"

"Drugs or alcohol?"

"The law?"

If yes: "Were there recurrent/major offenses?"

"Worrying much too much?"

"Not eating enough, or controlling their weight by throwing up or taking laxatives?"

"Hearing or seeing things that weren't there, or having strange ideas that didn't make sense to other people?"

Summary

The process of defining mood symptoms and detecting patterns of comorbidity helps to facilitate diagnosis and to start a child and family on the path toward good treatment. For this reason, PEP begins by educating parents and their children about mood symptoms and disorders. Part II is a session-by-session description of conducting PEP.

Psychoeducational Psychotherapy
Session by Session

Chapter 5

Discussing Mood Symptoms with Children

IF-PEP Child Session 1
MF-PEP Child Session 1

Session Outline

Goals:	1. Introduce the child to PEP.
	2. Help the child recognize depression and mania symptoms in general.
	3. Help the child recognize and rate his/her own particular mood symptoms.
Beginning the Session:	Do a check-in.
	Introduce the child to PEP.
	Establish rules, set up a reward system, and describe session structure.
Lesson of the Day:	Feeling and mood symptoms/patterns
	Teach the child to identify and rate feelings (Handouts 1, 2).
	Help the child identify his/her mood symptoms (Handouts 3, 4, and 5).
	Discuss mood swings and the child's pattern (Handout 6).
	Discuss comorbid symptoms (Handout 7).
	Present the PEP motto (Handout 8).
	Help the child generate a personal Fix-It List (Handouts 9 and 10).

Breathing Exercise:	Belly Breathing (Handout 11)

Session Review with Parents

Take-Home Projects:	Belly Breathing practice (Handout 11)
	Family Project: Fix-It List (Handouts 12 and 13)

Handouts:	
	1. Feelings
	2. Strength of Feelings
	3. Symptoms
	4. What Is Depression?
	5. What Is Mania?
	6. The Highs and Lows of Mania and Depression
	7. Other Symptoms That Cause Problems
	8. PEP Motto
	9. Fix-It List Areas (Sample)
	10. Fix-It List Areas
	11. Belly Breathing
	12. Family Project: Fix-It List (Sample)
	13. Family Project: Fix-It List

Session Overview

The goals of this first child session are threefold: to introduce children to PEP; to help them begin to understand depression and mania in general; and to help them to start to recognize and rate their own mood symptoms in particular. Each subsequent child session will begin with children's self-identification and self-rating of mood. This session also introduces the first take-home project, the Fix-It List, which asks children and parents to collaborate on identifying goals to work on over the course of PEP.

Beginning the Session

The session begins with the child (in IF-PEP) or children (in MF-PEP) and parents together briefly for introductions. In some cases, the parents and child have already met you for assessment sessions; in other cases, assessments will have been conducted by a different mental health professional. If you are meeting a family for the first time, this is an opportunity to get consent-for-treatment forms signed, and to spend a few minutes on introductions and getting to know each other. Parents then leave for the majority of the session. They will return at its end for a recap of the session content. The recap is typically led by the child, so that his/her comprehension can be demonstrated and understanding consolidated.

Do a Check-In

After the parents leave the room, spend a few minutes learning about the child. If this is your first session together, you might ask about the child's likes and dislikes, strengths, attitude toward parents and siblings, and feelings about school, as well as the breadth and quality of the child's peer network. If you have already met, check in on how the child has been doing since the assessment session. The goals are to begin establishing rapport and to gain some knowledge about how the child sees the world and what types of problems typically arise for the child.

Introduce the Child to PEP

The next step is to give the child an overview of PEP. A great way to start is to ask the child whether he/she knows why the family is participating in PEP and whether the child has any questions about it. Some children will come to PEP aware of their diagnosis and ready to develop coping skills. Others will have minimal knowledge about, and no insight into, their moods. It is important for children to understand that the purpose of PEP is to help them and their families understand more about mood disorders and learn to cope with the symptoms. It's helpful to start by taking a problem a child has identified and connect that to the child's mood symptoms, as shown in the following vignette.

Ten-year-old Jake came to the first child session of PEP with a sullen look on his face. He had been in therapy with a social worker for a while. From his perspective, they had mostly been talking about his "meltdowns" and everything else that he did wrong. Everyone seemed mad at him for getting angry and out of control, even though he couldn't help it. The last thing Jake wanted was to listen to more people telling him what he was doing wrong. He was really surprised when, after a few minutes of introductions, his new therapist asked his parents to wait out in the waiting room—and no one had said anything yet about his "fits." He was even more surprised when the therapist asked him why he thought he and his parents had come to see her. He told her, "It's because I have a lot of fits." What she said next surprised him a little.

THERAPIST: How do you usually feel before you have a "fit?"

JAKE: I don't know.

THERAPIST: Well, people usually don't have fits when they are in a good mood, right?

JAKE: I guess not. I guess I'm usually in a bad mood when it happens. Usually because my mom tries to make me start my homework or something, when I just want to chill out after school.

THERAPIST: Do you ever feel grumpy after school?

JAKE: Yeah. Usually.

THERAPIST: Well, PEP is about helping you understand the way you feel and figuring out ways to keep the way you feel from messing up your life. Like when you have one of these "fits"—does anything good happen when you have one?

JAKE: No. I usually lose something, like my iPod.

THERAPIST: Usually when kids have "fits," it is because something is wrong. Sometimes what is wrong is being grumpy or in a bad mood a lot.

JAKE: That might be me. I feel grumpy pretty often.

Jake's therapist picked up on his family's term "fits" and used a discussion about them to begin making a connection between his "fits" and being "grumpy," which is a common way for children to describe the mood symptom of irritability. This provided an opportunity to walk Jake down the path toward understanding both what his mood disorder was and how it affected his life.

The therapist then explained that PEP would teach Jake skills to help him have fewer "fits," and to get along better at home with less conflict. The skills could also help him perform as well as possible at school, and be successful making and keeping friends.

Establish Rules, Set Up a Reward System, and Describe Session Structure

Next, establish a few basic rules: participating actively in sessions, doing the take-home projects, and (for MF-PEP) confidentiality about what happens in group sessions. Write the rules down and post them in subsequent sessions. The rules can include the system of rewards to be used for encouraging the child's attention—for example, earning points at planned intervals to be redeemed for prizes, as described in Chapter 3. The general session structure can be introduced to the child in this context.

Common Issues Children Raise and Helpful Responses

After hearing about PEP, children may have concerns or raise objections. The following are comments we often hear from children, followed by responses we have found helpful.

CHILD: This takes too much time.

THERAPIST: What we've learned from other kids we've worked with is that after working hard in PEP, kids usually find they come out ahead in the end. By that, I mean they have told us that putting time and energy into PEP helps them feel a lot better about themselves, and if they've been having trouble getting along with other kids or with their family or teachers, those relationships start to get better, too. Does that seem worth it to you? Are there things that you wished would go differently? PEP is also about your goals-not just your parents'. Maybe if you put the time in you'll like the way things are going better!

CHILD: I don't want to miss any other after-school activities.

THERAPIST: You tell me what you don't want to miss, and we will try to schedule around it.

CHILD: I don't want other people to know about my symptoms.

THERAPIST: Do you know what the word "confidentiality" means? It means that everything you say here is private and that no one else will know. We only need to tell your parents something you've told us if we are concerned about your safety.

THERAPIST: [In MF-PEP] It's important that everyone here respect "confidentiality." This means that everything you say and everything you hear in here is private.

Lesson of the Day: Feelings and Mood Symptoms/Patterns

Mark the transition to this part of the session by naming it for the child. For example, you might say, "Let's start the Lesson of the Day. Today it's about feelings and mood symptoms. Are you ready?"

Teach the Child to Identify and Rate Feelings

Children with mood disorders frequently have difficulty recognizing how they are feeling—a critical step in coping with emotions. To manage their feelings, children need to be able to identify them. This session helps children name their feelings, rate how strong an emotion is, and consider why they are feeling that way.

First, children are given Handout 1 (Feelings), a set of kid-friendly pictures depicting emotions. Ask, "How are you feeling right now?", and then ask, "Do your feelings match any of the feelings shown here?" They can choose a feeling not pictured and may choose more than one feeling, as people often experience several emotions at once. For instance, on the first day of PEP, a child might say he/she is feeling scared and excited. You might then ask, "Why do you think you feel that way?" Alternatively, you could point out a possible connection between the feelings and the situation—for example, "Many children feel scared about meeting new people and starting therapy, but are also excited to start learning new ways to manage their problems and feel better." Helping children thinking about the link between their current emotion(s) and recent events starts them on the road toward future discussions about the links among thinking, feeling, and doing—the foundation of CBT.

Next, children are taught to rate the intensity of their strongest emotion on Handout 2 (Strength of Feelings). You can demonstrate how to use the feelings thermometer in this handout by describing your own current feelings and talking through what your actions would be at different emotion levels. A low rating on the thermometer means that a feeling does not affect a person's actions much. A high rating on the thermometer means that the feeling is really intense; when feelings get that strong, it is hard to control them and make good choices about how to act. That's when people start to get into the "Danger Zone," where feelings and actions get out of control. You can then color in the thermometer on the left to rate your own feelings. Here is one example of a therapist's description of his feelings and thermometer rating at the first PEP session:

"Today I am feeling excited. I'm feeling almost halfway up on the thermometer for excited. The reason I'm feeling that way is because it's our first session of PEP, and I'm excited to meet you, and I'm glad that you're here and ready to go and be involved in PEP. I'm not at the bottom of the thermometer, just a little excited, because I have some extra energy because I'm excited. I'm not at the top of the thermometer, the Danger Zone, because if I were that excited I would be having trouble staying in my seat and focusing on what we are doing. So I am about halfway up between low and high on my feeling of being excited."

Children are then asked to write their strongest emotion on the line below the right-hand thermometer, and to color in the scale to show how strong the feeling is. From this point on, children will label and rate their own feelings at the beginning of each session. Doing this can (1) quickly reestablish rapport; (2) help you take the child's current mood into account when completing session tasks; (3) open discussions about specific emotions and related events; and (4) help you gather specific examples to use to illustrate PEP concepts. Over time, children should get better at labeling and rating their feelings, so that this can be done more quickly.

Help the Child Identify His/Her Mood Symptoms

It is important to find out how much children know about mood disorders in this first session. Children who know little else will usually know the problems they have been experiencing. You can build on that knowledge to help a child develop a language for discussing his/her mood disorder. Children need to know that "symptoms" are feelings or behaviors that go together and are part of an illness or diagnosis. A cold can be used as an example; children are usually able to name cold symptoms (e.g., runny nose, coughing, sneezing, headache). Similarly, depression, mania, and other syndromes/disorders have their own symptoms, which involve difficulties in managing feelings or moods. With guidance from the therapist, children are typically able to come up with examples of symptoms they have experienced.

> Latisha, a 9-year-old girl, was diagnosed with MDD after completing a diagnostic assessment at a community mental health agency. She had never been in therapy before, and her mother told her that she just hadn't seemed like her happy self for the past month. During the diagnostic assessment, Latisha talked about how she had been feeling sad and grumpy a lot lately. She had also been spending a lot of time alone in her room lying on her bed listening to the radio and munching on potato chips. She didn't have much energy and usually asked her mom to say she wasn't home when her friends called. She felt pretty self-conscious because she had gained weight and her clothes had gotten too tight. She used to like school, but she was having a hard time paying attention lately, and she had gotten low grades on assignments because of careless mistakes or daydreaming in class and not finishing her work.

Although Latisha had not had any formal training on mood disorders, she knew how she felt. She was reporting several symptoms of depression, including feeling sad and grumpy, not having much energy, appetite increase, difficulty sustaining attention, social withdrawal, and loss of interest in things she usually liked to do. Latisha was an expert on her own depression; the challenge in this session was to give a name to the syndrome that was plaguing her and to begin to instill hope.

Using what she already knew about Latisha, her therapist, June, began to help Latisha develop a language for discussing her mood disorder.

JUNE: Latisha, you have already described some of the problems you have been having, like feeling sad and grumpy and not having much energy. Right?

LATISHA: Yeah …

JUNE: Well, we have a name for those problems—they are called "symptoms."

LATISHA: You mean like when you have a cold, having a sore throat is a symptom?

JUNE: Exactly, and instead of having symptoms of a cold, you are having symptoms of depression. Can you think of some other symptoms that are causing problems for you?

LATISHA: Well, I'm tired a lot and never want to do anything. Is that what you mean?

JUNE: Are you usually someone who has energy and wants to do things?

LATISHA: Yeah, I usually always want to play with my friends.

JUNE: What about at school? Are any symptoms causing you problems at school?

LATISHA: Yeah. School is usually easy, but now I keep getting in trouble for not getting my work done.

JUNE: Let's take this worksheet [Handout 3] and make a list of all of the symptoms that are causing problems for you.

Once children understand what symptoms are, they are typically quick to make connections with their own experiences. With their therapists' help, most children are able to generate a list of current or past symptoms of depression, mania, and/or other syndromes/disorders. Box 5.1 lists ways in which children have described their own mood symptoms. You can provide prompts about what happens (to sleep, appetite, energy level, etc.), or make suggestions based on information provided by the parent or child during the assessment. The symptoms can be written down in the child's language on Handout 3 (Symptoms), in the appropriate columns for depression and mania. If children list symptoms of other disorders, these can be recorded as well but discussed after the mood symptom discussion.

Using the children's language to record and talk about feelings and symptoms builds rapport and helps them understand the concepts. For this reason, we usually do not provide Handouts 4 (What Is Depression?) and 5 (What Is Mania?) until after the children have made their own lists. If a child is not familiar with the terms "depression" or "mania," or is struggling with identifying his/her symptoms, you can provide these lists of common symptoms and ask the child to circle the ones he/she has when feeling depressed or manic. There is also space on the bottom of these handouts for children to write down symptoms in their own words. Even children without a bipolar diagnosis may benefit from hearing about symptoms of mania, as approximately 25–50% of prepubertal children with depression develop BD. For children without manic symptoms, Handout 5 can be reviewed briefly rather than discussed.

BOX 5.1. Ways Children Describe Their Mood Symptoms

Depression

- Feeling upset or sad all over my body
- I don't wanna do nothing, I just wanna sleep
- Feel like yelling at my dad and mom and for no reason
- Bored with everything
- Feel like my family would be better off if I weren't here anymore
- Really tired, but I can't fall asleep
- Easily overwhelmed

Mania

- My thoughts are jumpy
- Really high happy
- Hyper
- I feel like something good's gonna happen to me today
- Real crazy, bouncing off the walls
- Sometimes I can get through almost the whole night without going to sleep
- Calling out the answers in class without waiting
- Thinking about girls' bodies too much and saying inappropriate things
- Like I can do dangerous things and not get hurt
- Everything is funny
- Super, super angry

Discuss Mood Swings and the Child's Pattern

To increase a child's understanding of depression and mania, discuss Handout 6 (The Highs and Lows of Mania and Depression). Some children have several days in a row where they feel manic or depressed; and other children's moods change more often, even several times in one day. Children can talk about their experiences of slow mood swings or rapidly fluctuating moods. The difference between the small fluctuations in mood due to everyday circumstances and the major mood swings seen in mood disorders can be discussed. Children may note that sometimes they feel super-happy when their baseball team wins, their favorite relatives are coming to visit, or they do really well on a school assignment. Explain that these time-limited, minor changes happen to everyone, but that depression and mania are characterized by mood swings that cause problems or last much longer than the precipitating event. A manic episode can be triggered by a big event, like going on a trip for a vacation or a visit to relatives; what distinguishes it from typical "ups and downs" is the "over-the-top" nature of the excitement or irritability.

Discuss Comorbid Symptoms

Comorbidity is closer to the rule than the exception among children with mood disorders. Therefore, it's helpful to take a few minutes to discuss symptoms of other common comorbid conditions, such as ADHD and anxiety disorders. Use Handout 7 (Other Symptoms That Cause Problems). Less frequently, children with mood disorders may have psychotic symptoms. Most often, psychotic symptoms in children are mood-dependent and go away when a mood episode is treated; in rare cases, however, the psychotic symptoms occur without mood symptoms and have to be specifically treated. Reviewing the "Other" category on Handout 7 may give children words to label these psychotic experiences or encourage them to share these symptoms. Experiencing them can be unsettling or embarrassing to discuss. Helping children describe and categorize their symptoms can boost their understanding and thus make it easier to improve their functioning. It also aids in differential diagnosis and certainly facilitates treatment. Mood disorders are episodic; symptom recognition greatly enhances the ability to treat mood episodes when symptoms first emerge and are most responsive to intervention.

Present the PEP Motto

Improving functioning is the goal of PEP; thus the PEP motto is "It's not your fault, but it's your challenge!" Children need to understand that their depressive, manic, or other symptoms are not their fault; that is, they did not cause the symptoms. Rather, their symptoms indicate a problem in their brain, and they were probably born like this. Even so, it is their challenge, meaning that they need to work to level out their moods, as shown by the arrows on Handout 8 (PEP Motto). PEP is about working to raise mood when a child is depressed (too sad, worried, or grumpy) or lower mood and energy when a child is manic (too high, too angry).

In explaining this motto, it is also important to make sure that the child understands what he/she can and cannot control.

Kayleigh crossed her arms, started staring at her shoes, and looked increasingly tense as her therapist, Gina, talked about the PEP motto. Gina saw this and commented, "You look like something is bothering you." Kayleigh took a breath and then burst out, "My teacher keeps telling me that I can control myself, and now you are too, and I don't feel like I can!" Gina immediately sensed that this was a crucial moment for Kayleigh and PEP. "You're right! You don't have control over your mood right now, do you? I know that your parents and your psychiatrist have been working hard to find helpful medicines for you, but the medicines aren't helping enough yet. Our motto doesn't mean that you can control the way you feel, and it doesn't mean that you can control yourself all of the time. It means that you need to be part of the team that is working on helping you manage your mood. On helping you feel better. And right now that means learning new ways to help yourself and really practicing them. Does that sound okay to you?" Kayleigh began to relax. "Yeah, I'd like to be part of the team, and I really want to feel better."

Children with mood disorders, especially those in the midst of acute mood episodes, can be very sensitive about adults' implying that they have more control than they feel they have. It's helpful to validate the child's concern, as illustrated in the example above. PEP is all about helping a child and family develop strategies for leveling mood, which, along with medication, can help them feel better and give them some control. When children understand this goal, and realize that PEP activities are steps to reaching that goal, they can be highly motivated to work in therapy. This discussion leads into the introduction of the Fix-It List, the first take-home project, in which they and their parents will develop concrete goals they will work toward for the duration of PEP.

Help the Child Generate a Personal Fix-It List

The point of the first take-home project is for children and parents to come up with an agreed-on list of three problems they would like to work on or "fix" during the 24 weeks of IF-PEP or 8 weeks of MF-PEP. In preparation, each child, with therapist guidance, first creates his/her own list in this session. The parents are instructed to create their own separate list (described below). From these two lists, a single Family Fix-It List is negotiated.

In this session, the discussion has three components: First, introduce the project to the child, explaining that you and the family are going to work with him/her to help the child gain better control over his/her feelings and have fewer problems.

Next, help the child generate a list of problems he/she would like to work on. You can prompt for ways that the child's feelings are causing problems with parents and siblings, or getting him/her into trouble at home, at school, or with friends in the neighborhood. Drawing from information gathered during assessment, you can also provide ideas to get the child started. This discussion should be structured so that the child is able to identify problems but not become overwhelmed by them. The focus should be on problems that are specific and thus much more solvable. Handout 9 is a sample list of child problems in the three areas. Handout 10 is a blank version that can be filled out during this part of the session.

Finally, the child's list of problems is narrowed down and used to help the child develop three realistic goals for improving behavior. The child should be guided to list goals that can be realistically achieved within the time frame of treatment. These three goals become the Child Fix-It List in the take-home project (see Handouts 12 and 13).

We typically present the Fix-It List to the children separately, as described above, and bring parents into the discussion about the list as a family project at the end of the session. However, in IF-PEP, depending on your clients, you may choose to work with parents and children together. Some children will benefit from having their parents' feedback during this discussion; others will not need it or will have a harder time doing this task with their parents in the room. MF-PEP does not allow for such flexibility.

Breathing Exercise: Belly Breathing

Three breathing techniques are taught during PEP: Belly, Bubble, and Balloon Breathing. Belly Breathing is introduced in this session. At least one of the three breathing exercises should be practiced briefly at the end of each child session.

Belly Breathing is taught first, because it helps children understand the physiology of deep breathing and lets you double-check the children's form while breathing. An exaggerated demonstration can be a great way to start. You can begin by placing one hand on your upper chest and one hand at your waist. Then demonstrate how, as you take a shallow breath, your shoulders and chest move up and down and your belly does not move much. This means that the air is just going to the top of your lungs and not deep into your lungs. Next, demonstrate how, if you take a deep breath, your belly expands and your shoulders and chest do not move much. Explain, "deep breathing is a way to help ourselves calm down and even out our moods."

After the explanation, have children practice Belly Breathing in the session. Lying down or bending over helps children learn how taking a deep breath feels. If space permits, have them lie down on the floor. This allows for the best feedback on whether the technique is being accurately applied. If the space does not permit or a child is unable or unwilling to lie down, have him/her practice while bending over at the waist. This second option, however, will not work if the child's clothes are tight around the waist. Deep breathing is not very portable or inconspicuous if you have to lie down or bend at the waist to do it. For this reason, children also should practice while sitting and standing, so they can take the technique anywhere and use it when they are upset. Each method is described below.

- *Lying-on-the-floor practice.* Ask the children to place one hand on the chest and one hand on the belly or at the waist. Then demonstrate how the hand on the chest does not move much and the hand on the belly does move when the children take a deep breath. Explain that it is hard to move the shoulders up when lying down, and so the air goes deep into the lungs more naturally. Guide the children through taking a deep breath in and blowing it out slowly. It may be helpful to count by saying something like this: "Take a slow, deep breath in—one, two, three, four.... Now breathe out—one, two, three, four.... Breathe in—one, two, three, four," and so on. It is important for the children to slow down their breathing and notice where in the body the breath goes. Children may find it helpful to count in their heads to make sure they take their time. After practicing for a few minutes, the children should stand up slowly so as not to become dizzy.

- *Bending-over practice.* Ask the children to relax and bend over at the waist, limply, like a rag doll. The arms should hang down limply at either side of the head. The children need to be relaxed when they are bent over, so that the breath then goes deep into the lungs. Otherwise, they will take shallow breaths, and the shoulders will move up and down.

- *Standing or sitting practice.* If time allows, or if neither of the other two options is possible, you can guide children in Belly Breathing while standing or sitting. The children should practice with one hand on the chest and one on the belly, to help them notice where the air is going.

Between sessions, children should practice deep breathing while sitting and standing up, so that (as noted above) they can use it anywhere. It is also useful for them to practice lying down or bent over, so that they can double-check that they are breathing deeply rather than taking shallow breaths. Give out Handout 11 (Belly Breathing) and ask each child to complete one to two sets of breathing practice on at least three different days. The child and/or parents should then log the practice dates on the handout. Rewards can be given in session for practicing between sessions. Also, children can teach their parents about deep breathing as a way to consolidate their learning, and to give the parents a coping strategy they can use themselves. Handout 11 provides space for parents to log their own practice times.

Session Review with Parents

With about 10 minutes left in the session, parents should be invited to join children. In MF-PEP, depending on the room sizes, children may join the parent group or vice versa. Children are asked to describe three topics to their parents: the Lesson of the Day, the take-home projects, and the breathing exercise. In MF-PEP, it is good to have three volunteers share the three topics. You should reinforce important concepts and add key points a child may have left out. The review should include a child's completed Fix-It List of three goals on Handout 10. Ideally, this list has been completed by the end of this session, but parents should help their child finish the list if necessary.

Take-Home Projects

Belly Breathing Practice

Explain Handout 11 to the parents. Encourage them to help children complete Belly Breathing practice and log their practice dates on the handout, as well as to learn and practice the techniques themselves.

Family Project: Fix-It List

Explain to parents that they and their child should together develop a Family Fix-It List. Give parents copies of Handouts 12 and 13 (the completed-sample and blank Family Project: Fix-It List). The parents will need first to generate their own Parent Fix-It List of three problems they would like to work toward solving. Emphasize that these should be problems that can be partially or fully "fixed" over the 24 weeks of IF-PEP or 8 weeks of MF-PEP. The parents' list should include items that are within parental control, such as speaking, not yelling, taking time for stress management (e.g., exercising for 30 minutes daily), and improving communication between parents. Rather than "Tom will listen to me," a parent might list, "I will be sure to gain Tom's attention before asking him to do something." The more specific the items, the easier they will be to accomplish and track.

The Family Fix-It List should be developed together. Problems should be phrased for the whole family (e.g., "No one in the family will hit anyone else," rather than "John won't hit anyone"). Again, families should be encouraged to develop specific goals for which progress can be tracked. Review this list at the beginning of the next child-focused session, when parents and children meet together.

Staying Organized

In closing the session, let children and parents know that they will be accumulating many handouts over the course of treatment. If you have not chosen to use the pre-made workbooks (see *www.moodychildtherapy.com*), and will be making individual copies of handouts from this book, it will be very important for a child to have his/her own folder for storing the child handouts. Parents also need to maintain a folder or binder for their child's treatment information and for their own handouts, as they will refer to them frequently.

Chapter 6

Reviewing Symptoms and Disorders with Parents

IF-PEP Parent Session 1
MF-PEP Parent Session 1

Session Outline

Goals:	1. Introduce general framework of PEP.
	2. Help parents recognize symptoms of depression and mania, particularly those their child is experiencing.
	3. Give parents hope and motivate them to work hard in PEP.
Beginning the Session:	Do a check-in (Handouts 12 and 13).
	Provide orientation to therapy.
	Present overview of PEP (Handouts 14 and 15).
	Discuss the importance of take-home projects.
Lesson of the Day:	Mood symptoms and disorders
	• Myths and facts about mood disorders
	• Why do people get mood disorders? (Handout 16)
	• Understanding mood disorders in general

- What are depressive spectrum disorders? (Handout 17)
- What are bipolar spectrum disorders? (Handout 18)
- Suicide risk (Handout 19)
- The impact of season on mood (Handout 17)
- Co-occurring symptoms (Handout 19)

New Take-Home Project: Mood Record (parents only; Handout 20 or 21)

Ongoing Take-Home Project: Family Project: Fix-It List (Handouts 12 and 13)

New Handouts:
14. PEP Parent Session Topics
15. PEP Child Session Topics
16. Brain Differences in Mood Disorders
17. Tracking Mood Changes: Depressive Spectrum Disorders
18. Tracking Mood Changes: Bipolar Spectrum Disorders
19. Additional Concerns
20. Mood Record: Tracking Three Moods, Three Times per Day
21. Simple Mood Record

Handout to Review:
13. Family Project: Fix-It List

Session Overview

This first parent-only session is heavily content-laden, but it also needs to set the tone for open communication and support. As you start by giving parents an overview of the entire program, point out that subsequent sessions will shift more to skill building. A basic PEP premise is that education, support, and better problem solving skills lead to better understanding of mood symptoms and behavior, less family conflict, and more effective treatment.

Information about mood disorders and their symptoms is presented in this session. By the end of this session, parents will have learned about the myths and facts of mood disorders; causes of mood disorders; mood symptoms and diagnoses; and comorbid disorders. Parents will go home to complete a Mood Record and to continue working on the Family Fix-It List. Your role is to help parents take a step back and learn the background information they will need as a foundation for the skills they will learn during the rest of PEP. Parents should come away with a much clearer idea of why their child has a particular diagnosis. This is critical in order for them to be effective, active participants in their child's treatment.

Beginning the Session

Do a Check-In and Provide Orientation to Therapy

Begin each session with a quick check-in on how the family and child have been doing since the last session. Parents in IF-PEP may wish to do some brief problem solving about issues that have arisen with the Family Fix-It Project from the first child session. For MF-PEP parents, begin with a general introduction of group members, as discussed for MF-PEP children in Chapter 5. If you have not already obtained information on the parents' efforts and frustrations in managing their children's mood disorders during the assessment, you can ask now for a brief review. This aids in empathically connecting with parents during this and subsequent sessions.

Give parents a brief orientation to basic therapeutic guidelines. This includes discussing the limits of confidentiality and the importance of developing a no-fault, guilt-free atmosphere, so that parents feel comfortable discussing their deepest fears and most devastating moments. Some basic courtesy rules also apply (e.g., arriving for sessions on time and turning cell phones off or to the vibrate-only setting).

In an ideal world, all of a child's caregivers would attend each session. The reality is that families often need to send one representative. The parent or caregiver who attends the session should set aside time to review session content and discussions with his or her partner. Reviewing this material with other caregivers will increase the benefit families get from PEP. As a therapist, your goal is to encourage as much attendance and between-session participation as possible from all caregivers without instilling guilt or adding undue pressure.

Present Overview of PEP

Parents need to have a sense of what they will gain from PEP, as well as what their children will gain. A brief review of parent and child session topics will help parents know what to expect. Give parents copies of Handout 14 (PEP Parent Session Topics) and Handout 15 (PEP Child Session Topics). As the handouts show, there is considerable overlap between what the children learn and what the parents learn. You can then highlight what parents, as well as their children, have to gain from PEP. Parents can benefit from the following:

- Learn about depression and manic–depression (bipolar disorder) in children.
- Learn about the biopsychosocial treatment of childhood mood disorders.
- Learn how to work with the school system and the mental health system regarding your child.
- Learn new communication and problem-solving strategies to manage mood symptoms and improve family life.
- Become educated consumers and be the best advocates for your children.

In this and other sessions focused on symptoms and disorders, parents sometimes express concern about their children's being "labeled." If this issue is raised, it presents a great opportunity to introduce the PEP motto: "It's not your fault, but it's your challenge!" The more children understand what their illness is, how their medications work (if applicable), and why they should use coping strategies, the more they will be able to accept the challenge and become part of the solution to the many problems that mood symptoms create. The same holds true for parents, who often begin PEP overwhelmed and confused.

> PARENT: It seems like everyone is giving me different advice, and it's so overwhelming. I know that things are bad, but I don't know how to help Anna and our family.
>
> THERAPIST: It sounds like things at home have been really difficult over the past several months, and that it has been really hard to figure out what to do. My goal is to help you to understand more about Anna's mood disorder, so that you are in a better position to set priorities. In sessions, we will work on developing some skills that will help you avoid some difficult situations and be better equipped to handle others.

A common struggle for parents is differentiating between times when a child's mood symptoms are out of control and causing problems, and times when a child is just exhibiting difficult behavior. We think of this as "can't" versus "won't." Parents are often faced with trying to figure out what a child "can't" control versus what a child "won't" control. For example, a manic child is likely to flit from activity to activity, leaving messes in his/her wake and a sense of chaos throughout the household. This is different from the child who drops his/her backpack, coat, and lunch box in the middle of the kitchen each day before racing off to watch TV. As parents learn to recognize mood symptoms, distinguishing "can't" from "won't" becomes somewhat easier. (This important concept is discussed further in Chapter 12.)

Discuss the Importance of Take-Home Projects

At the first child session, parents and children have been instructed on how to complete the Family Fix-It List. (For parents in IF-PEP, this session will have preceded the present session. For MF-PEP families, this instruction usually comes at the end of the current session, since parent and child sessions in MF-PEP ideally run simultaneously.) Explain that each session will have a project associated with it, including this one. Later in the present session, parents will be instructed on how to keep records of their child's mood. Some projects will be just for the child to complete (with occasional parental assistance), some just for the parents, and some for the family. These projects are designed to increase participation in PEP between sessions.

Prepare Families to Set Aside Time for Projects

Encourage families to make PEP projects a priority. Explain that the projects are key to developing solutions. Taking time to complete the projects now will mean less time spent on problems later. Families will need to set aside at least 15 minutes a week to complete written work and then discuss it. Suggest that family members plan when they will do their project as they go home from each session.

Troubleshoot Potential Obstacles to Completing Projects

Families may initially complain that they don't have time to complete projects, that projects don't seem helpful, or that they had difficulty understanding how to complete an assignment. Part of your job is to "sell" the projects to parents and to troubleshoot obstacles to completing them. For example, new ideas presented in a session may sound like something families have tried before without success, or parents may think that these ideas would be unlikely to help. Explain that new ideas often help in unexpected ways. Projects help put ideas into action and may help to break old, ineffective patterns. Encourage families: "Try it. You might like the results!"

Discuss Parent and Child Roles in Family Projects

You should help parents determine their role in coaching their child through family projects. In some cases, only parental support and encouragement will be necessary. In other cases, parents will play the role of scribe. However, some families have a long history of parent–child struggles over homework, and they may have difficulty developing a smooth working relationship. Putting this issue on the table with parents can be useful. Defining roles at this early point may help to reduce conflict and increase success. However, if family members are in open conflict about working on projects, the therapist may need to mediate a family discussion at the end of one of the child's sessions when projects are discussed. In some cases, a discussion with only the parents may be more helpful.

Answer Parents' Questions and Provide Support

Sometimes parents think they understand a project as it's explained in the session, but when they get home, they aren't sure where to start. Tell families they can refer to the handouts they reviewed during the session or contact you between sessions for clarification if needed. Encourage parents to try something new and to practice new skills between sessions. Part of your job is to create a comfort level that allows family members to ask questions during a session or to call between sessions for clarification. The following dialogue illustrates how this discussion can unfold.

> THERAPIST: At the end of each session, I will send you away with a project to work on between sessions. When the session is primarily focused on Jaquan, the project will be for him to do, sometimes with you and sometimes independently. Other projects will be just for you to work on or for the whole family to do together.
>
> PARENT: How long will these projects take? We get really busy during the week, and our schedule is so hectic.
>
> THERAPIST: Some projects will take only a minute or two each day. For example,

this week's project asks you to rate and record Jaquan's mood on a chart each day. Other times, you'll need 15–30 minutes at some point during the week to do it. I promise you that the projects will be relevant to what is going on in your family and with Jaquan. Families have usually found projects to be doable and ultimately helpful when they put the time in to do them fully.

PARENT: What happens if we don't get to one?

THERAPIST: Jaquan gets points that he can turn in for prizes for doing his project. You may find that he pushes you to get yours done! I certainly understand that sometimes things happen that make it hard to do these projects. If you don't get around to one, I will probably suggest that we carry that project over to the next session and maybe try to double up on projects so we stay on track.

PARENT: What should I do if Jaquan refuses to do his project?

THERAPIST: Don't battle with him about it! Give me a heads-up before the next session with an email or phone message, and I'll troubleshoot with him about it. If you ever have questions or concerns about the projects between sessions, please contact me! We can also talk about it during your check-in time at Jaquan's next session.

Lesson of the Day: Mood Symptoms and Disorders

Frequently families come to PEP after many months or years of therapy without any improvement. Parents know that they are dealing with a significant problem, but often do not have a good definition of the problem and are lacking a sense of what to expect. They want the problems to go away, but need to learn how to recognize and manage the symptoms. Introduce the session's main topic: what we know and what we do not know about mood symptoms and disorders.

Myths and Facts about Mood Disorders

First and foremost, tell parents that mood disorders are treatable illnesses. However, some common myths and attitudes can get in the way of treatment. Address these first.

Myths

Two common myths about mood disorders are "It will go away (soon) on its own" and "Everybody gets this way." Yes, everybody has a bad day every now and then. Kids are irritable the day after a sleepover due to lack of sleep; kids get sad when something disappointing or upsetting happens. However, "typical" moodiness (e.g., sadness, irritability) does not disrupt family functioning, peer relationships, and school functioning. Childhood depression or BSD can be long-lasting and can cause significant negative consequences for a child and his/her family. A child who is sad or irritable across a long period of time (e.g., 6 months, half a school year) misses out on a lot of developmental opportunities, such as experiences with friends.

Other myths and misunderstandings about mood symptoms create some unhelpful but widespread attitudes in our society:

"You ought to just snap out of it."
"Getting treatment is a sign of weakness."
"Moody kids are bad or lazy."

Both adults and children can carry these attitudes, and they make it more difficult for children to get treatment.

Facts

We do know that mood disorders are relatively common among psychiatric disorders. At any given time, 9% of adults and 8.3% of adolescents are depressed (Centers for Disease Control, 2010; National Institute of Mental Health [NIMH], 2010a) and 3.7% of children aged 8–15 have a mood disorder (NIMH, 2010b). Depression does not discriminate on the basis of physical, political, religious, or cultural characteristics; it occurs across all ages and groups of people, and can even occur in animals. Partly because of the myths and negative attitudes described above, only about one-quarter of the estimated 19 million Americans with depression actually seek help.

The misconceptions described above increase stigma. Parents can also be judged and blamed for their children's moodiness or acting out. All of these factors make childhood depression and BSD difficult for families to recognize as problems needing treatment.

Why Do People Get Mood Disorders?

Explain that research points to genetics and biology as causes of mood disorders. Parents need to think of mood disorders as "No-fault brain disorders." People don't get to choose the genes they inherit or the genes they pass on to their children. To underscore this point, the following figures on genetic risk (from Tsuang & Faraone, 1990) can be presented to parents:

If one parent has a mood disorder, there is a 27% chance of a child's having a mood disorder.
If both parents have a mood disorder, there is a 74% chance of a child's having a mood disorder.
If one twin has depression, there is a 56% chance that an identical twin will have depression, and a 14% chance that a nonidentical (fraternal) twin will have depression.

In addition, research has found differences in brain structure and brain chemistry between those with and without mood disorders (see Chapter 2). Refer to Handout 16 (Brain Differences in Mood Disorders) as you review these concepts with parents, to help them understand the biological bases for their child's struggles.

Biologically based problems are no one's fault. But while the *cause* of mood disorders is probably biological, the *course* of illness is strongly influenced by psychosocial events. The goal is to treat the symptoms, since we do not currently have ways to cure the illness.

Understanding Mood Disorders in General

In order for parents to sort through the advice they get, they need to have a clear understanding of what mood disorders are and how to recognize symptoms. Explain that mood disorders are diagnosed according to the following general characteristics:

- Each mood disorder has key mood states.
- Each has a particular cluster of symptoms.
- The symptoms are severe enough to cause problems for the child or family.
- Those symptoms have to occur across an established time period.

In depressive disorders, for example, the mood is sad, low, anxious, or irritable. In BSD, mood changes from too low (depression) to too high (mania or hypomania).

To help get the best treatment for their child, parents need to keep track of their child's mood symptoms over time in four important ways: how frequently mood symptoms occur; how intense or severe the symptoms are when they occur; how long the symptoms last; and how much impairment the symptoms cause. As noted in Chapter 4, FIDI is an acronym for *F*requency, *I*ntensity, *D*uration, and *I*mpairment. The child's problems can be quantified within each of the FIDI areas as follows:

- *Frequency*:   Most days in a week?
- *Intensity*:   Mild (clearly noticeable but tolerable), moderate (between mild and severe), or severe (extreme display of symptoms)?
- *Duration*:   Four or more hours a day?
- *Impairment*: Extreme disturbance in one domain (e.g., home, school, peers)? moderate disturbance in two or more domains (e.g., home, school, peers)?

The next part of the session covers specific mood disorders and their symptom pictures. Parents can keep the above-described general characteristics in mind as they learn the details of specific disorders. Referring to Handouts 17–19, link the symptoms the child has experienced to the mood diagnosis he/she has been given, to help parents understand how the diagnosis was made.

What Are Depressive Spectrum Disorders?

Refer to Handout 17 (Tracking Mood Changes: Depressive Spectrum Disorders). Explain that there is a spectrum of depressive disorders, and that these vary according to the number of symptoms, their intensity, and their duration as follows:

- *Major depressive disorder (MDD)*: at least 2 weeks; sad or irritable mood or loss of interest plus at least four other symptoms (e.g., too much or too little sleep, too much or too little appetite, no energy, trouble concentrating, anxiety).
- *Dysthymic disorder (DD)*: at least 1 year; sad or irritable mood plus at least two other symptoms.
- *Depressive disorder not otherwise specified*: clearly impairing depressive symptoms that do not meet criteria for either of the two disorders above.

Parents need to understand that MDD involves at least 2 weeks of mood disturbance occurring at the same time as four or more other symptoms of depression. In contrast, DD is like a low-grade fever: It lasts a long time (at least 1 year), but requires fewer symptoms (two or more). Although the symptom picture is not as severe, the long-lasting nature of DD results in significant functional impairment, and so this disorder should definitely be treated.

What Are Bipolar Spectrum Disorders?

Refer to Handout 18 (Tracking Mood Changes: Bipolar Spectrum Disorders). Explain that BSDs are more complicated than unipolar depressive illnesses and thus harder to diagnose, particularly in children. In addition, the current standard definitions below are based on research on adults with BSD. Our understanding of these illnesses in children and adolescents is expanding rapidly, but is not yet reflected in the definitions. BSD all involve some combination of depressive mood symptoms and manic or hypomanic mood symptoms.

- *Bipolar I disorder* (BD-I): at least 1 week of mania—that is, euphoric or irritable mood, plus three (four if the mood state is irritable) or more other symptoms (e.g., exaggerated self-esteem, little sleep, racing thoughts, talkativeness, easily distractible).
- *Bipolar II disorder* (BD-II): at least 4 days of hypomania (i.e., less severe mania) plus at least 2 weeks of major depression.
- *Cyclothymic disorder*: at least 1 year of cycling between hypomania and depressive symptoms.
- *Bipolar disorder not otherwise specified* (BD-NOS): clearly impairing manic and depressive symptoms that do not meet DSM-IV criteria for BD-I, BD-II, or cyclothymic disorder)

It is helpful for parents to understand that in BD-I, depressive and manic symptoms can occur simultaneously. This is called a "mixed episode."

BD-II involves alternations between depression and hypomania. Explain to parents that although people with hypomania (less severe mania) can often continue functioning, their behavior is clearly out of character and their altered mood and behavior are noticeable to others and impairing. Cyclothymic disorder involves cycling between hypomania and periods with depressive symptoms (the number or duration of symptoms is not enough to meet criteria for major depression). Symptoms are more subtle but cause ongoing disruption in the person's life.

It is important to have some discussion about the BD-NOS diagnosis. Many parents will have come across this diagnosis and may need help understanding what it means and why it is used. It's a category for individuals whose bipolar symptoms have a negative impact on their functioning but do not fit the descriptions of other BSD. (See also the discussion of BD-NOS in Chapter 4.)

Suicide Risk

Refer to Handout 19 (Additional Concerns). As you discuss symptoms of mood disorders, it is important to cover suicidal thoughts and actions. These symptoms are particularly terrifying for parents, who need to know when to look for them, and how to recognize them and any other risk factors they should be prepared to mitigate.

- Suicide risk is highest:
  - During or just following inpatient treatment
  - During a crisis
  - Following the suicide of a friend or relative
  - When positive or negative life events happen
- Warning signs:
  - Talking about death/suicide
  - Saying goodbyes, making wills, giving away belongings
  - Increase in suicidal thoughts when medications are being changed
- Other risk factors:
  - Depressed/hopeless mood
  - Drug/alcohol use
  - Impulsivity/anger
  - Physical/sexual abuse
  - Running away
  - Past attempt
  - History of self-injury
  - Self-destructive behavior
  - Perfectionism
  - *Access to guns* (see below)

The most important risk factor for completed suicide is access to guns. Any clinician working with youth at risk for suicidal ideation or behaviors should ask clear questions about access to guns. Gun cabinets are not sufficient for removing access. Even locking ammunition separately from the locked guns is not enough to prevent suicide. We strongly urge families to remove guns from their homes if they have a depressed family member living there. It is important to emphasize to families that this is not an anti-gun statement; it is a pro-safety statement.

The Impact of Season on Mood

Families also need some understanding of how seasons might interact with symptoms. Return to Handout 17 on depressive spectrum disorders to discuss seasonality. For children, there are two reasons why symptoms can be affected by seasonal changes. One reason is biological: Changes in the amount of light can trigger either depression, as in seasonal affective disorder (SAD), or mania. The second reason is environmental: The level of structure and degree of academic and social pressure a child experiences differs significantly, depending on whether school is in or out of session. SAD refers to depression that typically begins in the fall or winter, when the amount of sunlight decreases. It can be thought of as a "hibernating" depression, with increased sleep and appetite, carbohydrate craving, and decreased activity along with increased sadness or irritability. Children who are unhappy in school (e.g., children who have a learning disability that complicates their ability to function in that setting) typically perk up over the holiday break and on weekends. This is *not* SAD. Those with SAD show little mood reactivity until spring or summer, when they experience a reduction in depressive symptoms. For some, the increase in sunlight that occurs in the spring can trigger mania or hypomania. Families of children with mood disorders need to be aware that seasonality can either trigger or worsen mood episodes.

Co-Occurring Symptoms

The final set of issues to address is that of co-occurring symptoms and diagnoses. Refer to Handout 19 during this discussion. Children with mood disorders often have co-occurring problems, as discussed in Chapter 4. These may include (among others) behavior disorders, anxiety disorders, eating disorders, and developmental disorders (especially learning problems or autism spectrum disorders). The diagnostic and treatment planning process should involve identifying those problems and making plans to manage them. Parents then need to understand how these problems fit into the child's treatment. It is important for you as the therapist to have a clear understanding of the symptoms a child is experiencing in addition to mood symptoms, so that you can help parents understand them and how they will be addressed. In some cases, treating the mood disorder is the primary focus, and this can sometimes also remedy co-occurring problems. In other cases, especially when the mood disorder has been effectively treated with medication, co-occurring symptoms may become the focus of treatment.

As described in Chapter 4, it is helpful to sort co-occurring symptoms into related groupings or "piles" when talking with parents. In some cases, the co-occurring symptom "pile" will respond to the same treatment as the mood disorder. For example, anxiety may be treated with antidepressants. Sometimes other medications are necessary, and in most cases specific therapy and environmental interventions are necessary. The following illustrates how one child's multiple problems and treatments can be discussed in terms of "piles" of symptoms.

"Many of the struggles you have at home are a direct result of Yoko's mood disorder. Her irritability, her periods of intense interest when she gets super-excited and can't settle down, her difficulty getting to sleep when she is so excited, and the times when she is so sad that she can't stop crying are all symptoms of her bipolar disorder. Those symptoms make up the 'bipolar pile'—problems that are directly related to bipolar disorder. However, that isn't Yoko's only pile. She also gets very anxious whenever she has to separate from you—whether to go to bed at night or to go to school. This anxiety creates its own problems—crying in the morning before school, delaying so she is ultimately late to school, coming in your room at night—and makes up the 'separation anxiety pile.' To complicate things further, Yoko has a learning disability in math. This is its own pile because it causes its own set of problems. Another pile that Yoko may have is difficulty sustaining attention, avoiding distraction, and keeping herself organized. These problems come under the 'ADHD pile.' We'll have a clearer idea of whether she also has this pile after her mood stabilizes with treatment. It can be overwhelming to look at all of the problems at once, but once the problems are in piles, we can make a plan to work on one pile at a time. Together, we will work to find ways to manage each of these piles, starting with the bipolar pile."

Psychotic Symptoms

Perhaps most frightening for parents are times when their child experiences psychotic symptoms. Psychotic symptoms frequently occur when a child is at the highest or lowest point of a severe mania or a severe depression, respectively. In most cases, when the mood is treated successfully, these symptoms go away. Give parents an overview of these symptoms, as listed below, but emphasize that they are most likely to be part of the mood disorder.

Psychotic Symptoms

1. Hallucinations are sensory perceptions that aren't based on reality. Examples:
   a. Hearing voices
   b. Seeing things
   c. Smelling or feeling things (less common)
2. Delusions are beliefs that aren't based on reality. Examples:
   a. Special messages (e.g., a child's listening to the TV for personal messages from a particular character)
   b. Special powers (these are different from grandiosity; e.g., a child's being sure he/she can see the future)
   c. Unusual thoughts/ideas (e.g., a child's being sure that a world leader wants advice from him/her)
3. These symptoms tend to occur when mood symptoms are severe.
4. They typically go away when the mood symptoms are treated.
5. *They are very unlikely to be schizophrenia.*

Take-Home Projects

Be sure to allow adequate time for discussing the weekly projects as they are explained, and for reviewing them in the subsequent session.

New Project: Mood Record (Parents Only)

The parents' new project for this session is to start keeping a Mood Record. The goal is to get parents to think systematically about their child's symptoms and responses to intervention. The Mood Record can be very detailed or simple. Handout 20 provides a Mood Record for family use that provides spaces for recording up to three times a day whether a child is sad, angry, or euphoric. Handout 21 is simpler; it calls for recording the child's general symptom level—doing well or not well along a 10-point scale—only once each day. On either version, information can be recorded about medications, coping strategies, and life events that may have an impact on the child. At this point in the program, parents need only record the child's mood (in the next parent session, you will discuss how to use the Mood–Medication Log to track the child's response to medication; see Handouts 31–32). Decide with the parents which version of the Mood Record will work better for the family. This will be determined by the nature of the child's mood (e.g., a child with long-lasting sadness but no irritability or euphoria won't need to have three moods monitored), as well as by the estimated ability of the family to keep detailed records. Although more detail is useful, there is no benefit in overwhelming a parent who simply gives up because a handout is too intimidating.

Tell parents to bring the completed Mood Record to their next session, so that mood symptoms can be reviewed and so that observations of their child's mood can be linked to any interventions being tried. The goal is to help parents more objectively monitor "the enemy" so that they, in conjunction with their child, can learn skills to manage the symptoms. Emphasize to parents the importance of monitoring mood consistently over time, particularly when their child is not doing well or when they are switching treatment options (e.g., type or dose of medication, a new school placement, frequency of therapy visits).

Tips for Parents on Keeping a Mood Record

The Mood Record fits with an ongoing goal of PEP: to increase children's awareness of their moods and feelings. Parent–child interactions during the week can encourage progress in this area. Parents can ask questions such as "Where is your mood right now? Is it up high, down low, or going up and down really fast?" Or "How are you feeling? How strong is that feeling?" However, it is also important for parents to check in with their children regarding how best to monitor mood. Some children may find this level of querying highly annoying. Others will find it useful—particularly if it is done in a low-key, supportive way—as a cue to think about their mood and what they can do if they are feeling sad, angry, or too high.

Parents can emphasize that symptoms, including the child's feelings, are not the child's fault. Feelings are never right or wrong. They just are what they are. Parents have the task of helping children to face two challenges:

1. *Returning to a calm state.* If a child is manic, the child's challenge to choose activities more likely to bring his/her mood down. If a child is depressed, it's the child's challenge to choose activities that might bring his/her mood up.
2. *Taking responsibility for his/her actions.* Feelings are what they are; actions are the result of choices. For example, it is okay to feel mad, but it is not okay to punch a sibling.

Parents can help a child meet these challenges by noticing emotional buildups, making the child aware of them, and indicating the choice the child has in how to respond (e.g., "You seem to be getting angry. What's your challenge right now?"). Children will learn tools they can use to manage their moods in their next session.

Ongoing Project: Family Fix-It List

Parents in IF-PEP have learned about the Family Fix-It List (see Handouts 12 and 13, Family Project: Fix-It List) at the end of their child's first session. MF-PEP parents will hear about it at the end of this session. As this first parent-only session is wrapping up, remind parents that they should be prepared to discuss both their Parent Fix-It List and the Family Fix-It List at the next session, and that progress on the Family Fix-It List will be evaluated periodically throughout PEP. These updates will provide opportunities for the therapist to help the family members fine-tune their goals, based on the skills being taught throughout PEP. For example, as the focus shifts to problem solving, better definitions of problems and more focused problem solving might really facilitate progress on the Fix-It List.

Remind parents to keep all the materials from therapy sessions in one folder or binder. Children will also bring home several handouts from each of their sessions. Encourage parents to review those handouts with their child, so that they will know what their child learned. They should also help their child keep his/her handouts organized in a binder or folder and make sure that the child brings this to each subsequent session.

Finally, remind parents that you will need a list of their child's medications and dosages/administration times at the child's next session.

Chapter 7

Teaching Children How to Separate Symptoms from Self and How Treatment Helps Symptoms

IF-PEP Child Session 2
MP-PEP Child Session 2

Session Outline

Goals:
1. Help the child separate symptoms from self.
2. Educate the child about treatment, the treatment team, and his/her role on the team.
3. Educate the child about medications.

Beginning the Session:
Do a check-in and review Mood Record (Handout 20 or 21).

Review Belly Breathing practice (Handout 11).

Review Family Project: Fix-It List (Handout 13).

Have the child identify and rate feelings (Handouts 1 and 2).

Lessons of the Day:	Differentiating symptoms from self and understanding treatment

Lessons of the Day: Differentiating symptoms from self and understanding treatment
- Naming the Enemy (Handout 22)
- Get Help to Put the Enemy behind You (Handouts 23 and 24)
- How medications can help (Handouts 25, 26, 27)

Breathing Exercise: Bubble Breathing (Handout 28)

Session Review with Parents

Take-Home Projects: Family Project: Naming the Enemy (Handouts 29 and 30)
Bubble Breathing practice (Handout 28)

New Handouts:
22. Naming the Enemy
23. Get Help to Put the Enemy behind You (Sample)
24. Get Help to Put the Enemy behind You
25. My Medicine
26. Summary of Medications and the Enemies They Target
27. Common Side Effects and What to Do about Them
28. Bubble Breathing
29. Family Project: Naming the Enemy (Sample)
30. Family Project: Naming the Enemy

Handouts to Review:
1. Feelings
2. Strength of Feelings
11. Belly Breathing
13. Family Project: Fix-It List

Session Overview

Children with mood disorders have not had time to develop strong self-identities before grappling with depression and/or mania. Therefore, they may begin to identify the mood symptoms as their traits. A goal of this session is to help increase children's awareness of their strengths and positive characteristics as distinct from their symptoms. A further goal is to help them understand that treatment can push their symptoms into the background so that their strengths and interests can be dominant. A final goal is to orient each child to his/her specific treatment team and show the child how to play an active role on that team. This may include discussing medication. Prior to the session, you should have an up-to-date list of a child's medications and doses from the parents.

Beginning the Session

Do a Check-In and Review Mood Record

Begin the session with parents and children together for a brief check-in on how the week has gone, and then review each child's Mood Record and the other take-home projects. Some children feel supported by having parents stay in the room throughout the review of projects; for others, this may feel infantilizing, and/or the children may not open up with their parents in the room. In still other cases, some review of projects can be done with the parents in the room, but then can be finished when the parents leave.

Review Belly Breathing Practice

Ask the child about between-session practice of Belly Breathing. Check to see whether the practice log in Handout 11 has been kept. If it has, and if a reward system has been set up for breathing practice, give the reward. Has the child had any trouble practicing? If so, make a note to address problems during the breathing exercise practice at the end of the session.

Review Family Project: Fix-It List

Review Handout 13 (Family Project: Fix-It List), which should now be completed. Check to make sure that family goals are worded to include everyone, rather than focusing only on the behavior of the referred child. Help the family rephrase the goals if this is a problem. Also check that the goals can be realistically accomplished within the treatment's remaining time frame. If the goals seem unrealistic or too difficult, help the family modify them. The Family Fix-It List will be revisited in later sessions; seeing progress on their three goals helps keep family members motivated. It is preferable for a family to meet a goal and set another than to set a difficult goal, make little progress, and become disheartened. The following case illustrates how a therapist can help refine a difficult goal into a more achievable one.

> Conrad was an 8-year-old boy with BD-II. When he and his parents came to their PEP session, Conrad proudly handed his personal Fix-It List to Stephanie, their therapist. Conrad had listed "getting along better with my brothers," "having more friends," and "not yelling at my parents as much" for his part of the exercise. His parents, Judy and Paul, had listed "being more patient with Conrad when his mood is too high or too low," "spending less time yelling," and "having more fun together as a family." The Family Fix-It List included, "everyone talking out problems without yelling," "all kids accepting 'no' for an answer," "having family game night once a week," and "everyone picking up after themselves." For the most part, the goals the family came up with could reasonably be accomplished. There was one exception.

STEPHANIE: Conrad, which goal do you think will be easiest?

CONRAD: Probably yelling at my parents less.

STEPHANIE: Okay, which goal do you think will be hardest?

CONRAD: Making more friends.

STEPHANIE: Why do you think making more friends will be so hard?

CONRAD: Because I've been trying for a long time and it isn't working.

STEPHANIE: Making new friends can be really hard, and it is an important goal. I wonder if we can figure out some goals for you that might help you on your way to making new friends, but that wouldn't be quite so hard. What do you think?

CONRAD: I guess that would be Okay.

STEPHANIE: (*turning to Judy and Paul*) When you watch Conrad with the neighborhood kids, what problems do you notice?

JUDY: Sometimes he gets really silly, and it seems like the other kids get annoyed at him. Other times, he gets really excited about a game he wants to play and tries really hard to get everyone to play his way. When the kids don't play his way, he gets upset and usually ends up storming away.

CONRAD: But it's not fair! They never listen to me!

STEPHANIE: Sounds like you get really frustrated when you play in the neighborhood. Do you get frustrated during recess at school, too?

CONRAD: Yeah. No one ever wants to play what I want to play.

STEPHANIE: Okay, Conrad. We are getting really close to some goals that you could put on your Fix-It List that I think you could make some good progress on, and that would probably help you make more friends. You want to hear what I think?

CONRAD: Okay.

STEPHANIE: What's more important to you—getting kids to play games your way, or making more friends?

CONRAD: Making more friends.

STEPHANIE: Good. So then we need to really listen to what your mom said. She said that sometimes you get too silly and this seems to bother kids, and that sometimes you try really hard to get kids to play your way even when they don't want to. What do you think you could do that might help other kids want to play with you more?

CONRAD: Try not to be too silly?

STEPHANIE: And what else?

CONRAD: Don't try so hard to get kids to play my way?

STEPHANIE: Yes. Now do those sound like goals you might be able to work on? Trying not to be too silly when you are playing, and not trying so hard to get kids to play your way?

CONRAD: I think so.

STEPHANIE: Which one would you like to choose to put on your Fix-It List?

CONRAD: Not trying so hard to get kids to play my way.

STEPHANIE: That sounds like a great Fix-It List goal. Maybe we could write it like this: "Be willing to play games that other kids suggest." I think that might help you get more friends!

Your role as the therapist in situations like the one above is to help guide the child or family toward goals that they can control and that can be accomplished during the course of PEP. It is also helpful to model, whenever possible, turning negatively worded language (e.g., "not trying so hard …") into positively worded language (e.g., "be willing …").

Have the Child Identify and Rate Feelings

In the first child session (Chapter 5), the child was asked to identify what he/she was feeling and to rate its strength, using Handouts 1 and 2. The child is now asked to do that again. There are three steps. Ask the child:

1. "How are you feeling now? Do your feelings match any of the feelings shown here [on Handout 1]?"
2. "Why do you think you feel that way?"
3. "Write the name of your strongest feeling under the thermometer [on Handout 2], and then color the scale to show how strong the feeling is."

This exercise can be done while the parents are still in the room or after the parents leave the session. If a child has a difficult time articulating his/her feelings, it can be helpful to do this with the parents in the room, particularly early in treatment. You can then model for the parents how to help their child be aware of internal emotional states. It can also help parents provide more information to the therapist on how the child's week has gone. As sessions progress, however, this exercise becomes quite routine and makes a nice transition to the child-only portion of the session.

Lessons of the Day: Differentiating Symptoms from Self and Understanding Treatment

Naming the Enemy

The Naming the Enemy exercise involves making two lists; the first is of the child's positive characteristics, and the second is of the child's symptoms. Use Handout 22 (Naming the Enemy) to write down what the child lists, as described below (in MF-PEP, generate group responses on a whiteboard or on butcher-block paper). Children complete the exercise with your guidance during the session, and then again at home with parents as a family project. The activity was developed to help all family members externalize mood disorder symptoms and see them as a separate entity rather than as qualities of the child (Fristad, Gavazzi, & Soldano, 1999). This concept, borrowed from narrative therapy, helps the parents and child view the symptoms as less rigid and restricting than if they view them as fixed attributes of the child (Fristad et al., 1999). When mood disorders develop in childhood, it can be difficult to differentiate normative developmental changes from mood symptoms, as children are in the process of developing their personalities and individuality.

In session, show the child Handout 22. Depending on the child's preference, you can be the scribe, or the child can do the writing. For the family project, either the parent or child can do the writing. The page is divided into two columns. In the left column, the child's positive characteristics are listed (e.g., "funny," "kind to others," "excellent soccer player," "good singer"). In the right column, the child's symptoms are listed in the child's (and family's) words (e.g., "cranky," "can't fall asleep," "bored with everything," "hyper"). The right column can be divided into sections depicting various disorders or sets of symptoms (e.g., depression, mania, anxiety, ADHD). As children generate a list of their symptoms, they demonstrate what they learned about symptoms of mood disorders from their previous session.

After the lists have been generated, the paper is folded down the center so that the child's positive qualities are hidden behind the symptoms. Then discuss with the child how the mood disorder has been covering the child's positive qualities. For example, a girl who is generally kind may make mean comments or yell at friends or family members when she is feeling very irritable because of depression or mania. A boy who in general is a good soccer player may be struggling to make it to practice or to practice on his own because of his depression-related fatigue and loss of interest. Then unfold the paper and refold the symptom list behind the child's positive traits. Point out that the right treatments can help children's positive qualities shine through and actually put their symptoms behind them (literally, in this case). The child's project this week is to make his/her own individual list of personal characteristics and symptoms, and to discuss it with the parents.

This exercise is designed to accomplish several purposes. First, it helps children develop a critical understanding of themselves as separate from their mood disorders. Second, it conveys the message that strategies are available to "put the symptoms behind you." This exercise illustrates how, throughout treatment, both verbal and visual representations of therapeutic concepts are presented, with the intention of connecting with the wide variety of learning styles children and their parents bring to treatment. In this instance, the hopeful message that symptoms truly can be managed can help motivate families to continue working hard in therapy. This activity leads into a discussion of specific interventions and the treatment team members who can help children put the enemy behind them.

Get Help to Put the Enemy behind You

Children need to understand that they are important members of the treatment team, which also includes their parents, school personnel, therapists, doctors, and other treatment providers. When children understand their treatment and realize that they have an active role to play in it, they are more likely to comply with treatment.

Children with mood disorders often get help from several different sources. Treatment may include a three-pronged approach, including school-based interventions, therapy, and medication, as indicated by the graphics at the top of Handouts 23 and 24 (Get Help to Put the Enemy behind You). Interventions at school may include talking to a counselor or supportive teacher, or educational plans allowing extra time to complete assignments, a reduced workload, or tutoring in specific subjects. Therapy may include group, individual, and/or family therapy, depending on the family's needs and resources. Medication may also be included as part of the treatment plan. Children can be active members of their own treatment teams by reporting and discussing their symptoms and helping to determine whether an intervention is working the way it's supposed to work.

Using Handout 23 (which is a filled-in sample), go over key aspects of the child's treatment plan, including who provides what kind of help and how the child can know whether the help is working or not. For example, a child who knows how his/her medication should be helping can report on whether or not it is working. Then, using Handout 24 (the blank version), help the child complete the form as it relates to him/her.

How Medications Can Help

Discussing medication will be most meaningful to children already taking it, but such a discussion can also be helpful when medication is being considered or may in the future be recommended as part of treatment. For any of these reasons, it is important to have a good sense of how severe the child's symptoms have been. If symptoms have been mild, discussing medication may not be relevant. However, if symptoms have been severe, this may be a timely opportunity to lay the groundwork for good adherence. As the child's therapist, you will need to know what other team members are thinking and doing about this issue. Are parents in the midst of a cost–benefit analysis regarding medications? Are they waiting for an appointment with a psychiatrist, or are they significantly opposed to medication? If they are dealing with less severe symptoms, a decision about medications may not be a critical one at this juncture.

Some of the medication issues that children must deal with are illustrated in the following case.

Chris was 11 and had experienced significant depression, followed by manic symptoms. When his PEP therapist, Julie, began talking about medications, Chris began recounting his last few months. He talked about how much he hated the way he used to feel, but also how annoying it had been finding the right medicine for him. He said that some of the medicines made him really hungry all the time. He gained weight and his clothes stopped fitting, and he felt funny around his friends. One medicine made him feel really jumpy, and another one made him feel really tired. When Chris was almost ready to give up on medication, he started taking lithium, and they switched giving him the medicine that made him so tired from the morning to the evening; the latter had the added benefit of helping him to fall asleep more easily. After a few weeks, Chris noticed he could pay attention longer in school and was not getting in as much trouble at home or in school. He was starting to believe that medication could actually help him, but he was still feeling cautious. He also wasn't crazy about the blood draws he had to have done to monitor his medicine.

Chris had a common experience: It had taken several trials to find a helpful medication regimen, and he now had to adjust to some bothersome side effects, along with periodic blood draws. His case is proof that there is no free lunch when it comes to medications. As a therapist, you will need to be comfortable talking about these issues with kids. Part of supporting adherence—especially with a child like Chris, who is approaching adolescence—is to provide clear, straightforward information. Such children need to come to their own understanding that mood episodes are worse than the nuisance of medications.

Some children will already know their specific medications when they come into this session, while others will need to be taught. In order to guide this part of the session you should refer to the list of medications and doses obtained from the parents prior to, or at the beginning of, this session. Start by asking the child, "Do you know what medications you take?", and, if the answer is yes, "What is each one supposed to help with?" Prompts may be helpful, such as "Does it help you sleep better?" or "When you take the medication, what differences do you notice?" Using Handout 25 (My Medicine), ask the child to write down their medications (or to name them while you write), along with what symptoms each medication targets. You can help rephrase the reason for the medication if the child's response is not consistent with the typical use of the medication. If the child does not know, you can share Handout 26 (Summary of Medications and the Enemies They Target) with the child and provide examples or suggestions for what each medication is known to target.

Children who are not taking medication may have questions about it that can be answered during this discussion, as in the case of Kyle.

Kyle was 10 and had been experiencing increasingly intense depressive symptoms for the past 4 months. So far, he was managing to keep up at school and was not having any significant peer problems, although he was spending more time alone than usual. He had seen a psychiatrist for a consultation, and although he had not yet been prescribed any medication, he knew that it was a possibility.

KYLE: My parents think I might need medicine. What would medicine do?

THERAPIST: That's a really important question. Let's think about the symptoms we have been talking about. What are some of the problems you have been having?

KYLE: I guess I've been grumpy a lot, and I get sad sometimes.

THERAPIST: What else?

KYLE: School is kind of harder, because I can't pay attention as well, and I don't really want to play with my friends as much.

THERAPIST: Okay. So medicines target symptoms like the ones you describe. Some medicines help you feel less sad and grumpy, and when you feel less sad and grumpy, you want to play with your friends more. Right?

KYLE: Yeah. But how long would I have to take the medicine?

THERAPIST: Well, first we have to get you to the point where you really feel better.

Once you are really feeling better, your doctor will probably want you to keep taking the medicine for a while. You can always keep talking to your parents and doctor about your medicine. Once you've been feeling better for a long time, like 6 months, then you, your parents, and your doctor might talk about whether it is time to try stopping the medicine.

KYLE: When I take medicine when I get strep throat, the medicine makes my stomach hurt. Will these medicines make my stomach hurt?

THERAPIST: Sometimes medicines cause problems, like making your stomach hurt. These are called "side effects." Before you start any medicine, your doctor will talk to you about the possible side effects. Not everyone gets side effects. If you do get them, there are sometimes things you can do to make them better. For example, if you always take your medicine with food, that often helps your stomach.

When children ask questions about medications, they often focus on three themes: the effectiveness of the medications in making them feel better; the impact of side effects; and the length of time they will need to take medicine. With the first two, your role as therapist is to instill hope and encourage a child to be an active part of the team. A child who is actively engaged in sharing how he/she is feeling makes it easier to judge the effectiveness of medications or the impact of side effects. Questions about the length of time a child will need to take medicine are easier to answer when the child is doing well without significant side effects. When medications are not proving to be very helpful, answers that focus on teamwork, patience, and the importance of clear feedback from the child and parents to the prescriber are more appropriate.

Other medication-related topics to discuss with children include which strategies for remembering to take medication may be helpful; why adherence to medication regimens is important; what to do if it seems that a medication is not helping (i.e., talk to their parents and prescribers about it); how to conduct a cost–benefit analysis (i.e., evaluate both the good and bad effects of taking medication, and discuss the pros and cons with their parents and providers); how to deal with stigma; how to manage side effects; and, as children get older, how to reconcile themselves to the idea that they "need" to take medicine to be healthy. Some suggestions for discussing adherence and side effects in particular are provided next.

Addressing Medication Adherence Issues

Adherence is a concern for anyone taking medication regularly. Assessing adherence and the reasons for any nonadherence are critical first steps. Adherence may be poor because family members forget the medication, because children do not want to take the medication, or because one or both of the parents are opposed to medication as part of the solution.

There are a host of possible reasons when parents forget the child's medication. For example, when a child is diagnosed with ADHD, there is a greater likelihood that a parent may also have it, making consistent routines a challenge. Strategies to combat forgetfulness include using "pill-minder" boxes, putting the pills in a visible location (e.g., by the toaster or coffee maker for morning medication), and setting the alarm on a parent's watch or cell phone as a reminder of the medication. If there are young siblings in the home, it is important to store medication where they will not be able to find it and take it by accident. Some parents may fear addiction, and will benefit from education regarding psychopharmacological interventions. The second parent session provides a detailed discussion of this issue (see Chapter 8).

Children's motivation to remember their medication often increases when they learn they can have bothersome withdrawal symptoms if they miss even one dose. Finding out why a child does not want to take his/her medication (or why a parent does not want the child to) is critical to increasing adherence. A common reason for problems is a loss of faith: The child begins to fear that no medicine will bring symptom relief, and thus becomes increasingly resistant to taking any medication. This is especially likely if the child has experienced particularly uncomfortable symptoms after starting out very hopeful that medication would help him/her feel better.

Michelle was 9 and came to PEP with a history of intense depression (sadness, irritability, and lack of energy), mixed with periods of agitation, mood elevation, and increased activity. Although medication had now taken the edge off her manic symptoms, she was still experiencing bouts of sadness and feelings of intense insecurity. When Jen, the therapist, quickly checked in with Michelle's parents at the beginning of the session to get an update on current medications, she learned that taking medicines each evening was becoming increasingly stressful. In addition to achieving only partial symptom relief, Michelle had had trials of multiple medications, several of which had actually led to a worsening of symptoms.

When Jen began discussing medications with Michelle during the session, she sensed irritation in Michelle's tone. She quickly validated what she interpreted as frustration on Michelle's part by saying, "Finding helpful medicines has been hard, huh?" Michelle nodded. "I have an idea," Jen said. "Let's go through the handout we just did [Handout 22, Naming the Enemy] and mark what symptoms are still bothering you. Okay?" As Michelle and Jen went through her symptoms on the Naming the Enemy handout, it became clear that symptoms of depression were still significantly problematic for Michelle. They then used that information to fill out Handout 24 (Get Help to Put the Enemy behind You) and Handout 25 (My Medicine). For the question "How do you know if it's working?" on Handout 24, Michelle immediately blurted out, "I won't cry at school and ask to see the nurse because I want to go home!" In response to the question "How will you know if it's not working?", Michelle again vehemently responded, "When I stay up all night because I'm so jittery and full of energy!" Michelle was more subdued when Jen asked the third question—"How can you be a team player to fight the Enemy and reveal more of Me?"—until Jen reminded her how willingly she was coming to her PEP sessions. Jen praised Michelle for being such an active team member, and told her that the kind of information she had provided was exactly the kind of information that would help with finding medicine for the symptoms that were still bothering her. Jen also assured Michelle that she would be talking with Michelle's parents and psychiatrist to make sure they all knew how Michelle was feeling.

Side Effects

Many medications have side effects. Children may not know what a side effect is or how to spot one. Some side effects start before the medication starts helping the symptoms; many side effects go away once the body gets used to the medication. Children need to know that some side effects can be serious and others are merely unpleasant. Children are coached to talk to their parents about any side effects they have, especially potentially serious ones (e.g., breathing difficulties, vomiting, or major sleep problems). Some annoying or uncomfortable side effects can be made more tolerable with a few environmental changes. If this is an issue for some children, you and the children can go over Handout 27 (Common Side Effects and What to Do about Them). The children can then talk to their parents and/or teachers about making accommodations. Learning to conduct a cost–benefit analysis helps children realize that tolerating unpleasant (not serious) side effects may be preferable to experiencing symptoms; that is, the benefits outweigh the costs or hassles (as depicted by the balance scale on Handout 27). At other times, the side effects may be worse than the condition they were initially prescribed to treat. Children need to understand the importance of talking frankly with their parents and prescribers if they have questions about medications. After all, the children are the ultimate consumers of care, and if they don't experience benefits that outweigh the costs, it is doubtful that they will (or should!) adhere to the treatment. Side effects often can be managed, but first they need to be communicated to parents and prescribers, so that strategies can be developed to deal with them.

Sometimes refusing medication has a hidden benefit for children, such as getting attention from parents. This is particularly common with anxious children, who may really like having their parents' attention focused on them. Many children with mood disorders also have disruptive behavior disorders; some of these children may use not taking their medication as a way to annoy their parents or to defy authority figures. Clearly, strategies to address these disparate reasons for nonadherence will differ according to the reasons why the children are not taking the medication. Helping children become active team members can significantly improve medication adherence.

Breathing Exercise: Bubble Breathing

First, briefly review Belly Breathing with the child and introduce him/her to the second breathing exercise, Bubble Breathing. Begin by asking whether the child can easily imagine blowing bubbles. Ask the child to demonstrate (or pantomime) holding the bottle, dipping the bubble wand, forming his/her mouth, and blowing air to blow bubbles. As the child does this, carry on a monologue with vivid imagery about blowing bubbles.

> "Now imagine holding your bottle of bubbles, and dip your bubble wand in. Now take a deep breath, and hold the bubble wand in front of your mouth. Purse your lips, like you are going to say 'oo,' and gently blow the air through the bubble wand. As you blow gently, you see several bubbles float away. You can see the shimmery colors reflected on the surface of each bubble. You watch a bubble float gently on the wind,

up into the air. Now dip your bubble wand in again, and take another deep breath—fill up the bottom of your belly with air. Blow out the air very gently. Imagine blowing softly enough that you make a big bubble. You see the bubble getting bigger on the bubble wand. You see a rainbow of shimmering colors on it as it grows and grows. You are outside on a warm, sunny day, and you watch as the big bubble floats away on the breeze. One more time, dip the bubble wand in again, and take a deep breath. Fill the bottom of your belly with good bubble-making air. Softly blow the air out through your mouth, shaped like you were saying 'oo.' Admire the shimmering bubbles that you are blowing. You are fantastic at this! This time we are going to try it without acting out dipping the bubble wand. Just use your imagination. Take a deep breath, and gently blow the air out through your lips."

Such a monologue can aid in relaxation, and the multisensory description tends to elicit positive emotions and memories. Because deep breathing should be as transportable as possible, a child eventually needs to learn to imagine blowing bubbles without pantomiming the action. Some children find this imagining easier if they close their eyes. Remind children to take deep breaths way down in the bottom of their bellies when they breathe in, to blow the biggest bubble they possibly can. Encourage each child to practice Bubble Breathing three or four times between sessions, and keep a record of it on Handout 28 (Bubble Breathing). Remind the child that these breathing exercises can be tools for helping to manage moods.

Session Review with Parents

With about 10 minutes remaining, invite parents to join the session. This provides an opportunity for the child to describe what he/she has learned and to review any medication questions that came up during session. Letting the child "teach" the parents allows you to monitor the child's learning and correct any errors in understanding that may still be present. Prompt the child, as needed, to review the copy of Handout 22 (Naming the Enemy) completed during the session with the parents. This process can be very emotional and touching for some parents. At times, it serves as hope that they will "get back" their "lost" child. This leads into discussion of the week's take-home family project.

Take-Home Projects

Family Project: Naming the Enemy

Between sessions, family members are to carry out the Naming the Enemy exercise together by filling in Handout 30 (Family Project: Naming the Enemy). The child shows his/her parents the copy of Handout 22 completed in this session, and solicits additional suggestions for each column. The child demonstrates to the parents how to fold the paper so that the symptoms cover who he/she is, and then how to refold the paper in the opposite direction to uncover his/her positive characteristics and to put the symptoms behind those characteristics. This can lead to discussion of all family members' goals and reasons for doing PEP. Handout 29 (a completed sample of this family project) can be used as an additional reference. Remind the child and the parents to put the completed exercise in the child's binder or folder and bring it to the next session.

When parents list the child's positive traits as part of this take-home project, it can give the child much-needed positive feedback. It also gives the family a common language to discuss symptoms. Parents who have been arguing about how to handle the child's behavior can unite with the child to combat the common Enemy. Likewise, children who have heard themselves described as "bad kids" can come to see the disorder, and not themselves, as the problem. Making this attributional shift often results in all family members' being able to deal more matter-of-factly with the child's symptoms and to reduce emotional intensity in the home. The list can be used in future sessions to examine progress toward symptom management, as well as to maintain a nonblaming perspective.

Bubble Breathing Practice

Have the child demonstrate to the parents how to do the Bubble Breathing. Remind the child to practice Bubble Breathing on at least three different days, three sets at a time, and to log the practice on Handout 28 (Bubble Breathing). Ask the parents to do the same.

Chapter 8

Discussing Medication with Parents

IF-PEP Parent Session 2
MF-PEP Parent Session 2

Session Outline

Goals:	1. Explain to parents how to use cost–benefit analysis to make medication decisions.
	2. Overview the medications used to treat mood disorders—their classes, symptom targets, and common side effects.
Beginning the Session:	Do a check-in and review Mood Record (Handout 20 or 21).
	Review Family Project: Naming the Enemy (Handout 30).
Lesson of the Day:	Medication and other biological treatments for childhood mood disorders

- Types of treatment
- Medication and the treatment team
- What medication can and cannot do
- The cost–benefit analysis
- Know the facts, share the facts
- Adherence: Taking medication as directed
- Tracking the child's response: The Mood–Medication Log (Handout 32)
- Tracking the child's response: Laboratory tests
- Managing common side effects (Handout 33)

- After a medication works, when should it be discontinued?
- Selective serotonin reuptake inhibitors (Handout 33)
- Atypical antidepressants (Handout 33)
- Herbal interventions for depression
- Mood stabilizers (Handout 34)
- Atypical antipsychotics (Handout 34)
- Antihypertensives (Handout 34)
- Stimulants (Handout 34)
- Nonstimulant ADHD medication (Handout 34)
- Nutritional interventions
- Light therapy

New Take-Home Projects: Understanding My Child's Medication (parents only; Handout 35)

Mood–Medication Log (parents only; Handouts 31 and 32)

Ongoing Take-Home Projects: Mood Record (parents only; Handout 20 or 21 unless replaced by Handout 32)

Family Project: Naming the Enemy (Handout 30)

New Handouts:

31. Mood–Medication Log (Sample)
32. Mood–Medication Log
33. Medication Summary for Depression and Anxiety Disorders
34. Medication Summary for Bipolar Disorder and ADHD
35. Understanding My Child's Medication

Handouts to Review:

20. Mood Record: Tracking Three Mood States, Three Times per Day *or*
21. Simple Mood Record
30. Family Project: Naming the Enemy

Session Overview

The second parent-only session educates parents about biological treatments for children with mood disorders. These interventions consist primarily but not exclusively of medications. General principles of medication utilization are reviewed, including how to determine whether medication should be considered for a child; which classes of medications are used and which symptoms they target; how to conduct a cost–benefit analysis of medication use; how to keep the Mood–Medication Log; how to manage side effects; and how to communicate most effectively with the prescribing professional (physician, nurse practitioner, or physician assistant), referred to as the "prescriber" or "provider" throughout. The session is *not* intended to provide prescriptive information for parents (e.g., "From what you've told me, I think your child should be on *X* mg of *Y* medication"). Parents should come away from this session feeling equipped to be active members of the treatment team when it comes to medication. In MF-PEP groups, a guest (e.g., a psychiatry resident, physician assistant, or nurse practitioner) can be invited in to lead the portion of the session focused on specific medications.

Beginning the Session

Do a Check-In and Review Mood Record

Parents should arrive at this session with their folder or binder and a completed Mood Record in hand. This is a great opportunity to link observations from the Mood Record with content from the first parent session on mood disorders and symptoms. Keep this discussion brief (about 5 minutes), as this session has considerable content to cover. If parents come in with significant questions, it may be worthwhile to jot them down and return to them at the end of the session. Many of their questions may actually be answered during this session; if many questions remain at the end, consider using an in-the-bank session of IF-PEP to address these. (For MF-PEP parents, consider referring them back to their children's prescribers.)

Review Family Project: Naming the Enemy

Review with family members how the discussion went with the Naming the Enemy project. In some families, siblings will have been included in the discussion; in other families, just the parents and child will have continued the discussion at home. Now that this exercise has been completed, it allows you to gently provide corrective feedback to any family member who slips back into "old" language of referring to the symptoms as a core feature of the child (e.g., if a father comments that his son is being a "royal pain in the neck" you could comment that his son's irritability is getting more intense and take a few minutes with the family to evaluate that symptom and develop a management plan for it).

Lesson of the Day: Medication and Other Biological Treatments for Childhood Mood Disorders

Types of Treatment

Briefly introduce the three basic types of intervention for children with mood disorders: biological, psychological, and social. Medications are the primary biological interventions, but others include nutritional interventions, electroconvulsive therapy, and light therapy. This session focuses on biological treatments. Psychological interventions include individual, family, and group therapy as well as parent guidance; social interventions include school-based interventions, home-based interventions, respite care, and out-of-home placements. The next parent session (see Chapter 10) will focus on psychological and social interventions. Also review the most common providers for biological and psychological interventions. Parents should understand the roles of psychiatrists, psychologists, social workers, physician assistants, and nurse practitioners in particular. Be sure to clarify the differences between psychologists and psychiatrists. (For guides to who's who in the mental health system, see Table 10.1 in Chapter 10, as well as Handout 49.)

Medication and the Treatment Team

Ideally, if medication decisions are to be made, a board-certified child/adolescent psychiatrist should be on the treatment team of each child with a mood disorder. In some geographic areas, it is reasonable to expect this standard of care. In other areas, a general psychiatrist, a developmental/behavioral pediatrician, a primary care physician, a physician assistant, or a nurse practitioner may fill that role. Regardless of the prescriber's training and background, well-informed, actively involved parents who keep careful records about their child's moods are very important members of the treatment team. Making the decision to start medication can be extremely hard. It is important to acknowledge the struggles parents experience, and to provide them with help to get through these.

What Medication Can and Cannot Do

Explain that medications do not cure a mood disorder, but they can help to manage it by stopping symptoms or lessening symptom severity. In addition, medications can prevent future episodes or decrease their severity. However, medications cannot solve every problem; other interventions will probably be necessary. For example, medications are not likely to change a child's tendency to argue with or refuse parental requests. However, when mediation decreases a child's irritability, it is more likely that good behavioral strategies will work to solve these other problems.

The Cost–Benefit Analysis

It is a risk to decide to go forward with medication. Medication might help or it might make things worse; it might work partially and bring unpleasant side effects. Parents need to know the available facts and then weigh a number of pros and cons, acknowledging that some of these factors are unknowns.

Costs of Symptoms

The symptoms of mood disorders have costs for children and their families. How much are symptoms negatively affecting the child at school, with peers, and in family relationships? What is the impact on parents and siblings? If symptoms have been mild, medication may not need to be considered.

Potential Benefits of Medication

The potential benefits of medication are that it will decrease disturbed mood and related symptoms. Different medications target different symptoms, and some symptoms may be more important to target than others.

Potential Costs of Medication

The potential costs of medication include the possible side effects; the expense and the inconvenience of multiple doctor visits; and, quite possibly, the need for blood draws and lab tests to monitor safety. Some, but not all, common side effects can be easily managed by adjusting the dose or timing of a medication. A few medications can have serious side effects. To weigh these factors adequately, parents need to get the facts about the medications under consideration. They can request fact sheets from the prescriber, or obtain them from a pharmacist or reputable website (e.g., *www.webmd.com*).

One of the most feared "cons" is that medications will change the child's personality. Reviewing the Naming the Enemy exercise (Handouts 22 and 30) can be helpful, as this exercise illustrates how mood symptoms can cover up or mask a child's positive features. If medications successfully reduce mood symptoms, the child's positive traits can once again show through. Some parents also fear that medications will be addicting like street drugs. This myth often requires some discussion as well.

> Patti and Ron were referred to PEP by their 10-year-old son's social worker. They had sought mental health treatment for Jonathon about 6 months earlier, when he began having difficulty at school. Prior to that, he had been irritable and often explosive at home, but had managed to get along with teachers and classmates at school. He had always had periods of giddiness at home, but they were typically brief (under an hour) and did not cause significant problems. Recently, however, Jonathon had been disruptive at school—making inappropriate sexual comments, calling out in the middle of instruction, needing to be sent out of the room to settle himself down, and having more trouble than usual focusing on his work. Their social worker had suggested a medication evaluation, but Patti and Ron were extremely hesitant. They had heard many horror stories and could not imagine "drugging" their son. Patti listened intently during their PEP session about conducting a cost–benefit analysis.
>
> PATTI: So how do we figure out if Jonathon needs medicine?
>
> THERAPIST: Well, the first thing you need to ask yourselves is this: What is the cost of Jonathon's symptoms? Is he having problems in the important areas of his life, such as his peer relationships, his functioning at school, and his family relationships?
>
> PATTI: I hate the idea of putting him on medicine—but he is losing friends right and left; he isn't learning anything; and I'm afraid that he is going to get placed in a special program at school if something doesn't start to change.

THERAPIST: Are there costs at home?

RON: I worry constantly when I'm at work that something really bad will happen. I'm really worried that Patti will get hurt. We walk on eggshells all the time and are afraid to plan any family activities because of his moods.

THERAPIST: Sounds like the cost of his symptoms is very high.

PATTI: But I have heard such horror stories about medications and kids.

THERAPIST: Keep in mind that while there is a lot of information out there, some of it is accurate and some is not. What is important to understand is that although there is no magic pill that can erase all symptoms without any cost, medications can often provide significant symptom relief.

RON: I'm scared for Jonathon now, but I'm also scared that if we do start medication, he will end up drugged out and not the exuberant kid that we love so much.

THERAPIST: Many parents share your concerns about medications changing their child's personality, but I have actually heard the opposite from parents—that once medication begins to reduce the mood symptoms, they are able to enjoy their child again. Do you remember the project Jonathon did [Naming the enemy] where he listed all of the good things about him on one side and his symptoms on the other? When medication successfully reduces the symptoms, a child's strengths and interests can begin to dominate again.

PATTI: But there are so many side effects to worry about!

THERAPIST: The goal for any prescriber is to get as much benefit from medicine as possible with as few side effects as possible. Some side effects go away as the body adjusts to the medicine, or can be easily managed with small changes in dose and timing of the medicine. Some side effects need a careful management plan or indicate a need to change medications. The process of finding the right medicines at the right doses is not easy. It can take a lot of time and patience.

PATTI: I want to do what is best for Jonathon, but I get so overwhelmed.

THERAPIST: This is clearly a very emotional issue for you, and you don't need to make a decision right now. What we will do during this session is provide you with accurate information about medications. You can then put that together with what you now understand about mood symptoms and mood disorders. Then you will be in a position to make an informed decision about this difficult topic.

In an ideal world, after a family makes the difficult decision to try a psychiatric medication for a child, a good response is achieved on the first medication tried with minimal side effects. In reality, life is imperfect. Partial responses often occur, and side effects have to be tolerated and managed. Trials of several medications may be needed before the best one is found. Parents need to be prepared for this process. It's important to know the facts about the medication, and then to keep track of the child's symptoms and any side effects on a Mood–Medication Log (see below).

Know the Facts, Share the Facts

Most psychiatric medications do not work right away; in fact, many take up to several weeks to work. Families need to know what to expect and how to track symptoms during that time period. Some symptoms improve before others; for example, physical symptoms such as insomnia often improve before mood and thinking do. It is important for parents to ask questions and to request and keep fact sheets about medications from their prescriber. They should also get and retain the medication sheets available from their pharmacist. Encourage parents to keep this information in their child's treatment binder, so they can have "one-stop-shopping" for all necessary information regarding their child's treatment. Parents should be familiar with a medication's common side effects, so that they will be equipped to manage them. It is particularly important to know what to do if a serious side effect should develop. Plans for such medication-related emergencies may vary among providers and among geographic regions. Whether the plan is to call the prescriber (or his/her emergency line) or go directly to the local emergency room, knowing what to do beforehand will allow family members to act as calmly and quickly as possible.

It is also important for information to be shared with key people. Primary care physicians should be kept up to date on medications, including any herbal remedies, over-the-counter medications, or nutritional interventions the child is taking. There are many reasons for this, but drug interactions are a concern. For example, Biaxin (an antibiotic) and Tegretol in combination can lead to dangerous side effects. Information should be shared with all professionals involved in a child's care.

In addition, parents should be encouraged to share medication information with their school team, particularly the school nurse. The most common reason parents resist or refuse to tell school personnel about medications is stigma. If parents withhold information about medications and a side effect manifests itself at school, school personnel will not know what is wrong with the child or how to help. If information about medications and the targeted symptoms is shared with the school staff, overall coordination of treatment may prove to be more effective. Teachers can also play an important role in tracking mood and behavior during the school day, when parents typically cannot consistently observe their children. This feedback can be very useful in fine-tuning doses and timing of medications.

Adherence: Taking Medication as Directed

Families need to be proactive about adherence. That is, family members need to have a plan and a backup plan for helping a child remember to take medicines on time. Some effective strategies include pill boxes and well-established rituals, such as taking morning pills with juice right after breakfast and evening pills just after toothbrushing. Even the best plans sometimes fail, so families also need to know what to do about missed doses. In some cases, the medicine should be taken as soon as the missed dose is remembered; in other cases, doubling up on medication is not safe. Rules are needed for every medicine being taken. Parents are often embarrassed about missed doses. It is important to remind them that honesty with their prescriber will help to generate a fair evaluation of the child's medication response, and that admitting to problems with remembering doses is the first step in determining how to prevent future missed doses. Parents also need to master getting refills on time. This should include a discussion of the time needed to contact the doctor, to call or mail in the prescription refill, or to take whatever other steps are necessary to obtain a child's refills.

One other issue occasionally arises regarding adherence: Some parents expect their children to be responsible for taking charge of their own medication. This is certainly a goal worth striving toward; however, for children 12 and under, and especially for those struggling with mood disorders, this goal is unlikely to meet with much success. It's important to discuss developmentally appropriate expectations with such parents, and to guide them in how they can gradually increase expectations over time as their child improves.

Tracking the Child's Response: The Mood–Medication Log

Following the last session, parents should have begun using a Mood Record (Handout 20 or 21). This will have caused them to start paying attention to their child's mood fluctuations over time. Now parents will be asked to track their child's mood symptoms in response to medication or changes in medication. Items to record on a Mood–Medication Log (Handout 32) include the date a medication was started; the child's weight; other co-occurring notable life events; the dose and timing of medication; side effects; and the child's mood and treatment response. Record keeping can help parents notice patterns, such as more good days creeping in among the bad days. Benefits from medication sometimes start slowly and progress in a subtle manner. This can be illustrated by reviewing Handout 31 (the sample Mood–Medication Log) with the parent; it shows slow improvement in mood over the course of a month. Here is another example:

> Hiroaki, an 11-year-old, had an extremely difficult winter and spring; he first experienced significant depression and later developed manic symptoms. After trials of two antidepressants that both resulted in a worsening of symptoms, two atypical antipsychotics that resulted in rapid weight gain with minimal benefit, and a trial of valproic acid that caused an escalation of symptoms, he started a trial of lithium. Hiroaki's parents kept a careful Mood–Medication Log during all these medication trials. Although they initially reported that things were still terrible, after 3 weeks on lithium they noticed that their ratings had shifted from mostly "8's" (on a scale where 10's are "terrible") to "7's". This realization gave them hope to keep trying. A few weeks later, "7's" had become "5's". Although Hiroaki still had a long way to go to get back to his previous level of functioning, life was becoming more livable for all of them.

By the same token, record keeping may help identify a lack of progress, and thus help to spur changes in the medication regimen.

During the medication discussion, Teri, mother of 9-year-old Anna, raised a question. Her daughter had initially begun taking a stimulant medication because she was having significant difficulty maintaining attention, resisting distraction, and suppressing impulses at home and especially at school. Anna had begun taking the stimulant medication 2 years ago in second grade, and at the time, her teacher had been very involved in providing feedback about how Anna was doing, which had helped determine the effectiveness of the stimulant medication. Over the past year, Anna's diagnosis had become less clear. Part of the reason her family was participating in PEP was to help them figure out which of Anna's problems were related to her mood and which were related to other problems. Anna could be explosive, was impulsive at times, and in general was difficult to manage. At times she was very irritable and got into conflicts with her parents and siblings almost constantly. Anna's psychiatrist had added an atypical antipsychotic, but Teri was concerned because it was unclear to her whether Anna's medications were helping at home. Although her second-grade teacher had been involved in giving feedback about Anna's attention, distractibility, and impulsivity, her current fourth-grade teacher had not been asked about Anna's mood during the school day. Since her mood had never been discussed with school personnel, her teacher did not know to offer feedback, and thus large chunks of information about Anna's days were missing. Anna had also gained 10 pounds since she started on the atypical antipsychotic 4 months ago. This was concerning, as she had never had a weight issue prior to starting the medication. Their therapist encouraged Teri to start using the Mood–Medication Log to keep track of Anna's symptoms. She also suggested that Teri begin working on scheduling a meeting at school, and that they include the issue of Anna's mood during the school day as a topic for that meeting (see Chapter 16).

Keeping records and noting questions can help parents make efficient use of brief medication appointments with their child's prescriber, which in many practice settings last no more than 15–30 minutes. Maintaining the Mood–Medication Log should be an ongoing project for parents. It also helps parents report on the entire interval since their last appointment, not just the preceding few days. This helps parents avoid focusing exclusively on the negative events that have occurred.

Over time, the Mood–Medication Log becomes a record of what medications were tried, what the response was, and why particular medications were stopped. This information may help to guide treatment at a later point in development, and can be particularly useful if the child and family switch providers, as it can often be difficult to obtain complete records from previous service providers.

Tracking the Child's Response: Laboratory Tests

Laboratory tests represent another important set of tracking tools. Many psychopharmacological treatments require lab tests prior to starting the medication, and some require monitoring while taking the medication. Blood tests are important for some medications, to help identify proneness to some of the more serious side effects, to track the development of side effects, and in some cases to help determine how much of a medication a particular person should take. For example, lithium and valproic acid levels are important to obtain, as too little medication in the blood will be ineffective, but too much will be dangerous. In such cases, blood work is very helpful in guiding dosages of medication.

After a thorough evaluation and a couple of other medication trials, Kara began a trial of lithium. After the first 2 weeks, her parents were still walking on eggshells, but Kara was able to make it through a day of school (albeit with a lot of support). Her parents were fearful that things were as good as they were going to get, and this thought distressed them very much. They called Kara's prescribing physician, who asked them to have blood work done. The blood work confirmed that Kara's blood level of lithium was at the low end of the therapeutic range. Her doctor increased her dose, and also raised her parents' hope that lithium might provide even more benefit and that life might shift from just barely manageable to comfortably livable.

These blood tests are important aids to taking medications safely and using them effectively. If Kara's blood level had turned out to be at the top of the therapeutic range, her doctor might have suggested adding a second mood-stabilizing medication or switching to an atypical antipsychotic, rather than increasing her lithium dose. For children who struggle with blood draws, topical numbing creams can be very helpful and are easily accessed through the prescriber.

Managing Common Side Effects

Parents need to know the potential serious side effects of their child's medications, as well as what to do if a medication-related emergency does occur. But most side effects are mild, although annoying. It is very important for parents and children to approach managing side effects as a problem-solving task; many can be effectively dealt with if parents and children work together. Some side effects go away as the body adjusts to the medication. A problem-solving approach might begin with tracking the symptoms to see if they go away or improve. When the side effects do not disappear, the most common can be helped by the strategies listed below. These strategies are also listed in Handout 33. If these are relevant, given a child's particular medication, be sure to point them out to the parents.

Side effect	*Management strategies*
Increased thirst/ urination:	• Drink six to eight glasses of liquid/day. • Avoid high-calorie beverages. • Make school plan to use bathroom often.
Tremor:	• Take medication with meals or in divided doses. • Avoid caffeine.
Increased appetite/ weight gain:	• Develop and maintain balanced diet and regular, developmentally appropriate exercise. • Avoid drastic diets and/or diet pills.
Skin sensitivity:	• Use sunscreen. • Wear protective clothing. • Avoid sunlight/sunlamps.

Impaired sleep:	• Have routine sleep habits.
	• Don't let the weekend disrupt these by more than 1 hour.
	• No exercise/caffeine in the evening.
	• Wake at regular times, even if tired.
	• Do not nap during the day.
Dizziness:	• Stand up slowly.
Dry mouth:	• Drink water.
	• Use sugarless gum/candy.
Constipation:	• Eat high-fiber diet.
	• Drink six to eight glasses of water/day.
Persistent nausea:	• Take medicine with meals or in divided doses.

Some side effects (e.g., dry mouth) are easily managed (e.g., with sugarless gum or hard candy). Others present a greater challenge; for example, increased appetite requires careful eating and an increase in activity level. Weight gain from increased appetite is associated with a number of mood-stabilizing medications, and it can lead to serious chronic health problems, such as diabetes and other metabolic disorders. The next child session in IF-PEP (Chapter 9) focuses on healthy habits and provides ideas about how to handle this issue.

When parents are in the midst of trying medication for their child, these are critical points they need to remember:

- Don't despair.
- Communicate clearly with your prescriber.
- Work as an active partner in evaluating the treatment.
- Encourage your child to be an active partner.

After a Medication Works, When Should It Be Discontinued?

When symptoms are eliminated by medication, a different set of problems arises: When, if ever, should medication be discontinued? A full response is not necessarily a reason for a child to stop taking a medicine. Some medications are useful in preventing future episodes. Particularly for children with BSD, medication can prevent or lessen a future episode, which is a very important part of care. In many cases, it is easier to prevent an episode than it is to stop an episode already in full swing. Whatever the case, it is important for parents to plan with their prescriber when and how to stop or reduce medicine. With some medications, an abrupt discontinuation will result in unpleasant side effects, so a prescriber may recommend a tapering schedule.

The balance of the session focuses on what parents need to know about each type of medication. Refer to Chapter 2 for a discussion of the current research supporting medication for pediatric mood disorders, and keep in mind that research is progressing rapidly and that new, more effective medications are becoming available all the time. One good resource for parents is Timothy Wilens' (2009) book *Straight Talk about Psychiatric Medications for Kids,* currently in its third edition.

Selective Serotonin Reuptake Inhibitors

SSRIs are typically the first medications used to treat depression and some anxiety disorders, including OCD, generalized anxiety disorder, and social phobia. The SSRIs all work by increasing serotonin availability in the brain. Serotonin is one of several brain chemicals that enables communication between neurons. Medications in this class vary in their chemical structure, their half-life (a term describing the rate at which they are broken down by the body), and their side effects. Overall, the side effects of SSRIs are mild for most people and can be reasonably well managed and mitigated. Common SSRI side effects include the following:

Dizziness
Nausea
Stomachaches
Diarrhea
Nervousness
Changes in sleep/appetite
Drowsiness
Weakness
Dry mouth
Tremor
Perspiration

SSRIs have been given a "black-box warning" by the U.S. FDA. This means that parents and children need to be aware of significant risks these medications might pose. Current FDA guidelines state that children taking SSRIs should be monitored closely, particularly in the first 8 weeks, for suicidal behavior and manic activation. The only SSRI currently approved for pediatric depression is Prozac. Currently available SSRIs by trade name (listed first) and generic name are as follows (see also Handout 33):

Prozac   fluoxetine
Zoloft   sertraline
Luvox   fluvoxamine
Celexa   citalopram
Lexapro   escitalopram
Paxil   paroxetine

Atypical Antidepressants

The atypical antidepressants are sometimes used to treat pediatric mood disorders. These medications are called "atypical" because they work differently from the SSRIs.

TABLE 8.1. Atypical Antidepressants

Trade name	Generic name	Possible side effects
Wellbutrin	bupropion	Irritability, decreased appetite, insomnia, tics
Effexor	venlafaxine	Nausea, agitation, stomachaches, headaches, increased blood pressure, suicidal behavior (not recommended for children/teens)
Cymbalta	duloxetine	Nausea, dry mouth, stomach problems, metabolic and nutritional disorders, decreased appetite
Serzone	nefazodone	Sedation, agitation, dry mouth, constipation
Desyrel	trazodone	Sedation, agitation, dry mouth, constipation
Remeron	mirtazapine	Sedation, "heaviness," upset stomach

Table 8.1 and Handout 33 provide the trade and generic names of some of the atypical antidepressants; the table also lists their respective possible side effects. In some cases, a medication is used because of a helpful side effect; for example, a medication with sedation as a possible side effect may be prescribed to be taken close to bedtime to reduce insomnia. Black-box warnings have also been issued by the FDA for these medications.

Herbal Interventions for Depression

Supplements that target depression and related symptoms are widely available. The challenge is that many of these supplements have not been adequately studied in children, and in some cases not even in adults. St. John's wort has some empirical support for mild to moderate depression; however, it can result in side effects similar to those of SSRIs. An added caution with St. John's wort is that it can cause birth control pills to become ineffective. S-adenosyl methionine (commonly known as Sam-e) has also been used for depression, but without any research to support its use in children. One of the most commonly used supplements is melatonin, which can be helpful as a sleep aid. It can cause morning sedation and changes in dream activity. If parents are using or considering use of any herbal intervention for their child, they should be sure to tell all their prescribers. Emphasize that they need to keep prescribers informed about *all* medications (prescription and over-the-counter) and *all* herbal, natural, and nutritional remedies their child is taking. Encourage parents to seek research on a remedy's use in children from a reputable source (e.g., the National Center for Complementary and Alternative Medicine, *nccam.nih.gov*) before embarking on a trial.

Mood Stabilizers

Mood stabilizers are mostly used to treat BD, including mania and depression. The most common are listed in Table 8.2, as well as on Handout 34, by trade and generic names.

TABLE 8.2. Mood Stabilizers

Trade name	Generic name	Possible side effects	Research findings
Eskalith, Lithobid	lithium	Nausea, dizziness, thirst, increased urination, tremor, weight gain, acne, renal function over time	Decreased manic and depressive symptoms; effective as a maintenance treatment
Depakote, Depakene	valproic acid	Nausea, vomiting, drowsiness, weight gain	Superior to lithium and placebo in one study
Tegretol	carbamazepine	Nausea, dizziness, dry mouth, headache	Adult studies positive; no controlled studies in youth
Lamictal	lamotrigine	Skin rash, blurred/double vision, fatigue, insomnia, dizziness	Not advised for children; good data re: bipolar depression in adults

Lithium

The oldest mood stabilizer, lithium, is the most widely studied. It is used as a treatment for acute mania and recalcitrant depression, and as a maintenance mood stabilizer. There are many forms of lithium (e.g., Lithobid, Eskalith, Lithium Carbonate). Lithium is absorbed into the blood and processed by the kidneys. Blood needs to be drawn periodically to check the level of lithium in the blood (the therapeutic range is between 0.6 and 1.2 mmol/L), as well as to monitor kidney and thyroid functioning.

Anticonvulsant Mood Stabilizers

Valproic acid (Depakote, Depakene) carbamazepine (Tegretol), and lamotrigine (Lamictal) are antiseizure medications that are also mood stabilizers. Valproic acid is FDA-approved for the treatment of manic episodes in adults, as well as for the treatment of complex partial seizures and migraines. Although some results have been mixed, open-label studies, case reports, and a randomized placebo-controlled study comparing lithium and Depakote have suggested the efficacy of Depakote for treating pediatric BD (see a recent review by Kowatch, 2009a, pp. 139–142). A possible complication of valproic acid treatment in girls is the development of polycystic ovary syndrome. Common side effects include weight gain, sedation, nausea, and increased appetite. Valproic acid is metabolized by the liver and requires blood test monitoring.

Carbamazepine (Tegretol) is another anticonvulsant mood-stabilizing medication. Controlled studies have demonstrated the efficacy of carbamazepine as a monotherapy agent for adults with mania (Weisler, Cutler, Ballenger, Post, & Ketter, 2006). However, controlled trials have not been conducted in children, and carbamazepine has multiple drug–drug interactions, making it an unlikely first-line treatment for pediatric BD (Kowatch, 2009a). Lamotrigine (Lamictal) has had one positive open-label study in adolescents (Chang, Saxena, & Howe, 2006), but it has an FDA black-box warning for persons under 16 years of age, because of the higher rate of a potentially life-threatening rash (Stevens–Johnson syndrome) that can occur in this age group (1%, compared to 0.3% in those over 16 years of age).

Other anticonvulsants have been tested with no demonstrated efficacy in adults and/or youth. Gabapentin (Neurontin) is ineffective as a mood stabilizer, but may be beneficial in treating anxiety in persons with BD (Kowatch, 2009a, p. 147). Oxcarbazepine (Trileptal) worked no better than placebo in one controlled study of youth (Wagner et al., 2006).

Atypical Antipsychotics

The atypical antipsychotics control psychotic symptoms (hallucinations, delusions) and decrease anxiety, agitation, and aggression. They are an increasingly important set of medications for treating childhood mood disorders, especially BD. Their mood-stabilizing effects have been observed and increasingly demonstrated through research. They are called "atypical" because they work differently from older antipsychotics (e.g., haloperidol [Haldol]). Side effects include the following:

Drowsiness
Increased appetite and weight gain
Slowing
Tremor
Tenseness
"Mask-like" face (i.e., facial muscles become less expressive)
Headaches
Insomnia
Nausea

Compared to older antipsychotics, the atypicals carry a lower risk of the side effect called "tardive dyskinesia" (involuntary movement of facial and other muscles). They may increase risk for diabetes and hyperglycemia, as well as problems with movement, known as "extrapyramidal symptoms." These symptoms include "parkinsonism (tremor and other possible abnormal movements) and "akathisia" (intense feelings of physical restlessness accompanied by excessive movement). Prolactin levels have been reported to increase in persons taking atypical antipsychotics. Weight gain is a frequent concern and can lead to other problematic health issues.

The trade names (listed first) and generic names for atypical antipsychotics used with children are as follows (see also Handout 34):

Risperdal   risperidone
Seroquel   quetiapine
Zyprexa   olanzapine
Clozaril   clozapine
Geodon   ziprasidone
Abilify   aripiprazole
Invega   paliperidone

Antihypertensives

Two The antihypertensive medications, clonidine (Catapres) and guanfacine (Tenex, Intuniv), are sometimes used to decrease agitation, assist with sleep, reduce impulsivity, and reduce tics. Side effects include drowsiness and dizziness.

Stimulants

The stimulant medications are used to improve attention, reduce impulsivity, and lower hyperactivity in individuals with ADHD. They are controlled substances, which mean that prescribers can only write one 30-day prescription at a time. Common side effects include appetite reduction and weight loss, stomach pain, restlessness, dizziness, heart palpitations, insomnia, and headache. Given that some of the symptoms of pediatric BSD and ADHD overlap, children with BSD are sometimes initially diagnosed with ADHD. For these children, treatment with stimulants can sometimes trigger mania or psychosis. Stimulants used for children, listed by trade name (first) and then generic, are listed below. (The abbreviations in brackets indicated drugs that are available in various long-acting/extended-release forms, as well as in their standard forms.)

Ritalin [LA], Metadate [ER, CD], Concerta	methylphenidate
Focalin	dexmethylphenidate
Dexedrine, Dexedrine spansules	dextroamphetamine
Adderall [XR]	amphetamine–dextroamphetamine
Daytrana	methylphenidate transdermal system
Vyvanse	lisdexamfetamine

Nonstimulant ADHD Medication

Atomoxetine (Strattera) is a selective norepinephrine reuptake inhibitor. It works similarly to the SSRIs, but on the brain chemical norepinephrine instead of serotonin. It can be taken once or twice a day and works continuously (unlike the stimulants, which are short-acting, although longer-acting formulations work for up to 12+ hours). Strattera is less likely to cause tic, sleep, or anxiety problems than the stimulants are. Since it is not a controlled substance, filling prescriptions is easier, and there is no abuse potential. The most common side effects are weight loss, decreased appetite, nausea, vomiting, tiredness, dizziness, and mood swings.

Nutritional Interventions

As noted in Chapter 2, omega-3 fatty acids are receiving increasing attention as critical nutrients. Research has begun to demonstrate their benefit for individuals with mood disorders, cognitive decline, and a host of other health concerns (e.g., cardiovascular disease, rheumatoid arthritis). There is growing evidence for their benefit as an adjunctive intervention for both depression and mania in children.

Another potentially beneficial nutritional intervention discussed in Chapter 2 is a multinutrient called EMPowerplus (EMP+; *www.truehope.com*). Child and adult case studies, case series, and open-label trials of EMP+ are promising, but large-scale double-blind placebo-controlled trials are still needed.

Light Therapy

Light boxes, or phototherapy, can be beneficial for those struggling with SAD (see Chapter 6). Typically, a user sits in front of a light box first thing in the morning for 20–30 minutes. Some individuals benefit from a second treatment in the mid- to late afternoon. As too much of any physiological intervention for depression can do, too much exposure to the light can trigger manic symptoms in those with BD.

Take-Home Projects

New Project: Understanding My Child's Medication

The first new take-home project is a direct follow-up to the session's content. On Handout 35 (Understanding My Child's Medication), parents are asked to record each of their child's medications and doses, symptoms targeted by the medication, side effects, strategies for managing those side effects, and anything important they need to remember about the medication (e.g., a child should not take ibuprofen with lithium). Parents should bring the completed form to the next parent-only session (covered in Chapter 10).

New Project: Mood–Medication Log

Parents should continue to monitor their child's mood, but if the child is or soon will be taking medication, they should now do so with Handout 32. The Mood–Medication Log tracks mood in conjunction with medication and side effects.

Ongoing Projects

Parent Project: Mood Record

If the child is not on medication and not expected to be, encourage parents to continue monitoring their child's mood with one of the two versions of the Mood Record (Handout 20 or 21).

Family Project: Naming the Enemy

Remind parents that if they have not reviewed the Naming the Enemy exercise with their child, they should do this by the next child session.

This session is packed with information. If you feel rushed, or if parents have many questions and concerns about medications, this topic may be a good candidate for using an IF-PEP in-the-bank session to discuss the issues further. This may especially be the case for families who come to PEP needing to conduct a cost–benefit analysis of medication.

Chapter 9

Discussing Healthy Habits with Children

IF-PEP Child Sessions 3 and 7
Not a Session in MF-PEP

Session Outline

Goals:	1. Teach the importance of healthy sleeping, eating, and exercise routines in mood regulation. 2. Explain how to improve healthy habits. 3. Help the child select first- and second-priority healthy habits to address.
Beginning the Session:	Do a check-in and review Mood–Medication Log (Handout 32) or Mood Record (Handout 20 or 21). Review Bubble Breathing practice (Handout 28). Review Family Project: Naming the Enemy (Handout 30). Have child identify and rate feelings (Handouts 1 and 2).
Lesson of the Day:	Healthy Habits for managing mood • Therapist Overview • Introducing Healthy Habits (Handouts 36 and 37)

- Healthy sleeping habits (Handouts 38, 39, and 40)
- Healthy eating habits (Handouts 41, 42, 43, and 44)
- Healthy exercise habits (Handouts 45, 46, and 47)

Breathing Exercise: Balloon Breathing (Handout 48)

Session Review with Parents

New Take-Home Projects: Selected healthy habits chart (Handout 40, 44, or 47)

Balloon Breathing practice (48)

New Handouts:
36. Three Important Healthy Habits
37. Healthy Habits Worksheet
38. Sleep
39. Sleep Chart (Sample)
40. Sleep Chart
41. Healthy Eating
42. The Food Pyramid
43. Healthy Food Chart (Sample)
44. Healthy Food Chart
45. Exercise
46. Exercise Chart Sample
47. Exercise Chart
48. Balloon Breathing

Handouts to Review:
1. Feelings
2. Strength of Feelings
11. Belly Breathing
28. Bubble Breathing
30. Family Project: Naming the Enemy

Session Overview

This chapter focuses on building healthy habits (sleep, eating, and exercise), with the goal of increasing healthy coping and mood stability. Since sleep, eating, and exercise habits are important yet difficult to change, IF-PEP includes two child sessions (3 and 7) focused on these topics. This chapter should be used as a guide for both sessions. This topic is not covered formally in MF-PEP; however, concepts related to sleep, eating and exercise are often incorporated into treatment, particularly when participants are constructing their Tool Kits.

During the first IF-PEP healthy habits session (Child Session 3), a plan should be established for which habit will be covered first and which during the second session (Child Session 7). If all three areas need work, or if one of the areas needs additional follow-up, consider using an in-the-bank session to address these needs. The first healthy habits session presents a great opportunity for you, the clinician, to model problem-solving strategies—something you will specifically teach in IF-PEP Parent Session 5 and Child Session 6. In Child Session 7, you will then be able to coach the child and the family to work through issues relevant to healthy habits, using a problem-solving approach.

Parents may be more involved in this child session than is typical, depending on the child's age and the particular family's characteristics. For a young child who is struggling with healthy eating habits, it may make sense to spend much of the session with the child and parents together, working on how healthy habits might be incorporated into family life. On the other hand, an 11-year-old might do better making a plan alone with you, one on one. The plan can be shared with parents when they rejoin the child toward the end of the session.

Beginning the Session

Do a Check-In and Review Mood–Medication Log or Mood Record

Begin the session with parents and child together for a brief check-in on how the week has gone. Using the Mood–Medication Log as a resource (or Mood Record, if a child is not on medication), hear the parent and child perspective on how the week has gone. Explain in general the Lesson of the Day, to determine whether it will be more productive to have the parents remain in the entire session or whether working alone with the child for a portion of the session is preferable. Respond briefly to any parent questions about the Mood–Medication Log and the project involving Handout 35 (Understanding My Child's Medications).

Review Bubble Breathing Practice

Check briefly to see whether the parents and child have practiced Bubble Breathing since their last session. Ask whether they have any questions about how to do the deep breathing required. If necessary, give a pep talk on how useful deep breathing can be as a coping strategy to manage mood. Emphasize the importance of practice, so that the skill can be "taken out and used" when it is urgently needed.

Review Family Project: Naming the Enemy

Review child and parents' work with Family Project: Naming the Enemy (Handout 30). So much of treatment focuses on symptoms that it is refreshing to refocus attention on the child's strengths. Awareness of the child's positive attributes is beneficial in developing coping strategies in this session. In addition, referring to the child's positive attributes serves as a useful reminder to the family that treatment will help "bring back" their child.

Luke shared the Naming the Enemy project he had completed with his parents' help. He read the list of his strengths and positive attributes: "caring," "a good athlete," "funny," "loves dogs," and "smart." The family had divided the "Luke's Symptoms" section into three parts: one each for mania, depression, and ADHD. Symptoms listed for *mania* included "too hyper," "has a hard time following instructions," "silly," and "can't sleep." For *depression*, Luke's symptoms included "sullen," "argues with siblings, parents and friends," "wants to lie around," "wants to skip sports practices," and "grouchy." For *ADHD*, the family had listed "easily distracted," "too much energy," "acts before he thinks," and "trouble finishing homework." Luke's mom mentioned that Luke did a great job of explaining how his symptoms covered up his positive attributes, and named not wanting to go to sports practice as an example. He said that not going to practice covered up his trait "a good athlete," because when he didn't go to practice, his coach wouldn't let him play.

After Naming the Enemy has been reviewed and any related issues are discussed, the parents leave if it has been decided that the child will work with you alone.

Have the Child Identify and Rate Feelings

Using Handouts 1 (Feelings) and 2 (Strength of Feelings), ask the child to identify his/her current feelings, ask why the child feels that way, and then have him/her rate the strongest feeling. Prompt the child as needed to provide this information. Usually by this session, children are quite practiced at identifying and rating the strength of their feelings.

Lesson of the Day: Healthy Habits for Managing Mood
Therapist Overview

Positive changes to lifestyle can be a very important part of managing mood disorders. The three lifestyle issues we focus on for children in PEP are good sleep habits, healthy eating habits, and regular exercise habits. We consider these to be "free medicines": They support good health in general, as well as being important to maintaining healthy mood states and preventing mood episodes. In addition, since sleep, appetite, and energy changes are symptoms of depression and mania, tracking and managing these behaviors are especially important. Although some of the medications used to treat BSD and depression can help to regulate sleep, appetite, and energy, some can also cause fatigue, increase appetite, and lead to sluggishness. Thus managing sleep hygiene, weight, and daily activity levels can become an important part of side effect management as well as overall treatment. Prior to conducting the sessions on healthy habits, it can be helpful to review the information in Chapter 2 on how sleep, eating, and exercise are related to mood disorders.

Sleeping, eating, and exercising should be covered in the order that makes most sense, according to the family's priorities. If sleep has been an area of significant concern, it is a good place to start. If eating habits are causing significant problems or have been identified as an issue, start there. If neither of these have been "hot spots," begin with exercise, as it can be beneficial in terms of activity scheduling and social goals in addition to general health.

Improving healthy habits can be challenging and require creative problem solving. Initially, you might walk the family through defining a problem and agreeing that it is worth solving. Getting the child to "buy into" the need to solve a problem is very important. Without it, conflict between parents and children is likely and success unlikely. Once everyone agrees on the problem definition and agrees that it needs to be solved, you can walk the family through brainstorming potential solutions and making a plan.

Introducing Healthy Habits

Review Handout 36 (Three Important Healthy Habits) with the child. Discuss why sleep, eating, and exercise matter for the child's overall physical and mental health. Then, using Handout 37 (Healthy Habits Worksheet), elicit specific examples from the child on habits he/she (and the family) currently engage in that are healthy, and those that are not so healthy. Summarize by reviewing why healthy habits are so important; then ask the child to choose the area he/she thinks is the highest priority. Review that area first. If there is enough time at the end of the session, you can briefly review the other two areas, or you may need to save the entire discussion of those areas for a later session or two.

Healthy Sleeping Habits

Defining the Problem

Sleep can play an especially important role in managing mood disorders. It is critical for families to understand its importance and know how to maintain good sleep hygiene. Use Handout 38 (Sleep) to help children understand that getting too much or too little sleep has important consequences for them and their mood symptoms. The handout also helps children become more aware of their sleep habits and of the reasons why current habits may be a problem. Review a child's various sleep patterns—for instance, weekdays versus weekends; nights at Mom's house versus nights at Dad's house, if divorced parents share custody; sleep patterns now compared to when the child was doing well.

Nine-year-old Michaela and her parents came to their session looking incredibly stressed out. Joan, Michaela's mother, seemed to be at her wits' end. Robert, Michaela's father, sounded defeated. They described the past few days as very difficult. No one had been to sleep before midnight for the past several nights. Homework had been a constant battle, and Michaela had been in and out of her bedroom, repeatedly insisting that she needed to do "one more thing." Initially, her parents had tried to redirect her back to bed, but this resulted in a tantrum that seemed to take longer than just letting her do what she needed to do. Michaela had been up by 5 A.M. each day, waking the whole house (including her 6-year-old brother, who was getting increasingly whiny as the days progressed). When their therapist started reviewing the week with the family, she realized what a significant role sleep hygiene (or lack of it) had been playing. She suggested that they focus on sleep for the first healthy habits session. Using Handout 38 and the previous week's experience, the therapist helped Michaela fill out the section "How much sleep do I get?" Then the therapist asked Michaela how much sleep she used to get before the problems started. As they talked about sleep, the therapist helped Michaela recognize that when she didn't get enough sleep, she became "hyper," and then it was even harder to get to sleep, so the problem just got worse and worse.

Problem Solving

Children first need to see that their sleep habits are causing them problems. They can then be encouraged to take ownership of the solution by helping to set sleep goals and then tracking actual sleep times on a Sleep Chart. Handout 39 is an example of a filled-in sleep chart. At the top are written target goals for bedtime, falling asleep, waking up, and total sleep for both weekdays and weekends. The rest of the chart records actual times for each day of the week. Handout 40 is a blank Sleep Chart.

To help Michaela take more ownership of her sleep habits, her therapist taught her how to use the Sleep Chart. On her chart, Michaela wrote down goals for her bedtime, fall-asleep time, wake-up time, and total sleep time for both school days and weekends. In addition, they reviewed scheduling as a family. When they went back and looked, they realized that the downward spiral had started after Michaela slept over at a friend's house and didn't fall asleep until 2 A.M. They decided as a family that any sleepovers Michaela would attend would be held at their house for the time being, so that Joan and Robert could make sure Michaela got to sleep at a reasonable time.

Troubleshooting

For girls in particular, sleepovers can present a unique challenge (we like to tell families they are called "sleepovers" because a child sleeps when they're over!). Helping parents recognize such pitfalls is critical. Problems can be compounded when children spend different nights of the week with different parents. Moreover, as children approach the teenage years, their normal sleep patterns start to change; often this leads to dramatically different sleep patterns on the weekends compared to weekdays. Parents used to a young child's habit of waking up early on a Saturday morning to catch cartoons suddenly find that the child is sleeping until noon as adolescence approaches. If a child is having a manic episode, a medication adjustment may be needed before sleep will improve. Keeping a tight rein on sleep habits in the spring, especially around the onset of daylight savings time, may help to prevent or alleviate a manic episode.

Sleep habits can be hard to change, especially if bad habits have become entrenched. Children and parents may need a lot of support and encouragement to make these changes. Setting small, incremental goals for children and families to work toward can be helpful. Changing and improving sleep routines can be a multistep process.

Charlie, who was 10, had been difficult to get to sleep since he was a baby. He demanded a lot of parental attention around bedtime, which put a significant strain on his parents, who also needed to get his 5-year-old brother to sleep. Charlie's father traveled a lot for his job, so he often was not home to help with bedtime. When the family entered PEP, both boys were going to bed at the same time. This meant that Charlie's little brother was going to bed close to 9 P.M., and Charlie was not settling down until almost 10 P.M. (and sometimes not falling asleep until 11 P.M.). Charlie also tended to demand attention while his brother was being read to and trying to fall asleep; then his little brother wouldn't fall asleep and would get whiny and fussy while Charlie was trying to read with his mom. Overall, bedtime had become a mess.

When Charlie talked about sleep during a PEP session, he complained that he didn't get any one-on-one attention at bedtime. Although Meg, his mother, was focused on bedtime for 2–3 hours each night (leaving her stressed and frustrated), she wasn't getting much "quality time" with either boy. With their therapist's support, Charlie and Meg decided to try separating the boys' bedtimes. Charlie's little brother really needed to be in bed closer to 8 P.M.; for Charlie, being in bed by 8:30 and asleep by 9 P.M. would be okay.

Charlie agreed to find a quiet activity between 7:30 and 8:00 P.M. so Meg could get his brother to bed, and then he could have some one-to-one time with her between 8:00 and 8:30 P.M. Since Charlie really liked comic books, they agreed that Meg would get him a new comic book to start with, and that he would earn 50 cents toward a new comic book for every day that he followed the plan. Charlie would keep track of his bedtimes/amount of sleep on his Sleep Chart (Handout 40).

The initial check-in at Charlie's next session went as follows:

THERAPIST: How have bedtimes gone since I saw you last?

MEG: Well, I have to give Charlie credit. He has made it much easier for me to get his brother to bed. He has really done a good job of looking at his comic books while I take care of his brother. However, the mornings have still been a disaster.

THERAPIST: (*to Charlie*) How do you think things have gone?

CHARLIE: I've been going to bed, but I still can't fall asleep until 10:00 or later.

MEG: Maybe because you don't stay in bed? I know you have been going to bed at 8:30 or 9:00, but every other minute you are up telling me something else.

THERAPIST: It sounds like it has been really hard for you to get settled, Charlie.

CHARLIE: Yeah, I'm just not tired.

THERAPIST: Well, given how hard it has been for you to get up in the morning, you probably need the sleep. But it doesn't sound like you are relaxed and sleepy at bedtime, and we also know that every time you get up out of bed, you get your blood pumping and keep yourself from getting any closer to being sleepy. Sounds like we need to add to our plan! Half of our plan worked—Charlie, you aren't interfering with your brother's bedtime—but we still need to find a way for you to get to sleep sooner.

MEG: How about Charlie stays in bed?

THERAPIST: That is certainly the goal. Part of our plan was for Charlie to spend some one-on-one time with you at bedtime. How has that been going?

MEG: It seems like all of the time turns into me trying to get him to get ready for bed.

THERAPIST: Charlie, is that how you want to spend time with your mom?

CHARLIE: No, I'd rather show her some of my comic books.

MEG: I could spend more time with you reading or looking at comic books if you were ready for bed. It seems like all I hear from you is "Just a minute."

THERAPIST: It sounds like we are working toward a plan. What do you think, Charlie?

CHARLIE: I guess if I get ready for bed, my mom could sit with me for a while …

THERAPIST: We had said that from 8:00 to 8:30 would be your time with your mom. What if your mom set a timer to go off to remind you to brush your teeth and get ready for bed just before 8:00? Would that help you be ready to spend time with her?

CHARLIE: I think that would help.

MEG: I would like to try. If you were ready, I could read to you, or we could read comics together.

THERAPIST: Sounds like a plan. I think you might find that it is easier to fall asleep if you have been doing something quiet like reading. Next time, we'll check in to see how things are going.

It would be important for the therapist to continue to check in about the sleep routine with Charlie and Meg together, as well as with Meg alone. Sometimes difficulty in settling down to fall asleep is related to mood symptoms or medication side effects. If a child's mood tends to get elevated in the evening, shifting doses of medication so that sedation occurs close to bedtime can be helpful. If a child takes a stimulant medication for ADHD and it hasn't worn off by bedtime, the medication can interfere with sleep. Some children benefit from a nightly dose of melatonin to aid sleep. Encouraging parents to consult with their child's prescriber can be an important part of improving sleep.

Breaking down the sleep routine for every family member can be quite helpful. In doing this, parents should be encouraged to examine their own sleep habits. When parents are caught up in overly long, stressful bedtime routines, they often find that they need time to wind down after getting their children to bed, and then they themselves end up going to bed later than they should. Long, stressful bedtime routines also prevent parents from having time together as a couple in the evening. If children aren't settled until after 10 P.M. it may be time for parents to go to bed by the time the children are asleep.

Likewise, if a child has gotten into a rut of needing a parent in his/her room (or even in bed with him/her) to fall asleep, chaos can erupt if the parent isn't available on any given night. Learning to fall asleep independently is a necessary skill the child will ultimately need to learn. In addition, when the parent's lying down with the child is part of the sleep routine, the tired parent often drifts off to sleep while waiting for the child to fall asleep. This keeps parents from connecting with each other and can result in an early evening "nap" that leads to staying up too late.

Good sleep habits for the entire family support overall health. Even small changes can make a big difference. It is not unusual for families to feel so overwhelmed by everything they are dealing with that they do not break the situation down into component parts. By separating sleep out and helping family members to come up with small changes they can realistically accomplish, you can help them all achieve better health and better mood regulation.

Healthy Eating Habits

Healthy eating can be a challenge for children with mood disorders. When depressed, many children eat to comfort themselves. Some children lose their appetite and begin to lose weight. This can be particularly problematic for children with ADHD, who have already been struggling with appetite suppression due to their stimulant medication. Parents often describe strong carbohydrate cravings in their children with BSD. To make matters worse, many of the medications prescribed for BSD, increase appetite and lead children (or adults) to feel that they cannot get enough to eat, particularly, high-carbohydrate foods. Weight gain is a common medication side effect for children with BSD, and this weight gain can lead to serious health problems (e.g., high blood pressure, Type 2 diabetes, sleep apnea, high cholesterol). When children are eating too much of the wrong foods, they are also often not eating enough of the right foods.

Changes in diet are a family affair. Children typically cannot change their eating habits without the support of their parents, who do the grocery shopping and plan and cook the meals. Children, however, can be the impetus and inspiration for making major family changes in eating habits. This is particularly true for families in which parents struggle with their own weight issues.

Defining the Problem

The focus in PEP should be kept on developing healthy habits. "Dieting" should not be part of the discussion. Although considerable scientific attention has been paid to overweight children, there is not yet an evidence-supported method for reducing weight in children, aside from decreasing caloric intake and increasing exercise. If a child enrolled in PEP has a significant weight issue, the family should be referred back to the child's primary care physician. The focus in PEP should be kept on building healthier habits and not on weight loss.

To help children and parents identify unhealthy eating as a problem, use Handout 41 (Healthy Eating), in conjunction with Handout 42 (The Food Pyramid). Start by reviewing the prompts on Handout 41. Then bring out Handout 42 as a reference for the child, and review, as needed, standard guidelines about number and size of portions. Specific handouts and additional details can be found at a U.S. Department of Agriculture website especially for children (*www.mypyramid.gov/kids*).

Jimmy, age 10, came to PEP 20–30% overweight. His parents were also significantly overweight. According to the parents, Jimmy had been a skinny kid until he started on medication 3 years ago. Since then, he had gradually gotten heavier. Activities involving running had gotten harder and harder for him, and his asthma had become more difficult to control. Although Jimmy did not tell his PEP therapist directly, his parents reported that he often made disparaging comments about his weight as well as about his parents' weight. He also talked about wanting to be skinny like he used to be. In his first healthy habits session, Jimmy readily identified eating habits as the highest priority. To give both Jimmy and his parents a sense of what healthy eating habits would entail, the therapist started with a review of The Food Pyramid (Handout 42). Then they began to look at Jimmy's eating habits. His parents also began to talk about their eating habits, although the focus was not on them. They noted carbohydrate cravings that often resulted in snacking on high-carbohydrate foods like chips, crackers, and pretzels. Because of the way his school lunch was scheduled, Jimmy often came home from school starving, which led to extensive snacking after school. His favorite drinks were sodas, but he often drank juice because he thought it was better for him. Family mealtime had become chaotic: His mother felt like a short-order cook, because different people wanted different food and it was very hard to keep track of what anyone was eating. When asked about fruits and vegetables, Jimmy's mother sighed and said she knew it was important to eat fruits and vegetables, but that she had given up forcing her family to eat their vegetables at dinner.

Problem Solving

Once the child and parents agree that there is a problem and it needs a solution, problem solving can begin. This can start with a selection of healthy eating goals. The child can then keep track of the eating goals on Handout 44 (Healthy Food Chart). Handout 43 is an example of a filled-in Healthy Food Chart; for goals, it uses the recommended number of servings per food group from The Food Pyramid.

In the case of Jimmy (see above), he and his therapist identified the following goals for making his eating habits healthier:

1. More water and low-/no-sugar drinks, and fewer high-sugar drinks like juice and soda (Jimmy and the therapist talked about the added benefit that water is free! They calculated the amount of money the family would save by not buying soda and juice, and Jimmy and his parents agreed to spend it on a fun, physical activity the family could enjoy together—ice skating at a local rink.)
2. Adding healthy snacks to prevent Jimmy from feeling that he was "starving."
3. Getting the whole family involved with mealtime, and making meals calmer.
4. Finding fruits and vegetables that everyone would eat.

The therapist encouraged Jimmy to pick one change to try for the next week while tracking his eating habits on the Healthy Food Chart. Jimmy adamantly wanted to try two. He decided that he wanted to try adding some healthy protein to his snacks (including a snack to eat on his way home from school) and to try drinking more water and fewer high-sugar drinks. Jimmy couldn't wait to go skating!

Troubleshooting

A number of healthy eating pitfalls are described in Table 9.1, along with healthier options that can be suggested as solutions. As with sleeping problems, it can be helpful to use a multistep process of small, realistic changes and to follow up with the plan, troubleshooting obstacles as they arise.

Healthy Exercise Habits

Children with low activity levels enter into a negative cycle: They snack while sedentary and get heavier; this makes exercise harder, less immediately reinforcing, and often embarrassing. Increasing activity levels requires motivation from the child and possibly lifestyle change for the whole family. Your role is to get all family members energized about increasing their exercise, and to help both children and parents identify feasible ways of doing so. Although increasing all three types of exercise is the ideal endpoint for a child, starting with one or two new exercise strategies is more likely to meet with suc-

TABLE 9.1. Healthy Eating Habit Pitfalls

Pitfall	Why it's a problem	Healthier options
Sugary drinks (including fruit juices)	Lots of calories, lots of sugar, and no nutritional benefit. Fruit juices don't have all the fiber and other benefits of whole fruit!	Drink water, seltzer with a little juice added for flavor, or flavored water.
Getting to the point of "starving"	Being overly hungry tends to lead to overeating.	Eat small meals more frequently, or add healthful between-meals snacks that include lean proteins.
Not eating fruits and vegetables	The body needs the fiber, vitamins, and minerals in fresh fruits and vegetables. Fruits and vegetables are healthy sources of calories, and if you don't eat them, you tend to eat less healthy options.	Experiment with different fruits and vegetables. Try frozen fruits and make smoothies with low-fat yogurt. Try different ways of preparing vegetables, including raw with a low-calorie plain yogurt dip recipe.
Snacking on simple carbohydrates	You tend to eat more calories and burn through them quickly. Also, you don't get important nutrients.	Plan snacks with healthy proteins and healthy fats. Look for whole grains and fiber.
Nighttime munchies	These tend to lead to foraging in the kitchen and eating too many "empty" calories.	Make a healthy pre-bedtime snack part of the plan. Have the snack include healthy proteins, maybe some calcium, and fiber (e.g., a fruit smoothie made with yogurt; dry, slightly sweetened high-fiber cereal).
Eating food out of the package	You can eat several servings without realizing it.	Make it a habit to put a serving size in a bowl or baggie.

cess. The child can try additional exercises as the first additions become routine, or the child can change to a new set of exercises if the first ones lose their appeal.

Defining the Problem

Start by getting the child to assess problems he/she may experience as results of too little or too much exercise. Although too little exercise usually causes obvious problems, too much exercise can be a problem if it overly "revs up" a child who is already having a manic or hypomanic episode. It can also interfere with sleep if done too late in the evening, when the child should be winding down. Using Handout 45 (Exercise), review the problems the child acknowledges. Then discuss the different types of exercise and the qualities of each : Stretching can be a great way to relax the body; aerobic exercise works well to lift mood and can also help burn off agitated energy; strengthening is good for general health and can contribute to improved self-esteem. Help the child inventory his/her own exercise habits and determine personal goals in this category. For children who are demoralized by excessive weight gain, it can help to focus on how exercise can be beneficial to them for reasons other than weight loss.

Problem Solving

The plan for increasing exercise needs to be both financially and practically feasible, as well as enjoyable. There are many ways to increase activity, and these vary in terms of cost, time commitment, outdoor safety, and climate considerations. Many gyms and workout centers are becoming friendlier to families and have classes and workout times for children. But joining a workout center carries a financial cost and requires a time commitment from parents, since children are dependent on parents to get them there. Although tennis lessons may be prohibitively expensive through a private club, they may be affordable through community programs and local recreation centers. Families should be encouraged to look at how much, if anything, they want to spend on exercise. If the answer is "not much," then the plan should have zero financial cost.

The plan should be enjoyable and physically manageable. Children can brainstorm what they can do; for instance, running around in the yard with the dog is more active than sitting and watching TV. If going outside alone isn't an option, what are indoor options? Jumping rope (away from light fixtures!)? Encourage families to be creative. Can the child's exercise plan build on other areas of need? For example, martial arts are great for self-discipline and self-control, and yoga is great for relaxation and stress management. Team sports can provide social opportunities as well as exercise. Current guidelines recommend 60 minutes of physical activity daily (*www.mypyramid.gov/kids*).The following is a brief list of possible exercise options, ranging from mild to high-intensity:

Mild Activities
Walking with the family in the evenings
Playing chase with the dog
Swinging
Jumping on the trampoline

Moderate Activities

Playing neighborhood games (e.g., pick-up game of soccer or basketball, tag, hide and seek)

Riding bikes

Jump rope

Wii Fit

Exercise programs on TV (on demand)

High-Intensity Activities

Organized sports teams (football, baseball, gymnastics, swimming, etc.)

Dance team

Martial arts

Weight lifting

Will the plan work year-round, or are different plans needed for different seasons? In Arizona, a family can take walks throughout most of the year, but during parts of the summer heat needs to be taken into account. In Maine, seasonal plans are needed. The family members will also need to decide whether they want one activity plan for the whole family or whether the child will make his/her own plan. When a family is deciding to shift to a more active lifestyle, clearance from primary care physicians may be necessary for parents and possibly for children.

Troubleshooting

Several issues can get in the way of increasing children's exercise. Perhaps the most common is insufficient parental exercise. For a variety of reasons, most adults in the United States do not exercise enough; thus children do not see parents as role models who enjoy physical activity. Parents who are already burdened with long work hours and commutes may feel too tired to commit to an exercise regimen when they get home. In families of children with mood disorders, the parents have the added responsibility of helping their child negotiate the myriad issues resulting from the mood disorder. Increasing exercise in the child often requires a substantial rearrangement of family time and priorities.

Other common problems are the embarrassment and realistic restriction on exercise children can experience if they have had excessive weight gain following initiation of certain medications. These children are often acutely self-conscious and become less rather than more active as a result of their weight gain. For them, increasing activity level in a safe manner is particularly important.

THERAPIST: So, Zach, what happens to you when you don't get enough exercise?

ZACH: That's the story of my life! Ever since I started taking my new medicine, I've gained a bunch of weight.

THERAPIST: Do you ever have times when you get too much exercise?

ZACH: Well, it's probably not too much exercise, but when we have to run laps in gym class, I'm always the slowest. Even all the girls can go faster than me. My teacher told me last week that I should stop running, because my face had gotten so red and I was breathing really hard.

THERAPIST: Wow, that sounds pretty unpleasant. It sounds like running is especially difficult for you right now. There are three different kinds of exercise; let's see what you do in each category. Stretching is just what it sounds like—slowly stretching out your muscles to keep you loose and limber. Do you do any of that?

ZACH: My gym teacher sometimes has us start our classes that way. Lots of the girls like to show off how flexible they are, especially the ones who are into gymnastics. I don't like it. It just hurts.

THERAPIST: Hmmm ... sounds like maybe not your favorite part of gym class. Do you have a favorite part?

ZACH: When it's over!

THERAPIST: Okay—well, I know lots of kids who feel self-conscious or awkward in gym class. Let's keep brainstorming to see if we can come up with some ideas of exercise that sounds a bit more appealing to you. Another category of exercise is aerobic exercise. Running laps is one example of aerobic exercise, but there are lots of other examples as well—and maybe some that you would like better than running laps, and that wouldn't cause you to get out of breath and red in the face.

ZACH: That would be good.

THERAPIST: You've told me before how special your dog, Zoey, is to you. Now lots of dogs that I know think they never get enough playtime. Do you think Zoey would have fun if you played chase or fetch with her?

ZACH: (*smiling*) Yeah, Zoey's favorite time of day is when I come home from school. She usually comes to the door with a toy in her mouth, wanting me to chase her.

THERAPIST: And my guess is she could go on forever, but you would eventually get tired or bored of it?

ZACH: You got it!

THERAPIST: What would you think about setting the kitchen timer, say, for just 5 minutes at the beginning, and chasing her through the house? If you did that three different times in the day, that would be 15 minutes of aerobic exercise. Do you think you could do that?

ZACH: Yeah, probably. And Zoey would love it!

THERAPIST: Okay, great. Now, the third kind of exercise is strengthening. Your dad had mentioned before that he was thinking of signing you up for a martial arts class. Martial arts really combines several types of exercise. There is some stretching, usually at the beginning and end of class, some aerobic parts, and definitely some strengthening. What would you think about trying that?

ZACH: Aren't those the people who wear those funny white uniforms?

THERAPIST: Usually if you take a martial arts class, you wear a uniform, just like you would if you were playing any kind of team sport.

ZACH: I don't know. I wouldn't know anybody there.

THERAPIST: Do you think you might feel more or less self-conscious if you didn't know anybody?

ZACH: I guess maybe it's better that I wouldn't know anybody. At least the other kids from my class wouldn't be there laughing at me, like in gym class.

THERAPIST: Sometimes trying something new has some real advantages, just like you said. Not knowing anybody might allow you to feel more free to try the moves and techniques they teach in the class. Do you think you might be willing to try it? Usually these classes have a time limit, like 8 weeks or 12 weeks, so you could see what you think about it.

ZACH: I suppose so.

THERAPIST: Great! Let's fill out part of your Exercise Chart, then—the part about chasing Zoey every day. Then, when your dad comes back into the session, we can check with him on how soon you can sign up for the martial arts class. Once you know that information, you can add it to the Exercise Chart.

Breathing Exercises: Balloon Breathing

After the Lesson of the Day is completed, review the breathing techniques that were introduced previously: Belly Breathing (Handout 11) and Bubble Breathing (Handout 28). Then introduce the third breathing technique, Balloon Breathing (Handout 48).

Ask the child to think about how air seeps out of a balloon when it has a tiny hole in it or when it's not tied off tightly enough. Then ask the child to pretend that his/her lungs are a balloon. The child first takes in a deep breath, filling the lungs with air. Then the child purses his/her lips, making a small "pinhole," and gently blows the air out. This process is then repeated three or four times. Balloon Breathing can be introduced as follows:

"Today we are going to imagine that our lungs are a big balloon that we fill with air when we breathe in, and then gently blow the air out, like we had a little pinhole in our balloon. Just like with Bubble Breathing, purse your lips like you would to say 'oo,' and then let the air slowly seep out of your balloon. Okay, so take a deep breath and fill your lungs from the bottom up. Now make your lips like a pinhole and gently let the air out. As the air goes out, imagine that all the tension in your body goes with it. When a balloon loses air, it goes limp and loses the tension on the inside. Take in another deep breath and let the air and tension just seep out. (*Pause*) Did you notice your muscles feeling different before and after you let all the air out? Let's do that again. Take a deep breath in—fill up your big lung balloons from the bottom up. Now let's let the air come out slowly through that little pinhole. While the air escapes, notice how your muscles are starting to relax, as well. The air and the tension just seep out through the pinhole. (*Pause*) Okay, great. Let's do that one last time for today. Imagine your lungs are great big balloons. Fill them up with air from the bottom to the top. Now we're going to let those balloons go limp while we let the tension out of our bodies."

Children are encouraged to practice Bubble Breathing three times before the next session and keep track of it on Handout 48.

Session Review with Parents

In some cases, parents will have been present for the complete healthy habits session. If not, try to allow a little more time than usual (about 15–20 minutes) for them to rejoin the child and hear what he/she has learned about healthy habits. The child should explain the between-session plan for improving healthy habits to the parents. You should reinforce important concepts as necessary. To be successful, any habit change for the child will require considerable involvement by the parents; therefore, everyone should also determine what role the parents will play in the child's plans. For example, what help might the child need from the parents to carry out any planned change?

Take-Home Projects

New Project: Selected Healthy Habits Chart

This session's take home project will differ, depending on which set of healthy habits the child and family have chosen to focus on. It will be either the Sleep Chart (Handout 40), the Healthy Food Chart (Handout 44), or the Exercise Chart (Handout 47). Each chart is designed to raise the child's awareness of engagement in healthy habits. Discuss with the child and parents where the chart will be kept and who will take responsibility for completing it. Encourage the child to keep track of his/her healthy habit behaviors for the whole time until the next child session. Review what will be recorded in the chart, and make sure that the child has a good sense of his/her plan for increasing healthy behaviors.

If this is the first healthy habits session, remind the family members that later in treatment they will turn to the next priority on their healthy habits list. This allows the family to focus on building one healthy habit before adding another.

New Project: Balloon Breathing Practice

Ask the child and parents to practice Balloon Breathing—one to two sets each on three different days. They should record practice dates on the "Breathing Log" portion of Handout 48. If the parents and child do this together, it provides a nice reminder to the child that everyone in the family benefits from learning calming strategies.

End the session on a motivational note: Building healthier habits can produce life-long benefits for all family members. In particular, children with mood disorders can take positive steps to manage their own health. This can lead to a sense of empowerment, as well as to significant physical and emotional benefits.

Chapter 10

Teaching Parents about Systems: Mental Health and School Teams

IF-PEP Parent Sessions 3 and 6
MF-PEP Parent Session 3

Session Outline

Goals:

1. Give parents an overview of the mental health system, the range of mental health professionals, and ways to access different types of services.
2. Give parents an overview of educational services for special-needs children, who's who in the school system, and ways to build a coalition with the school.

Beginning the Session:

Do a check-in and review of Mood–Medication Log (Handout 32) or Mood Record (Handout 20 or 21).

Review completed Understanding My Child's Medication (Handout 35).

Troubleshoot problems with selected healthy habits chart (Handout 40, 44, or 47).

144

Lesson of the Day:	Building the mental health and school teams

- The mental health team and its services (Handout 49)
  - Evaluation
  - Medication management
  - Psychotherapy
  - Additional support
  - Levels of care
  - Parents' role on the mental health team
  - Troubleshooting access to care
- The educational system and team (Handouts 50 and 51)
  - How the school system works for children with special needs
  - Educational terms and acronyms: Knowing the lingo
  - Who's who in the school system
  - Building a coalition with the school
  - Stigma and other barriers to parent–school communication

New Take-Home Projects:

My Child's Treatment Team (Handout 52)
My Child's Educational Team (Handout 53)

Ongoing Take-Home Projects:

Mood–Medication Log (Handout 32) or Mood Record (Handout 20 or 21)
Support child's efforts on selected healthy habits chart (Handout 40, 44, or 47)

New Handouts:

49. Who's Who and What's What in the Mental Health System
50. Important School Terms and Abbreviations
51. Who's Who in the School System
52. My Child's Treatment Team
53. My Child's Educational Team

Handouts to Review:

35. Understanding My Child's Medication
32. Mood–Medication Log

Session Overview

The first part of the third parent session in both IF-PEP and MF-PEP orients parents to the types of mental health treatments for children with mood disorders, the range of professionals who may be on a child's treatment team, and the parents' role as treatment team members. The second part of the session focuses on the educational system and how it allocates services for special-needs children. Also covered are school personnel who may be on a child's educational team, and ways parents can be active and effective members of their child's educational team. It is important to be familiar with the nuances of both the mental health and educational systems in your own geographic area, and to incorporate those into your discussion.

Families enter PEP at all stages of treatment team and education team development. Some are new to a diagnosis (or a suspected diagnosis) and thus are at an early point in the team assembly process. Others may already have an effective team but want to fine-tune certain aspects of treatment. For families already knowledgeable about treatment, your discussion about the mental health team can be very brief. However, when you are a family's first point of contact in establishing mental health treatment for a child, or when the treatment team is not working effectively, the issues may be complicated and the discussion more lengthy. Your goal during this session is to make sure that parents walk away with an understanding of what mental health care is available and who provides the different aspects of care. In MF-PEP, anticipate many questions in the subsequent session from parents after they have checked their children's mental health and school resources. In IF-PEP, you will revisit these issues in the sixth parent session. At that time, parents may raise issues regarding their mental health treatment team, but there are almost always more issues to deal with regarding the school team. School is often a challenge for children with mood disorders, which means that developing a good educational team is critical. At the same time, building an effective coalition with the school can be very challenging.

Beginning the Session

Do a Check-In and Review Take-Home Projects

Ask how the family is doing, and briefly review the Mood–Medication Log (Handout 32) or Mood Record (Handout 20 or 21), depending on whether or not a child is taking medication. Parents should also arrive at this session having completed Understanding My Child's Medication (Handout 35). Respond to any questions raised by the exercise and any remaining issues about medications. A full review of whichever healthy habits chart a family in IF-PEP is working on (Handout 40, 44, or 47) will occur at the child's next session; however, parents frequently will have questions they wish to bring up without their child in the room (e.g., concerns about their child's recent weight gain upon starting mood-stabilizing medication). This parent-only session provides an ideal opportunity for such discussions.

Lesson of the Day:
Building the Mental Health and School Teams

The Mental Health Team and Its Services

Depending on your agency and geographic area, the players on the mental health team may vary slightly. Again, be sure to know the nuances of your particular geographic area and its local agencies.

The discussion should include information about levels of care, with details as appropriate (e.g., parents of a mildly depressed child will not need extensive information about residential treatment).

Families in PEP typically need at least two, and often benefit from all four, of the following mental health services:

1. An evaluation of the child, which can result in a diagnosis and a recommended treatment plan; this plan may include medication and/or psychotherapy.
2. Medication management.
3. Psychotherapy.
4. Additional support.

Although the same mental health professional may provide more than one type of service (e.g., evaluation plus medication management or evaluation plus psychotherapy), often one person does not provide all needed services. Frequently two professionals are involved, and sometimes more than two. These providers, along with the child and parents, form the mental health treatment team. Table 10.1 and Handout 49 (Who's Who and What's What in the Mental Health System) provide an overview of who does what in the mental health system, as well as information about varying levels of care.

Evaluation

Parents may not know that there are different kinds of evaluation (e.g., for diagnosis, medication, or cognitive/academic strengths and weaknesses), carried out by different kinds of mental health professionals—a psychiatrist, a psychologist, or a social worker, for example. If cognitive testing is necessary, a psychologist or school psychologist is likely to fill this role. Evaluation can be an ongoing, multistep process that may not result in clear-cut answers. A diagnostic evaluation often results in a preliminary or "working" diagnosis, or is used to rule out a particular diagnosis. As discussed in the parent session on medication (see Chapter 8), a medication evaluation may result in a recommendation for starting with a specific drug, but it often takes time to find the best medication at the right dose.

Medication Management

As discussed with parents in the medication session, it is usually preferable to have a child/adolescent psychiatrist evaluate and manage a child's medication. However, in

TABLE 10.1. Who's Who and What's What in the Mental Health System

Title	Degree/credentials	Role
	Who's who	
Psychiatrist	MD or DO	Completes evaluations; makes medication recommendations; monitors medication; sometimes provides therapy.
Psychologist	PhD, PsyD, or EdD	Completes evaluations; may do cognitive testing; provides individual/family/ group therapy and/or parent guidance; collaborates with prescriber; may collaborate with educational team.
Social worker	LSW, LISW, LICSW, or MSW	May complete evaluations; may serve as a "gatekeeper" for psychiatric services; provides individual/family/group therapy and/or parent guidance; collaborates with prescribing physician; may collaborate with educational team.
Therapist (various degrees)	PC, PCC, PCC-S, MFT, IMFT	Usually plays role comparable to a social worker's; these are professional counselors or marriage and family therapists.
Nurse with advanced training or physician assistant	APRN, RNCS, CRNP, MSN, PA	Completes evaluations; makes medication recommendations; monitors medication; sometimes provides therapy.
Case manager	MA, BA, or BS (may also have titles listed for "Therapist")	Helps coordinate services; makes home visits; works with child individually at school or home; may work with parents on strategies to manage problems at home; may work with educational team to coordinate services.
Others (e.g., Big Brother/Big Sister, neighbor, religious youth leader, family friend)	Varies	Respite; community mentoring
	What's what: Levels of care	
Wrap-around care	Varies	Provides support to child/family to improve communication and behavior; provides crisis management services; can provide home-based services; in some cases, provides one-on-one behavioral support at home and (when not provided by the school district) at school.
Inpatient care	MD, APN, RN, MSW/LISW, PhD/ PsyD, educators, various others	Provides safety when symptoms are severe and child is dangerous to self or others. Focus is on stabilization; child is usually discharged to less intensive care within

(cont.)

TABLE 10.1. *(cont.)*

Title	Degree/credentials	Role
		1 week; sometimes a few family therapy sessions occur; medications are probably adjusted; medical tests (e.g., drug screen, EEG, MRI) may be conducted; may coordinate return to school plan and evaluate academic needs.
Partial hospitalization program	MD, APN, RN, MSW/LISW, PhD/ PsyD, educators, various others	"Step down" from inpatient care: Child attends program during the day, goes home at night. Focus is on stabilization; child usually discharged to less intensive care within 1–2 weeks. Some family therapy is possible; medication adjustment may continue.
Residential treatment program	Similar to partial hospitalization program	Longer-term out-of-home treatment. Length of stay varies, depending on severity of symptoms (can be a year or more). School on site. Focus is on changing behavior to allow return to less restrictive setting.

reality, much prescribing will be done by general psychiatrists, pediatricians, family physicians, nurse practitioners, or physician assistants.

Psychotherapy

Psychotherapy varies, depending on who attends sessions, what the particular goals of treatment are, and what the therapist's theoretical orientation is. Individual therapy focuses on increasing self-awareness and improving coping and symptom management. Family therapy goals center on improving communication, problem solving, coping, and symptom management, and on resolving family conflict and other family problems. Parent guidance has goals similar to those of family therapy, but involves working only with parents. Group therapy for children with mood disorders tends to focus on improving social skills, coping, and symptom management.

These psychotherapies may provide a psychologists, a social worker, or another certified therapist, such as a marriage and family therapist or licensed professional clinical counselor. Parents should understand that these different modalities of therapy will be helpful in different circumstances and practice settings. In some cases, the same professional will work individually with the child, with the family as a whole, or with the parents separately. In other situations, one therapist may work with the parents, while a different therapist works individually with the child. Parents should be active participants in discussing the types of therapy that will be used, the frequency of sessions, and the goals. If parents are expecting to work as a family, but the psychotherapist intends to work individually with the child, the situation can become very frustrating. Clear communication on this issue is important.

Concerns about the course of treatment should be handled first through discussion with treatment providers and then, if that isn't helpful, through changes to the treatment team.

Additional Support

Many children benefit from having other types of mental health support. This support may be formal (e.g., case managers) or informal (e.g., regularly scheduled respite provided by an extended family member or a therapeutic summer camp). These resources should also be part of a child's overall treatment program.

Levels of Care

Some children, despite all the excellent lower-intensity care they receive, require more intensive levels of care. Availability of these higher-intensity resources in specific communities can vary widely; families may need to travel to access some of these services.

Most communities have some version of "wrap-around care." Wrap-around care is designed to provide support to the child and family, to improve communication and behavior, and to initiate crisis management services. In some communities, wrap-around care can include home-based services, including one-on-one behavioral support at home and, when not provided by the school district, at school.

Inpatient treatment is most commonly used when safety concerns are imminent (i.e., a child is dangerous to self or others). Such treatment focuses most commonly on diagnosis and stabilization. Medical tests such as drug screens, an electroencephalogram (EEG), or magnetic resonance imaging (MRI) may be ordered. Most inpatient stays are brief (approximately 1 week), after which the child is discharged to less intensive care. Inpatient treatment may include some family therapy sessions, and medications are usually started and/or adjusted.

Partial hospitalization provides a bridge between inpatient and outpatient treatment. In some settings, children can "move up" to partial hospitalization. In other communities, partial hospitalization is utilized as a "step down" from inpatient care. Children in a partial hospitalization program attend the program during the day but return home for the evening. Partial hospitalization provides additional support, but allows a child to spend a portion of each day with his/her family, with the ultimate goal of successful return to the home full-time. Partial hospitalization programs typically include a therapeutic school component; individual, family, and/or group therapy; and continued observation and medication adjustments.

Finally, residential treatment programs or therapeutic boarding schools provide longer-term out-of-home treatment. Occasionally school districts or insurance companies will pay for a portion of these stays, but for many families this will be a high out-of-pocket expense. Length of stay depends on severity of symptoms and can be a year or more. Both academic programming and therapeutic services are offered on site. The focus is on changing behavior to allow a child return to a less restrictive setting. The National Association of Therapeutic Schools and Programs website (*www.natsap.org*) can be used by families to begin to review these programs. This website is also listed in the Appendix. Some communities also have mental health practitioners who specialize in linking families with appropriate residential treatment programs.

Parents' Role on the Mental Health Team

Parents should be encouraged to approach all interactions with mental health providers as good consumers: They should arrive at sessions prepared, follow through on between-session tasks, and be active participants. Being prepared and active participants involves the following:

1. Understanding how the system works (discussed above).
2. Keeping good records and sharing them with the team.
3. Communicating honestly and openly.
4. Completing any assigned projects between sessions.

During the first few sessions of PEP, parents have been learning about tracking children's symptoms and keeping good records. These symptom records will allow parents to give a mental health professional a clear history with all critical details included. Parents' face-to-face time with each professional can be used most efficiently when parents arrive with these records and logs in good order.

Although parents may find some important information embarrassing or difficult to reveal, it can provide important clues on to how to proceed. For example, parents can be reluctant to share information about the level of family or parental conflict. Sometimes parents are embarrassed or even scared to admit that their children hit them. They can also be frightened of the consequences if they, or their child, mention that a parent has hit the child or caused accidental injury when an intense interaction escalated and the child needed to be restrained. Part of becoming an active participant is being open with treatment providers about the reality of the situation; if important information is left out, the team will be less effective.

Parents should expect to be treated by professionals as important members of the team. If they do not like the way they (or their child) is treated by a particular professional, they should try discussing the issue with this provider. If discussion does not improve the working relationship, it may be worth considering a change in providers.

During their sessions on medications and on building a treatment team, Cathy and Jeff listened intently and asked a number of questions about target symptoms for mood stabilizers and the impact of stimulants on unstable mood. They had begun seeing a child psychiatrist with their son, Erik, whose only current medication was a stimulant, and they were not feeling very comfortable with the way things had gone thus far. The doctor had asked them questions, but did not seem to listen to their answers. After the PEP session focused on medication, Cathy had questions about some specific medications and the reasons why the doctor was making particular recommendations. They had an appointment with the psychiatrist just after this session, and Cathy had written her questions down and brought a copy of the

Mood–Medication Log she and Jeff had been keeping. When she tried to show the doctor the log, he took the paper and put it on a pile on the desk. When Cathy started asking the questions she had written down (e.g., "Erik's mood seems to fluctuate between being very sad, being elated, and being extremely angry. Should we be considering mood stabilizers instead of stimulants?"), the doctor looked annoyed and said, "I guess you know everything you need to know and don't need me, huh?" When it came time to schedule the next appointment, Cathy told the receptionist she would call to schedule. She went home, called her PEP therapist, and requested some referrals for local psychiatrists who would value her input as an active and educated member of the team.

Troubleshooting Access to Care

Access to care is an important issue for many families. The factor interfering most frequently with access is finances. Child/adolescent psychiatrists tend to be in short supply, and in some communities they are not on insurance panels. For some families, this will mean that the cost of working with a psychiatrist is steep. This is one of the many times that families need to be creative problem solvers. Some families start with a psychiatrist for evaluation and establishment of a good medication regimen, and then move to their primary care physician (if this doctor is willing) for medication management. In addition to physicians, it is important to talk about nurse practitioners and physician assistants as medication managers. Depending on the state you live in, nurse practitioners may be required to work in collaboration with a physician or under the supervision of a physician, or may be certified to work independently. Physician assistants, as their title indicates, always work under the supervision of a physician. Although there still may be a significant cost associated with seeing a nurse practitioner or physician assistant, it may be more manageable. Families need to be honest about their financial status with their treatment providers; providers might have ways of working out an arrangement, but only if parents let them know they need help.

Geographic location is the second factor often affecting access to care. For families living in rural areas in particular, access to providers who are well versed in childhood mood disorders can be extremely limited. Again, creative problem solving becomes important. It may be worth the multihour drive to get a good evaluation. Armed with the information from that evaluation, a family may be able to assemble a good local treatment team, while maintaining the possibility of periodic consultation with the "remote" team that has provided the initial evaluation. For psychotherapy, families with long drives might explore the possibility of scheduling longer sessions (90 minutes rather than 50 minutes) but less frequently. Parents need to communicate openly about these difficulties and take a problem-solving approach. For example, a parent might say, "This drive is really tough, especially at rush hour. We like having you as part of our team, and we really want to make sure that our daughter has good continuity of care. How should we proceed?" There are usually several different ways to solve problems, but recognizing and stating the problem are critical steps along the path to a workable solution.

The Educational System and Team

Establishing an effective educational team and developing the best possible educational plan can be a source of great frustration for parents of children with mood disorders. The information presented in this part of the session can help lessen parent's frustration. It is very important for parents to understand the following:

- How the school system works for children with special needs.
- What educational terms and abbreviations mean.
- Who's who on the educational team.
- How to build a coalition with the school.

This part of the session should be shaped by the nuances of the school system in your own geographic area, as well as by any background knowledge that parents may already have.

How the School System Works for Children with Special Needs

Parents need to know about two U.S. federal laws that govern how schools help children with special needs. The first is Section 504 of the Rehabilitation Act, an antidiscrimination law. Section 504 requires that schools accommodate any identified disability, academic or otherwise. For example, if a medication side effect (e.g., dry mouth) distracts a child in the classroom, the school will accommodate this (e.g., the teacher will allow the child to have a water bottle in the classroom and take frequent bathroom breaks). The school's plan for accommodating a child under this law is called a "504 plan." Schools are responsible for establishing the plan; parents must be notified of the plan. The child's regular classroom teacher is the person who draws up the plan and implements it within the child's classroom during the school day. A 504 plan does not usually involve special staff or services outside the regular classroom.

The second federal law is the Individuals with Disabilities Education Improvement Act of 2004. (It is usually referred to as IDEA, the acronym of its former name, but sometimes as IDEIA.) IDEA mandates that children with particular disabilities (see below) are entitled to a free and appropriate public education (FAPE). It requires that a multidisciplinary team conduct a multi-factored evaluation (MFE). Based on that evaluation, an individualized education program (IEP) is written for the child by the school, with parental participation and approval. School districts receive federal funding for services provided under IDEA, and so they are likely to be more extensive than those provided under a 504 plan. An IEP may include special staffing and any other level of special services. Table 10.2 summarizes the key features of IDEA and Section 504.

Both laws have advantages and disadvantages. A 504 plan can usually be designed and implemented more quickly, and it is likely to be more flexible. However, its scope and implementation are dependent on what the regular classroom teacher can do. Under IDEA, a child usually receives more services, but the eligibility requirements are stricter and involve formally labeling the child as having one of the disabilities listed below. Specifically, to qualify under IDEA, a child must:

TABLE 10.2. Comparing IDEA and Section 504

Mechanism	Individuals with Disabilities Education Improvement Act (IDEA)	Section 504 of the Rehabilitation Act
Eligibility	Child's disorders must fall into one of the qualifying disability categories; the condition must adversely affect performance; child must need special education and related services	Eligible if physical or mental impairment is present and affects a major life activity (e.g., caring for oneself, performing manual tasks, breathing, seeing, hearing, walking, working, and learning)
Requirements	Written IEP based on an MFE	An agreed-upon 504 plan
Advantages	Federal money to the district; more extensive modifications/services	Expedient; often more flexible
Disadvantages	Requires more paperwork, time to complete, testing	No additional money to the district; adherence is dependent on the regular education teacher, as no time from specialized staff is allocated

1. Meet the criteria for one or more of the following categories as defined in law:
   - Autism
   - Deaf-blindness
   - Hearing impairment (including deafness)
   - Mental retardation
   - Multiple disabilities
   - Orthopedic impairment
   - Other health impairment
   - Serious emotional disturbance
   - Specific learning disability
   - Speech or language impairment
   - Traumatic brain injury
   - Visual impairment (including blindness)
2. Have a disability that adversely affects educational performance.
3. Need special education and related services.

Educational Terms and Acronyms: Knowing the Lingo

One challenging aspect of dealing with the educational system is mastering the "alphabet soup" that goes with it. Terms like "IEP," "IDEA," and "504 plan" are used by school personnel, but they can be difficult for parents to keep straight. Table 10.3 and Handout 50 (Important School Terms) list the most frequently used educational acronyms and terms.

Who's Who in the School System

Parents need to know who currently is, or possibly could be, part of the educational team serving their child. Table 10.4 and Handout 51 (Who's Who in the School System)

TABLE 10.3. Education Terminology and Abbreviations

Acronym (if applicable)	Term	Definition
—	Due process	Parental right to approve or disapprove of plans proposed by the school/district special services team, and to call for a review process if the parents do not approve of a plan.
FAPE	Free and appropriate public education	School districts must provide all eligible students with special education and related services, allowing personalized instruction and sufficient support services to permit the child to benefit educationally, at the public's expense.
FBA	Functional behavioral assessment	An evaluation, usually conducted by one or more school staff members, to identify triggers that precede losses of control or other significant behavioral problems.
—	Inclusion[a]	All special education services are provided within the context of the regular classroom with typical peers. A special education teacher coordinates services, oversees implementation of the IEP, consults, and sometimes teaches with the classroom teacher.
IEE	Independent educational evaluation	All parents have a right to obtain an IEE at the expense of the school if they are dissatisfied with the MFE and they have followed specific procedural requirements of the law.
IEP	Individualized education program	Specific plan devised by school personnel, with parental participation and approval. Establishes child's educational goals and specifies how they will be met.
LRE	Least restrictive environment	Placement that provides a child with needed educational services while maintaining his/her maximum participation in regular education services with typical peers.
—	Mainstreaming[a]	Children who have been placed in a self-contained classroom rejoin their regular class for particular subjects or time periods. Sometimes used as an incentive for children with behavioral challenges, or as a transition from a self-contained classroom back to a regular classroom.
MFE	Multifactored evaluation	An evaluation completed by the school (by a multidisciplinary team) to determine eligibility for special services. Ensures that no single procedure is the sole criterion for determining a child's eligibility for services.
OHI	Other health impairment	Classification for a child whose health problem adversely affects school performance and prevents the child's needs from being met entirely by regular education services. Some parents prefer this classification over SED for their children with mood disorders.
SBH	Severe behavioral handicap	Term (now dated, but still used in some districts) describing significant behavioral dysregulation.
SED	Serious emotional disturbance	Term used to describe significant emotional needs.
SLD	Specific learning disability	Term used to describe achievement in particular academic areas (e.g., reading, math) that is below expected level (often, but not always, based on tested ability level).

[a]Under IDEA 2004, which replaced the Individuals with Disabilities Education Act of 1997, the emphasis is on inclusion rather than mainstreaming

TABLE 10.4. Who's Who in the School System

Team member	Role(s)
Teachers (regular and special education)	Classroom teacher, school plan coordinator, case manager.
School counselor	Individual work with child; consultation with teacher, school plan coordinator; sometimes in charge of coordinating 504 plans.
School psychologist	Responsible for evaluation report; does testing with child; may provide direct intervention, consultation with teacher.
School social worker	Only present in some school settings; may provide direct intervention with child; may help families find resources.
Principal/vice principal	Administrator; may work directly with child; supports classroom teacher; attends IEP/504 meetings; has input into eligibility for services.
Special education coordinator	Works for the district coordinating special education services; knowledgeable about services throughout the district; consultation; sometimes attends IEP meetings; may help make eligibility determinations.
Local education agency (LEA) representative (may also be special education coordinator or another IEP team member)	Qualified to provide, or supervise the provision of, specially designed instruction to meet the unique needs of children with disabilities; knowledgeable about the general education curriculum; and knowledgeable about the availability of the LEA's resources.
Instructional support teacher	Title may vary from district to district; in charge of coordinating a team that meets to discuss children who may need academic or behavioral support prior to an evaluation's being initiated; may be in charge of developing 504 plans.
Occupational therapist	Direct intervention with students or consultation with teachers re: developing fine motor abilities/handwriting or making accommodations for fine motor weaknesses. Also provides consultation and intervention for children with sensory integration issues.
Physical therapist	Direct intervention with students or consultation with teachers re: developing gross motor abilities or making accommodations for gross motor weaknesses.
Speech–language pathologist	Direct intervention with students or consultation with teachers re: developing language abilities, developing compensatory strategies for auditory processing deficits, etc.
Other school personnel	A creative, flexible team uses all resources. Any staff members (attendance coordinators, in-school discipline specialists, custodial staff, secretarial staff, etc.) may become helpful members of an educational team.

summarize a full range of school personnel, including staffers whom parents may not initially consider as team members.

Building a Coalition with the School

Sometimes a child's entire team (i.e., parents, teachers, administrators, the child's psychiatrist/psychologist, etc.) agree on the services that the child needs at school, and those services are available and carried out effectively. Often, however, it takes significant effort to build a coalition with the school, develop a plan that is acceptable to everyone, and maintain the communication required to ensure that the plan works well. When parents and school personnel have a significant disagreement about the educational plan, maintaining a coalition becomes a challenge.

For many families, this is likely to be a topic of considerable importance. There are typically two types of parent–school disagreement: (1) School personnel recommend a more restrictive environment, and the parents do not believe it is necessary; or (2) parents believe that more services or a more restrictive environment are necessary, and the school disagrees. Helping parents understand, and reconcile, these discrepant views is an important component of developing an effective parent–school collaboration. In the following example, the parent disagreed regarding services recommended by the school.

During the PEP discussion on working with the educational system, Ellen, the mother of 9-year-old Jackson, said she had initially felt that Jackson's third-grade teacher was pretty good, but now she was getting really concerned. Jackson had a 504 plan that specified a behavioral plan. However, his teacher had recommended that testing be done and had said she thought that Jackson should have an IEP. Based on the results of testing, the school psychologist had written a report and labeled Jackson as having an emotional disturbance—one of IDEA's qualifying disabilities. Ellen had attended an IEP meeting about Jackson a few days ago and was still upset. The team had recommended that Jackson spend 1 hour each day in an emotional support class, where the focus would be on emotional and behavioral issues rather than on academics. This would mean that Jackson would be out of his regular classroom for science or social studies, depending on the day. Ellen was distressed by the label assigned to Jackson, and was also unhappy that he would be missing out on regular academics.

The therapist, Kathy, acknowledged the difficulty of Ellen's situation and articulated that coming to an acceptable plan that met Jackson's educational, social, and emotional needs could be extremely hard. Kathy asked Ellen to describe the behavior she thought had led to the school's concerns. Ellen described Jackson's ongoing difficulty getting along with classmates, behavior that disrupted instruction, and frequent refusal to do his work. In the nonthreatening environment of PEP, Ellen began to see that Jackson did have some significant emotional and behavioral needs at school. With Kathy's help, she was also able to identify why the school's specific plan concerned her: Jackson would be missing his favorite academic subjects, science and social studies, and these periods were the times he tended to have the least difficulty. This was an important issue that needed some careful problem solving. Ellen left the session ready to meet with the school team and discuss how to meet Jackson's emotional and behavioral needs without sacrificing his two favorite subjects.

If negative relationships between parents and school personnel develop, it is critical to help parents determine their child's needs and find points of agreement between the school's perspective and the parents' perspective. A small percentage of families can afford to move to a different school district, pay out of pocket for a specialized private school, or pay an educational lawyer to sue for services; however, the vast majority of families have to find a way to work with their present school districts.

When parents want additional services for their child, but the school denies that there is a need for them, parents often feel helpless or become frustrated; either way, they end up in conflict with the school district. An all-too-common scenario is this: Parents recognize that something isn't quite right by kindergarten or first grade, but teachers see the child as performing within the expected range and tell the parents that everything is fine. Parents often drop the issue, despite a nagging feeling, because they have been told by educators that everything is fine. However, by about fourth or fifth grade, the problems become more apparent. Sometimes the school then starts to recognize the problem, but sometimes not, as in the following example.

> Eric and Kelly's daughter, Ally, had been diagnosed with BD-NOS at age 7, and they had worked hard since then to establish an effective treatment regimen for her. Now age 10, Ally was quiet at school all day but was having increasingly dramatic tantrums each night that were often triggered by homework issues. She came home unsure how to proceed with her homework, struggled significantly with math, and did not know how to plan consistently and effectively for long-term projects. Through discussions with Ally's teachers, a 504 plan was developed. Some of the accommodations in the 504 plan proved helpful, but Ally's level of frustration seemed to be increasing nevertheless. Eric and Kelly had three primary concerns: that Ally's frustration would start to spill over into her behavior at school and her peer relationships; that she might have a learning disability in math that was not being addressed; and that the amount of strain incurred while getting through the school day might lead to an exacerbation of her mood symptoms. The school personnel were reluctant to initiate further assessment and were consistently telling Eric and Kelly that they thought Ally was doing fine.

Eric and Kelly were facing a common dilemma: In such cases, the school's perspective on the child is different from what the parents see at home. In other words, part of the educational team (the parents) has part of the data, and the rest of the educational team (the school staff) has another part of the data. The services ultimately recommended by the school will be considerably influenced by the information they have. You can help parents begin to think of themselves as part of an educational team that includes their children's teachers and other school personnel. Parents should be active team members. For example, in the case above, Eric and Kelly would need to make sure that the school had their information about Ally and that they had the school's input. To be effective, parents need to learn to be calm, well spoken, and organized in expressing their concerns to school personnel over time. It works best when parents are able to provide documentation and specific examples of a child's problems. The better their records, the more likely parents are to convince a school that more intervention is needed.

When parents have concerns about their child's school-based services, they can be most effective by proceeding as follows:

1. Request a meeting with teachers to share concerns.
2. Request in writing an evaluation of the child. (There is a "Permission to Evaluate" form; once this form is signed by parents, the evaluation must be completed within 60 school days.)
3. Keep well-organized, careful records.
4. Keep in mind that evaluation findings are not final and that conclusions may be appealed. (Documentation of parental rights is provided to parents at every IEP meeting.)
5. Always seek to build coalitions, not conflict, with the educational team.

Parents also need to be coached to be good consumers and to know their rights. Educational law (e.g., provisions relating to due process) protects their right as parents to disagree with decisions made by school personnel.

Stigma and Other Barriers to Parent–School Communication

As in the case of Ally, it is not uncommon for children to work really hard "keeping it together" at school, and then to come home and "let it all hang out." That is, symptoms may be relatively hidden at school but extremely troublesome at home. Parents are often hesitant to talk to the school about such a child's struggles. In some cases, they are embarrassed; they feel that if their child's troubles only appear at home, it must be their fault. In other cases, parents can't bear to reveal a child's problems when the teacher talks about how wonderful the child is at school. Whatever may be happening, you need to talk about stigma and encourage parents to share their worries and concerns with the school.

Parents sometimes have legitimate concerns about how school personnel might respond to information they share about their child. They and the school staff may already have a problematic history, possibly as a result of experiences with siblings. Parents may feel that the school does not like them or their child, or there may be an IEP or 504 plan in place that parents believe has not been followed. Sometimes the school personnel have good intentions but lack the resources to be able to carry out interventions well. Whatever the issues may be, they should be discussed between the parents and the clinician prior to a school meeting. If the situation is highly contentious, an in-the-bank session should be used before the school meeting to address these issues.

When a child's problems are evident in the classroom, schools can also fall into the trap of assuming that the parents are at fault, rather than the child's mood disorder. Moreover, some parents are affected by their own mood disorders, which can limit their ability to work effectively with the school. Their own symptoms may also create a chaotic home environment that makes it difficult for the child to come to school prepared. In some such cases, it can be hard for parents to see how significantly their own mood disorders affect their child. Part of your role as a PEP therapist is to increase parents' awareness of their own mental health concerns and to refer them, as appropriate, for their individual treatment needs.

Some parents who come to PEP are just beginning to grieve for the loss of the perfect, healthy child they always dreamed of raising. School personnel are sometimes the first to point out to parents just how serious a child's disability is. Your support and gentle guidance can help parents to move forward and prepare for action. Later in PEP, a session is scheduled that includes members of the school team. Parents' fears regarding stigma and other obstacles to working with school personnel should be addressed prior to this meeting.

Take-Home Projects

New Projects: My Child's Treatment Team and My Child's Educational Team

The new projects for parents this week are to write out the members of the treatment and educational teams on My Child's Treatment Team (Handout 52) and My Child's Educational Team (Handout 53). The act of completing these handouts may help parents recognize important people they do not immediately think of as being on one or both of these teams. These people include both the child and the parents. Completing the handouts may also help the parents to identify gaps in the team. Explain that not every team needs to include every type of member suggested on the form; teams should be constructed to meet the child's unique needs. Parents should bring the completed handouts to the next parent session.

As the family's therapist, you may be able to recognize additional services that could be helpful. For example, a case manager may be helpful for a family struggling to stay on top of mental health and educational issues; a privately hired tutor may be critical for school success.

Ongoing Projects: Mood–Medication Log or Mood Record; Selected Healthy Habits Chart

Encourage parents to continue monitoring their child's mood on the Mood–Medication Log or Mood Record, and to support their child's efforts (as appropriate) as the child works on healthy habits.

Chapter 11

The Child's Tool Kit
for Coping with Difficult Feelings

IF-PEP Child Session 4
MF-PEP Child Session 3

Session Outline

Goals:

1. Help the child identify situations that trigger difficult emotions (i.e., "mad," "sad," "bad" feelings).
2. Help the child recognize bodily signals for strong emotions.
3. Guide the child to develop a list of strategies for coping with feeling mad, sad, or bad.

Beginning the Session:

Do a check-in and review Mood–Medication Log (Handout 32) or Mood Record (Handout 20 or 21).

Review Balloon Breathing practice (Handout 48).

Review selected healthy habits chart (Handout 40, 44, or 47) (for IF-PEP only).

Have child identify and rate feelings (Handouts 1 and 2).

Lesson of the Day:	Building a coping Tool Kit for mad, sad, bad feelings

- My Triggers for Mad, Sad, Bad Feelings (Handout 54)
- My Body Signals for Mad, Sad, Bad Feelings (Handout 55)
- My Actions When I Feel Mad, Sad, Bad (Handout 56)
- Building the Tool Kit (Handouts 57 and 58)
- Explain the take-home project: Taking Charge of Mad, Sad, Bad Feelings (Handouts 59 and 60)

Breathing Exercise: Child's choice (Belly, Bubble, or Balloon Breathing)

Session Review with Parents

New Take-Home Project: Taking Charge of Mad, Sad, Bad Feelings (Handouts 59 and 60)

Ongoing Take-Home Projects: Selected healthy habit change with chart (for IF-PEP only)
Selected breathing practice

New Handouts:
54. My Triggers for Mad, Sad, Bad Feelings
55. My Body Signals for Mad, Sad, Bad Feelings,
56. My Actions When I Feel Mad, Sad, Bad
57. Building the Tool Kit (Sample)
58. Building the Tool Kit
59. Taking Charge of Mad, Sad, Bad Feelings (Sample)
60. Taking Charge of Mad, Sad, Bad Feelings

Handouts to Review:
1. Feelings
2. Strength of Feelings
40. Sleep Chart *or*
44. Healthy Food Chart *or*
47. Exercise Chart (for IF-PEP only)

Session Overview

In IF-PEP, this session begins with a careful review of the previous healthy habits session with the parent and child. Depending on how the selected habit change is going, more troubleshooting may be needed.

The main topic of the session—the Tool Kit for coping—represents the core of PEP. It helps to empower children with mood disorders by identifying effective tools they can use to cope with difficult emotions—"mad, sad, and bad" feelings. Note that although it is important to explain to children that feelings are neither "good" nor "bad" (they simply "are"), we use the phrase "mad, sad, and bad" in a mnemonic manner, to help children remember angry, dysphoric, and irritable and/or anxious moods—mood states children find unpleasant. Acknowledge that children don't always have control over their emotions and what triggers them. At the same time, you can help children understand that they do have choices in how they respond to those triggers and emotions.

The lesson begins with helping a child to identify situations that trigger strong emotions, and to recognize physical sensations that can signal a strong emotion. The child is then asked to consider how he/she reacts when feeling strong emotions, and whether a typical action is "helpful" or "hurtful." The child next works on developing his/her personal Tool Kit for coping with mad, sad, and bad feelings. These coping tools are grouped according to the acronym CARS (Creative, Active, Rest and relaxation, and Social. An angry mood may be soothed by shooting baskets out in the driveway, or a sad mood may be relieved by calling a grandparent to talk. Depending on the child's age and preferences, the Tool Kit may be a three-dimensional box filled with reminders and objects used in coping, or it may be a list on a note card stuffed in a backpack or desk drawer.

Beginning the Session

Do a Check-In and Review Mood–Medication Log or Mood Record

By this session, families are often in the "rhythm" of the session format. As always, the check-in begins with the child and parent together, and it should include a brief recap of the family's week and a check of the Mood–Medication Log or Mood Record and Balloon Breathing practice. (Note: Children in MF-PEP will move immediately after this to the Lesson of the Day, as they have not had a separate healthy habits session.)

Review Balloon Breathing Practice and Selected Healthy Habits Chart

While the parent is still in the session, review the child's selected healthy habits project. The child and family should have completed one of the three charts (either Handout 40, *Sleep Chart*; Handout 44, *Healthy Food Chart*; or Handout 47, *Exercise Chart*). Go over this chart, and then engage the child and parent in a discussion of any challenges encountered since their session on healthy habits. For some children, their parents will have been significantly involved in the plan to increase healthy habits; other children will have embarked on the project more independently.

> Kiara, an 8-year-old, was having a lot of trouble getting to sleep at night. She and her parents decided to focus on sleep first. Kiara was young, and although she was involved in the process, she needed significant parental support to begin to change her sleep-related behaviors. In this session, they discussed how her sleep had been going, and they reviewed what was recorded on the chart over the past 2 weeks. Kiara and her parents had been working as a family to keep the evening routine calm up to bedtime. One strategy they had decided on was to record their favorite TV shows so they could watch them well before bedtime. Although the routine had been a little better, the chart showed that Kiara was continuing to fall asleep late and was still having trouble getting up in the morning. Kiara's therapist encouraged them to keep working on the evening routine and to keep recording. He reminded them that sleep habits are difficult to change, and that it might take several weeks for them to start noticing changes. They all agreed that the issue of sleep should be brought up at their next appointment with Kiara's psychiatrist.

Although these family members had worked together on changing behaviors related to sleep, they hadn't seen actual improvement in Kiara's sleep yet. Having their therapist remind them that these things take time to change helped them to stay the course and continue working on healthy sleep habits.

> Beckah, 13, was very annoyed with her BD. Not only had it cost her friendships and led to poor grades at the end of the last school year, but now she was taking medication that caused her to gain weight rapidly. Her mood had improved and her behavior had settled down since she started taking the medication, but the extra 10 pounds around her tummy were not welcome. Before starting the medication, Beckah had been slender. When her therapist brought up the topic of healthy habits at her last session, Beckah decided to take action and focus on her eating habits. She tracked her food intake for the next 2 weeks and was surprised by how much she actually ate. She was ravenous, especially in the evenings. Dr. Hernandez used this opportunity to review with Beckah some food choice options she could try during her "carb-craving" moments that would help fill her up at a lower calorie cost. Beckah's mom, who knew that Beckah was concerned about her weight but hadn't known how to discuss it with her without making her feel worse, chimed in that she could buy more fresh fruit and veggies to keep the refrigerator stocked with healthy food choices. Beckah's mom also admitted that she had been struggling with her own eating habits, and suggested that she and Beckah could encourage each other to choose fruits and veggies at night, when they both tended to snack.

Beckah, an early teen, was very sensitive about her weight and wanted autonomy in dealing with it. Her mom was able to be supportive in the therapy session, although she had been at a loss about how to deal with the problem at home.

In the next example, Ron, like Beckah, was older and wanted a more independent approach.

During the session on healthy habits, Ron (11) decided that he wanted to work on increasing his exercise. He had made it clear that he wanted to do this by himself, and told his therapist he thought he might feel nagged if his parents were involved in reminding him. At the next session, Ron reported that it had been harder than he thought it would be to keep the chart. He decided part way through the week to ask for some help from his mom. They decided to move his chart from his room to the refrigerator, and also made an effort to have the whole family exercise more, which made it easier for Ron. In addition, they agreed that while his mom might make suggestions or provide opportunities, she wouldn't remind or nag him about the project. Both Ron and his parents thought that the exercise had been helpful, and Ron reported that he wanted to keep the chart on the fridge from now on.

Even with more independence, Ron found that he needed some parental support. He also found that changing healthy habits was hard and required concerted effort from him and from his family. He did appreciate how his mom was supportive, but at the same time wasn't nagging him when he didn't follow through with his plans.

Have Child Identify and Rate Feelings

After the parent leaves the session, complete a quick check-in with the child. By this session (the child's fourth in IF-PEP or third in MF-PEP), identifying feelings, determining their source, and rating the strongest feelings can usually be done quickly. If prompts are still needed, refer back to Handouts 1 (*Feelings*) and 2 (*Strength of Feelings*).

Lesson of the Day: Building a Coping Tool Kit for Mad, Sad, Bad Feelings

My Triggers for Mad, Sad, Bad Feelings

With guidance, children can identify situations at home, in school, and with peers in which they feel mad, sad, or bad; these situations are the "triggers" for these feelings. "Bad" is used to describe anxiety, fear, worry, or irritability, and is easier to remember than these other descriptors because it rhymes with "mad" and "sad." Again, however, remind children that feelings are not really "good" or "bad"; they simply "are." In the session, have a child generate a list of triggers from prompts about times when he/she has recently felt mad, sad, or bad. Use Handout 54 (My Triggers for Mad, Sad, Bad Feelings) for this list. It uses light switches to represent triggers, because they are events that "turn on" specific emotions. The light switches will also be used to indicate triggering events in later handouts.

It can be helpful to discuss how the same trigger can lead different people (or the same person at different times) to feel different ways. On one day, a child may say that he/she feels mad when friends do not want to play; on another day, the child may say that this makes her feel sad. One person can even have multiple feelings at the same time in response to a trigger. Ideas to convey include understanding that there are no "right" or "wrong" feelings; the key for children is learning what to do *in response to* the feelings they experience. Discussing the range of reactions a person might have to a specific event can help a child understand others' reactions and pay more attention to behavioral cues. This is a skill that many children with mood disorders need to improve; it is discussed further in Chapter 17 when nonverbal communication is addressed.

My Body Signals for Mad, Sad, Bad Feelings

The list of triggering events leads to a discussion of the signals in a child's body indicating that he/she is feeling mad, sad or bad. Most children feel certain emotions in places in their bodies, even if they don't initially recognize this when asked about it. For instance, some children describe their ears getting red when they get mad. Other children may tense up and make a fist when they feel provoked by another child. Knowing these bodily signals helps children identify their feelings, which gives them an opportunity to choose an appropriate coping strategy. With exploration, almost all children can identify at least several clues about their feelings from their bodies.

To prompt ideas, children may need to have some examples provided (e.g., "Your heart races if a car almost hits you on your bike," "Your palms get sweaty when a teacher announces a pop quiz"). Handout 55 (My Body Signals for Mad, Sad, Bad Feelings) shows an outline of the body. Ask the child to circle where on the outline he/she feels mad, sad, or bad emotions, using red, blue, and yellow for these emotions, respectively. For instance, if Lance says that his face gets very hot when he feels angry, he would circle his face in red. Many people have a "butterflies in the stomach" feeling when they are anxious. If Pei Lin feels that way, she could circle her stomach in yellow. If Noah feels sad when ignored on the playground, he may feel heaviness in his shoulders and arms, so those could be circled in blue. Again, having children reflect about where they feel certain emotions helps them label the emotions—a necessary step before choosing a coping strategy.

My Actions When I Feel Mad, Sad, Bad

Next, children reflect on what actions they tend to take when they feel mad, sad, or bad, and whether a specific action usually winds up helping or hurting them. The actions can be written down in the appropriate section of Handout 56 (My Actions When I Feel Mad, Sad, Bad). In discussing whether an action was positive or negative, children can think about the outcome in three ways: (1) "Does it hurt me?" (2) "Does it hurt someone or something else?" (3) "Does it get anyone in trouble?" These questions can be also used in future sessions to help a child examine whether an outcome was helpful or hurtful. Use these terms and focus on the consequences of the specific action. Avoid labeling actions as "good" or "bad," since a child may have been labeled as "the bad kid."

If a child has difficulty coming up with examples, you may be able to prompt the child to think about his/her actions after one of the triggers identified earlier occurs. You may also be able to offer examples from situations previously described by a parent. The discussion can include both effective ("helpful") and ineffective ("hurtful") actions. Examples of effectively handled emotions remind the child that he/she is capable of success. Talking about hurtful outcomes highlights where the child needs helpful strategies for handling strong emotions.

The following dialogue illustrates how the Lesson of the Day might unfold to this point. Josh was 12 and fiercely independent. Although medications had reduced the intensity of his mood swings, he continued to have periods of irritability and sadness.

THERAPIST: So your biggest triggers for feeling mad are your parents telling you to do something when you are in the middle of something you want to do; your brother bugging you; and having to do writing for homework. Right?

JOSH: Yeah.

THERAPIST: And your biggest trigger for feeling sad is not having any friends to hang out with.

JOSH: I guess so.

THERAPIST: It sounds like body signals are hard for you to notice, but from what you've mentioned before, maybe your stomach feeling tight lets you know when you are getting really mad, and feeling heavy all over your body is a signal that you are feeling sad. That sound about right?

JOSH: Yeah, I guess so.

THERAPIST: From what you and I have talked about and what your parents have told me, sometimes your actions when you are mad or sad are helpful and lead to you feeling better or to things going better. Other times they are hurtful, meaning that they make you feel worse or cause more problems for you, like getting in trouble. Let's go through this worksheet [Handout 56] and see if we can get a better idea of your helpful and hurtful actions, okay?

JOSH: What's the point?

THERAPIST: The point is that if your actions when you feel sad or mad are helpful, life will go more smoothly for you, and you might even be happier! Humor me, and let's see if we can come up with some examples.

JOSH: Okay.

THERAPIST: When you feel sad, what do you usually do?

JOSH: I usually just go in my room and lay on my bed.

THERAPIST: Is being by yourself when you feel sad helpful?

JOSH: No, but I just feel like being alone. Sometimes my dog comes to my room with me, and that usually helps, 'cuz he keeps trying to get me to play and makes me laugh.

THERAPIST: He sounds like a great buddy to have around! So being alone when you are sad is hurtful, but spending time with your dog when you are sad is helpful. Does this make more sense to you now?

JOSH: Yeah, I guess so.

THERAPIST: Okay. How would you feel if your mom asked you to turn off the TV and do your homework?

JOSH: I'd be really annoyed, probably mad.

THERAPIST: What do you think you might do?

JOSH: If I was having a good day, I'd probably set the DVR to record the rest of the show and then I'd try to get my homework done, but my homework sometimes makes me mad too.

THERAPIST: Okay, so using the DVR is a very helpful response. What helpful action could you take if your homework starts to make you mad?

JOSH: I could take a break from it, or I could ask for some help.

THERAPIST: Yes, those are both very helpful actions! The more that you make helpful choices, the better you will feel. What would you do on not such a good day—a day you were feeling grumpy?

JOSH: I'd probably ignore her, and then I'd probably yell at her or maybe throw something.

THERAPIST: So when you are grumpy, some of your actions are likely to get you in trouble, like ignoring your mom, yelling at her, or throwing something. Those are hurtful actions that tend to lead to more mad, sad, and bad feelings.

In such a discussion, you can once again point out that feelings are not "right" or "wrong," they just "are." How we handle our feelings, how we act, leads to positive or negative outcomes. By linking this to the PEP motto ("It's not your fault, but it's your challenge"), you can help the child understand the motto better and avoid self-blame for his/her emotions, while still taking action to manage the feelings.

After his therapist discussed the links among triggers, emotional responses, and subsequent behaviors, 9-year-old Jackson (who has been discussed in Chapter 10) said, "I get it. It's kind of like the time I got sent to the principal for yelling at my teacher." "Tell me about that time," the therapist encouraged. Jackson went on to describe how he had been working on his science questions when his teacher told the class to put away their science books and get out a sheet of paper to write down their spelling words. Jackson really wanted to finish the question he was working on and was hurrying to finish. He explained that having to hurry often made him cranky. When his teacher came over beside his desk, touched him on the shoulder, and asked him to put away the science book and get out some paper, he jumped when she touched him and yelled, "Quit it!" before realizing it was his teacher. He was sent to the principal's office. He talked about how hurrying had led him to feel frustrated. "So rushing is my trigger, and the feeling I was having was frustrated. It wasn't my fault that I was feeling frustrated, but I shouldn't have yelled at my teacher."

After the links among triggers, emotions, and subsequent behavior are discussed, it is time to help children identify strategies to manage their moods more effectively.

Building the Tool Kit

Strong emotions present challenges for children. The Tool Kit is a collection of strategies, or "tools," a child can assemble to use when his/her mood is too high or low. It may be either a physical collection of symbolic objects or a list. Children are reminded that it can be difficult to remember strategies to calm themselves in the heat of the moment; the Tool Kit makes these easy to recall and readily available. Children are asked to generate multiple tools, because (1) some tools cannot be used in certain situations; and (2) different tools are helpful for different feelings. Strategies for managing elevated mood, anger, irritability, sadness, and anxiety differ. For instance, a child who is feeling lethargic and sad may want to get energized by doing a few jumping jacks or going for a bike ride, but a child who is feeling too keyed up in an elevated or anxious mood may be overstimulated by these activities. A child in an elevated mood may benefit from listening to some soothing music, which could further decrease the energy of a lethargic, sad child.

Four categories of tools are discussed: Creative, Active, Rest and relaxation (R&R), and Social (the acronym CARS is used for these). Creative tools require a child to use his/her imagination (e.g., play with Play-Doh, build with Legos, draw). Active tools get the child's body moving (e.g., go for a bike ride, jump rope, tense and relax foot muscles). R&R tools help the child relax or calm down (e.g., take a hot bath or shower, lie in a hammock outside, breathe deeply). Social tools get the child engaged with other people or pets (e.g., call Grandma, play with the dog). Some activities can fit into more than one category (e.g., dancing is both creative and active), and can be listed in any category they fit into. Handout 57 (a filled-in version of Building the Tool Kit) shows examples of Tool Kit strategies in each of these four categories. Using the blank version of Building the Tool Kit (Handout 58), help the child generate and record several tools in each category. It is important that children generate enough tools to be used across a variety of settings (e.g., classroom, recess, at home during the day, at home when everyone is in bed and they need to be quiet, in the car). Children should also be encouraged to update their Tool Kit over time with new strategies. For children whose mood symptoms have a negative impact on them at school, it may be helpful to put together a Tool Kit especially for school, with input from the teacher. See Chapter 16 for further discussion of accommodations at school.

Explain the Take-Home Project: Taking Charge of Mad, Bad, Sad Feelings

Ask the child to make a Tool Kit before the next session. Depending on the child, decide whether the Tool Kit will be an actual collection of items in a box, or a continuation of the list of possible activities begun in the session. Older children may prefer simply to prepare a list of CARS strategies they can use to cope. An actual Tool Kit can be made with a shoe box or any other available container. It may be filled with a combination of pictures (e.g., of the family dog), other representational objects (e.g., Grandma's phone number, to remind them to call her when feeling bored) and actual objects (e.g., a bottle of bubble bath for a hot bath, an iPod). The Tool Kit should be kept in a location easily accessible to the child; it has to be readily available to be helpful.

Parents often have good ideas to include in the Tool Kit; encourage children to seek input from their parents. The family may also decide to generate multiple Tool Kits (e.g., one for the back seat of the car, one for the babysitter's house, one for home, one for school). For example, a child who often feels sad during indoor recess at school could have a Tool Kit with crayons and coloring pages, pictures of loved ones to look at, and a reminder to talk to friends to feel better. A child who gets angry with siblings or parents could benefit from a Tool Kit at home with modeling clay, a jump rope, a reminder to take deep breaths, and a picture of playing fetch with the family dog. When tools are gathered in this way, the child will require less prompting about ways to help him/herself feel better.

As part of the take-home project, the children should then write down the items in his/her Tool Kit in the top part of Handout 60 (Taking Charge of Mad, Bad, Sad Feelings), including one or more items from each of the CARS areas. The child is then asked to use the Tool Kit three times before the next PEP session, and to record those instances on the bottom half of Handout 60. The child should record the trigger for a mad, sad, or bad emotion; where on his/her body the feeling was recognized; how he/she remembered to use the Tool Kit; the tool he/she chose to use; and the outcome achieved. Handout 60 with the child's Tool Kit list may then be kept on the bedroom door or on the refrigerator as a reminder. Handout 59 is a completed-sample version of Handout 60, with the Tool Kit listed at the top and a recorded use of the Tool Kit at the bottom. Ask the child to bring the actual Tool Kit as well as the recording sheets to the next session. If you are using a point system for child sessions that includes points for project completion, you might offer bonus points for bringing in the actual Tool Kit.

Breathing Exercise

After the Lesson of the Day is completed, review the three breathing techniques that were previously taught: Belly, Bubble, and Balloon Breathing. Remind the child that these breathing exercises are great coping strategies, and that one or more of them can be included as tools in his/her Tool Kit—but for them to work well, the child will need to continue practicing with them. The child can choose to rotate the three types of breathing or can pick a favorite to use. Either way, the child should continue to practice on a daily basis. A good time to do this is before going to bed.

Session Review with Parents

Parents are asked to rejoin the session at this point, and the child presents a summary of the Lesson of the Day and the new take-home project to the parents, with your assistance as needed. A very important issue to discuss with the parents and child is how the child should be reminded about using the Tool Kit. We have found that if family members can develop a humorous cue, it often works better than a more direct reminder that a child might interpret as "nagging." For example, one boy would turn very red in the face when angry. The family had taken a vacation to Maine the previous summer, which they all had enjoyed very much. When the mother noticed the boy's face turning red, she would say "lobster"; this was a private cue to the boy that he was getting angry and should use his Tool Kit. When he heard the word, happy memories of delicious seaside dinners came to mind, which helped ease him into using one of his coping strategies.

Take-Home Projects

New Project: Taking Charge of Mad, Sad, Bad Feelings

The child should either build a three-dimensional Tool Kit, or develop a list and keep it in a convenient location to remind him/her to use the Tool Kit over the course of the next 2 weeks. Between now and the next session, the child should also keep a record on Handout 60 of how the Tool Kit worked.

Ongoing Projects

The child and parents should also continue to work at home on the selected type(s) of breathing practice (Belly, Bubble, and/or Balloon Breathing) and, if in IF-PEP, the selected healthy habit chart (Handout 40, 44, or 47).

Chapter 12

Discussing Negative Family Cycles and Thinking, Feeling, Doing with Parents

IF-PEP Parent Session 4

MF-PEP Parent Session 4

Session Outline

Goals:

1. Increase parents' awareness of how negative family cycles play out in their own family.
2. Help parents understand how thoughts, feelings, and actions interact in negative cycles, and how shifting to more helpful thoughts and actions can improve family functioning.

Beginning the Session:

Do a check-in and review Mood–Medication Log (Handout 32) or Mood Record (Handout 20 or 21).
Review My Child's Treatment Team (Handout 52) and My Child's Educational Team (Handout 53).

Lesson of the Day:	Negative family cycles and the role of thoughts, feelings, and actions
	• The typical negative cycle
	• How mood disorders "mess up" family life
	• The role of emotion in negative cycles: Parents' burdens
	• The role of thoughts in negative cycles
	• "Can't" versus "won't"
	• The importance of parental agreement
	• Breaking the cycle: Finding positive strategies
New Take-Home Project:	Thinking, Feeling, Doing (Handouts 61 and 62)
Ongoing Take-Home Projects:	My Child's Treatment Team (Handout 52)
	My Child's Educational Team (Handout 53)
	Mood–Medication Log (Handout 32) or Mood Record (Handout 20 or 21)
New Handouts:	61. Thinking, Feeling, Doing (Sample for Parents)
	62. Thinking, Feeling, Doing
Handouts to Review:	52. My Child's Treatment Team
	53. My Child's Educational Team

Session Overview

Any leftover business from previous parent sessions should be wrapped up in the first part of the fourth session. The main topics of this session are (1) common negative cycles that families of children with mood disorders face, and (2) ways parents can learn to interrupt those cycles and thus to improve family life. Interrupting the cycles starts with parents' becoming aware of them; of the situations that trigger them; and of the thoughts, feelings, and actions that fuel the cycles. Handout 62 (Thinking, Feeling, Doing), given as a take-home project, is intended to increase parents' awareness of the cycles and self-awareness of the role they play in them. It is challenging for parents to step back and examine their own role in these difficulties. Care must be taken that parents do not feel blamed for their child's symptoms.

By this session, the bulk of the "teaching" component of PEP has been accomplished, and a shift is made toward building coping skills within the family. Starting with this session, more time is spent facilitating discussion, and less time is spent conveying information.

Beginning the Session

Do a Check-In and Review Take-Home Projects

After a brief check-in and review of the child's Mood–Medication Log or Mood Record, review the parents' mental health and educational team handouts assigned in their previous session (Handout 52, My Child's Mental Health Team, and Handout 53, My Child's Educational Team). This often generates productive discussion about necessary changes to teams or changes in thinking about the roles of team members. Primarily, we want parents to understand that treating childhood mood disorders requires a team approach, and that they are critical members of the team as the child's primary caregivers and advocates. We want parents to feel empowered, not overwhelmed. If a team is missing a key member, we want parents to be able to identify the gap and feel that they can reach out to potential team members. This is also a good time to check in with the parents about how other projects are going with their child. They may have some observations or frustrations that are better discussed without the child present.

Lesson of the Day: Negative Family Cycles and the Role of Thoughts, Feelings, and Actions

The challenging behaviors that come with mood disorders make it very difficult for families to reach a comfortable equilibrium. As a result, family members often find themselves trapped in negative cycles. Begin the lesson by describing a common negative family cycle that rings true to most families of children with mood disorders. As you review this cycle with parents, they may nod knowingly or smile with recognition.

The Typical Negative Cycle

The typical negative cycle begins like this: The child becomes upset, and family members try to help by doing everything they can to help the child feel better—reassuring, coaxing, or protecting him/her. However, these efforts do not help the child feel better and do not result in behavior change. So parents keep trying different strategies to change things. They can vacillate among pushing, coaxing, and reassuring their child; this can result in strong negative reactions or withdrawal from the child. Parents then tend to shift among trying harder, giving up temporarily, or getting angry. Ultimately, the desire to help the child, sometimes fueled by guilt, tends to pull parents back into the cycle. The child can begin to feel hopeless and unworthy (i.e., "If I'm causing so many problems and my parents can't help me, I must be a really hopeless case!"). When the parents disagree on the approach and argue, everyone feels worse. As the cycle progresses, the child feels more alienated (causing mood symptoms to escalate), and the family members feel more rejected and more hopeless. Over time, the family burns out but still feels guilty and/or angry, and the child is thoroughly alienated, with the same or even worse symptoms.

This is why parents often feel they are "walking on eggshells" with their child. They have turned themselves inside out for their child, and the symptoms persist. They may feel they have already done too much. The way out of the negative cycle is not to do *more* for the child, but to respond *differently* to the child. It's not the parents' fault for trying to help, and it's not the child's fault when an attempt to help doesn't work. The true enemy is the mood disorder, not the child. Responding to the child differently means that parents must learn how to partner with each other and with their child to manage symptoms and stop the negative patterns that currently occur. The first step in interrupting these cycles is recognizing when a negative pattern is happening. The triggers tend to be the challenging behaviors caused by the mood disorder, such as the child's unpredictability, agitation, dangerous or violent outbursts, social failure with peers, or disengagement/ withdrawal. Highlight the challenging aspects of a particular child's mood disorder for the particular family. Your role as therapist is to help family members identify their patterns, starting with typical trigger situations. Later in the session, the focus should shift to parents' thoughts, feelings, and actions in response to the child's challenging behaviors.

How Mood Disorders "Mess Up" Family Life

Unpredictability

One of the most stressful aspects of having a child with a mood disorder is the child's unpredictable behavior. The lack of predictability caused by fluctuating mood makes it very difficult for parents to respond to the multiple needs of different family members.

Alice and Joe were the parents of 10-year-old Carly, who had been diagnosed with BD. They also had a 7-year-old and a 4-year-old. During their session, they talked about how hard it was to know how to plan family activities. On the one hand, Carly loved to go out and do things. On the other hand, they could never be sure how Carly would be the morning of a planned activity, or whether she would be able to manage getting ready to go and then to handle herself appropriately throughout the activity. Alice and Joe described family outings on two different Saturdays—one they had planned weeks in advance, and the other impromptu. According to Alice and Joe, Carly tended to do better with advance planning. They had gotten tickets for a special exhibit at the science museum, an outing that Carly would typically love. However, that morning Carly had multiple meltdowns. Her jeans didn't fit right; she couldn't find the right socks; everything her younger siblings did, including breathing, resulted in her screaming at them. After a great deal of stress and effort, everyone was in the car ready to go. Carly fell asleep in the car, which led her parents to think that she might be okay at the museum. Once at the museum, however, she became so whiny and demanding that Joe took her out of the museum so that the other children could enjoy it. Alice and Joe thus managed to salvage the excursion for their other two children, but it was hardly a fun and relaxing day. A few weeks later, a friend had given them tickets to a minor league baseball game at the last minute. Alice and Joe hesitated, because Carly often did not handle last-minute schedule changes well. This time, Carly got ready quickly without any issues and was pleasant throughout the game.

In this example, everyone did the best they could on both occasions, and the problem with the first activity was not Carly but her mood disorder. It helps parents to know that sometimes there is no correct answer, and that a conflict is a result of negative mood, not poor planning.

Agitation

Agitation also creates significant stress for families. Having a member of the household who is unable to settle down is very difficult. Often the agitated child needs one-on-one attention from parents, which can be very difficult to achieve, as it was with Carly in the vignette above. Related to agitation is the seeming "unreasonableness" that children with mood disorders can exhibit. By this we mean that although a problem may seem easily solvable, a mood-disordered child can become extremely upset and unable to discuss or solve the problem situation. Unlike situations in which a child's particular desire or demand causes conflict, an agitated child often does not know what he/she wants. At these times, parents can easily become frustrated and angry at the child, which in turn makes the child even more agitated.

Failure to Meet Family Expectations and Responsibilities

Children with BSD or depression often feel a need to be in control, but they are unsuccessful in their attempts. This is aggravating for parents and especially for siblings. Making matters worse, the child with the mood disorder often fails to meet his/her responsibilities within the family (e.g., taking out the garbage, walking the dog). This frustrates parents and infuriates siblings; they may all begin to feel as if they need to "walk on eggshells" in order to prevent crises.

Social Failures

There are few things more frustrating for parents than watching their child fail socially. Parents feel helpless as they watch their child constantly do the wrong things around peers and then get teased and ostracized as a result. These children fall increasingly behind their peers and tend to feel worse and worse about themselves as a result. School recess tends to be among the worst settings, as the structure is minimal and the level of stimulation is high. On family outings, parents often fall into a trap of admonishing their child for socially clumsy behaviors. It is important for parents to recognize this as a negative pattern that is unlikely to lead to social success. Instead of focusing on what a child should not do, the parents need to focus on how and where to achieve success. This particular problem is likely to need attention from both the mental health and the educational teams. A child struggling with mood states is definitely less aware of those around him/her and may need active coaching to notice and then appropriately address a situation.

Dangerous or Violent Outbursts

Violence is one category of behavior that often leads families to "walk on eggshells." Dangerous or violent outbursts are exceedingly difficult to manage and very distressing to families. The impact of violent behavior on family relationships is tremendous. Siblings often become frightened, regardless of whether they or their parents are the targets, or their mood-disordered sibling is simply destroying walls or objects within the house. Although both parents may see the behavior as unacceptable, they may disagree on how to handle it. This shifts the focus off the child's need for intervention and onto the parents' argument. Violent behavior affects family relationships in many ways; it is important to help parents begin to take a careful look, so they are able to recognize the impact in their own homes.

If violence is a problem in a family, the interventions needed to manage it will vary, depending on the intensity of the violence and the age/size of the child. A small child who throws toys during a rage may be managed by a parent's holding him/her or simply walking out of the room and ignoring the behavior. An older/larger child who picks up items to use as weapons and escalates this behavior if the parents try to intervene may need a more intensive intervention. There are few options when an emergency like the latter occurs; sometimes someone coming to the house (e.g., a close family friend, an uncle) breaks the interaction enough for the violence to end. Emergency response teams from crisis centers are not equipped to get to houses quickly enough to intervene in a situation like this. Other emergency resources require a child/family to come to a center. The police department is often the only rapid responder available to get to a home quickly if parents need help managing a violent rage. If parents do not agree about the best ways of managing and preventing violent behavior, considerable tension builds in the parental relationship, and this tension perpetuates the negative cycle.

Disengagement and Withdrawal

Some children with depression or BSD may be unmotivated, withdrawn, and disengaged. These "I don't care" kids can be especially challenging, because their lack of engagement makes family interactions a struggle, and their lack of interests makes it very hard to find healthy coping activities.

> Drew is 12. He has been on antidepressants since the age of 8. Although his parents remember him as a very active young child, he now resists most activities that do not involve a screen. He has reached an unhealthy weight and shows no interest in increasing his activity level or in eating a more healthy diet. When his parents limit his video time, he sulks in his room. Drew has two younger siblings. Family activities are extremely difficult to plan, because Drew tends to be withdrawn when they are out as a family. If his mother, Margaret, tries to draw him in, Drew gets irritated with her. His father, Bill, gets frustrated and tells Margaret not to bother. Tension rises between Bill and Margaret. Drew gets increasingly withdrawn and irritable. No one has fun.

Coaxing and pleading with a disengaged child is unlikely to be successful. With Drew's family, the therapist's role is to help his parents identify the following pattern: Margaret's coaxing followed by Bill's frustration leads to Drew's increased withdrawal. If they can see the pattern, they may be able to plan in advance to avoid it. Maybe on a family hike, instead of coaxing Drew to act more engaged, they can hand Drew the trail map and say, "Hey, you're good at following maps in your video games. How about being our trail map reader?" No coaxing—just a role that Drew can take on quietly. He doesn't have to be talking and smiling to be engaged. If Drew refuses the role, Margaret and Bill can accept his refusal and just say, "Maybe next time. You'd be good at it."

The Role of Emotion in Negative Cycles: Parents' Burdens

As a therapist, you need to validate the heavy emotional burden of parenting a child who has a mood disorder. Parents *routinely* experience a wide range of emotions, including guilt, powerlessness, denial, and anger. Anger can be directed at themselves, each other, the grandparents, the school, the psychiatrist, the world, deities/fate, the person driving in front of them, and anyone or anything else. Other emotions include anxiety, fear, uncertainty, confusion, blame, shame, and a host of others.

A very common experience is isolation. It becomes difficult for parents of children with mood disorders to share their experiences with parents of typical kids.

Cassie was the mother of 9-year-old Marie, who had been diagnosed with BD 2 years ago. During her fourth parent session, Cassie talked about a summer afternoon at the pool. Marie was mostly stable on her combination of medications, but each day still presented a significant challenge. Water play seemed to be one of the most soothing activities for Marie, so they had been spending a lot of time at the pool. When they arrived, Marie and her younger sister ran off to play in the water. Cassie sat down where she would be able to keep a careful watch, since Marie could develop signs of an approaching meltdown without much warning and might require rapid intervention. Another mother sat down near her and struck up a conversation. The other mother was talking about school, her daughter's participation in the swim team, and helping her daughter balance all of her activities with her desire to spend time with her friends. In her therapy session, Cassie talked about how isolated and sad she began to feel as she listened to this mother. Cassie had to deal with much more fundamental issues: How much activity could Marie handle before she would have a major meltdown? How could she help Marie make and maintain friendships when Marie so easily damaged them? How could Cassie intervene when she noticed the signs of a meltdown developing? Cassie talked about how sad it was to realize that her parenting world was so different from this other mother's world.

The example of Cassie and Marie also illustrates the grief that parents experience. During pregnancy, parents fantasize about all of the wonderful things they hope for their unborn child. During development, parents watch and wonder about how their children will develop different interests, what they will be like as they grow, and what they will become when they are adults. During these early musings, parents don't think about how they will handle medication decisions or what they will do when a specialized school is recommended by their IEP team. When these very difficult problems emerge, parents grieve for the healthy child they once fantasized about. Their expectations have to change. Their dreams have to be tempered. Sometimes they have to work hard to maintain hope.

Parents' emotions can add a lot of steam to the negative cycle. For instance, if a mother is sad, she may withdraw more easily. Irritability may contribute to impatience at her spouse/partner or the child, which can significantly aggravate the existing negative cycle. Your role as therapist is to help parents become more aware of their own emotions, so that they can focus on shifting the patterns rather than aggravating negative family cycles.

The Role of Thoughts in Negative Cycles

By now, you will have laid out some of the most challenging aspects of mood disorders for families. You've addressed parental emotions that need to be understood and accepted. Now your focus shifts to helping parents understand the role of their own thoughts, as in the following example.

> Marla and Rich had three children, including 10-year-old Eric, who was diagnosed with BD. Their younger children wanted to go ice skating. Marla thought, *"Family outings never go well. I don't know why we even try. Eric is sure to embarrass us once again, and I'm going to get stuck dealing with him."* Rich thought, *"We've got to stop letting Eric's issues control us. We're just going, and that's it."*

Marla's thoughts were fueled by feeling hopeless and irritated that she was always the one who dealt with Eric's meltdowns. Rich's thoughts were in response to feeling angry about the situation. In their private thoughts, they were already in conflict. Their therapist's role was to help Marla and Rich recognize their thoughts and respond differently to each other, to the situation, and above all to Eric.

THERAPIST: (*after talking with Marla and Rich about their thoughts*) It sounds like you have some pretty negative thoughts about family outings, Marla.

MARLA: Yes. I find it very frustrating to go into these situations, knowing things are going to go badly.

RICH: That's half the problem: You assume that things are going to go badly.

MARLA: But they always do ...

THERAPIST: Slow down for a second. This is a great example of how your thoughts can contribute to the negative cycle. You two are in conflict as a result of Eric's mood disorder. We could describe this situation a little differently, which might help how you both think about it. How about if we say that Eric's mood symptoms cause him to have a very difficult time adapting to new situations and dealing with a lot of stimulation? Is that fair?

MARLA: Sounds about right.

RICH: Sounds right to me as well.

THERAPIST: So you are both right—the way you have been doing family outings often leads to Eric melting down, and you still ought to have fun as a family. So we need to change the thinking, which will help change the cycle.

MARLA: How?

THERAPIST: Well, what if instead of "Family outings never go well," you think to yourself, "Rich and I really need to think about how to make this work for Eric and the rest of the family"?

MARLA: Okay. That makes sense, because then we could make a plan.

RICH: Makes sense to me, too. We could make a plan that might help Eric do better, but we could also make a plan for what to do if things don't go well.

THERAPIST: Great. Now you are using your awareness of your thoughts to change the family cycle.

Once parents learn to pay attention to their thoughts, there is an opportunity to change their thinking or to change their response to their thoughts. How parents think about their child's mood disorder is critical to this process.

"Can't" versus "Won't"

As parents understand what to accept and what to focus on changing in their own responses, they also need to understand what the child can and cannot change. For example, the child cannot help feeling agitated and irritable, but he/she can control whether to hang out in the kitchen and become increasingly aggravated by younger siblings, or to go to his/her room and listen to calming music. Teaching parents to differentiate between "can't" and "won't" is very difficult, especially since it can be difficult even for professionals to recognize the distinction.

Some kids give us signs to help us distinguish "can't" from "won't." With "can't" behavior, parents typically say things like "I see that look in his eyes, and then he's gone." In terms of "won't" behavior, parents note that they see "a naughty twinkle" or a smirk on the child's face. It has been our experience that when we focus on this concept with parents, nearly every parent has some sense of the difference between "can't" and "won't" behavior. Even though their baseline skill in making this distinction varies widely, nearly every parent can get better with practice.

The Importance of Parental Agreement

The following example illustrates a negative cycle fueled by parental disagreement on how to respond to the child.

As Anita listened to the description of the negative family cycle, tears welled up in her eyes. It sounded so familiar, and in a way, it was a relief to hear it described as a common pattern. Her 11-year-old daughter, Caterina, had always been a challenge to parent. Anita was typically the "sympathetic" parent: She tried to coax and reassure Caterina during times of high stress. Her "soft" approach often resulted in arguments with her husband, Caterina's stepfather, who thought that Caterina was getting away with too much and should be punished for her refusal to do chores and homework. Anita went back and forth between feeling sorry for her daughter and wanting to fix things for her, and agreeing with her husband and thinking Caterina's problems could be fixed with tougher discipline. In the meantime, Caterina seemed to be getting more and more depressed and was pulling away from the family. Every time Anita tried pulling back, she felt intensely guilty and ended up trying even harder; this typically created significant conflict with Caterina, who had started saying, "Mom, I'm not a baby!" a lot.

When parents disagree on approaches and work against each other, outcomes tend to be worse. This is not to say that only one parent's approach is ever going to work. Parents can often discern that they have different styles, and that one parent's style works better in some situations while the other's style works better in other situations. When this happens, parents can often determine in advance which approach to use when. Problems occur when parents disagree about what approach to take and work against each other. If parents have recognized their differences and agreed when to disagree, but still support each other, things tend to go better. A large body of research supports the benefit of parental agreement for both symptom reduction and healthy child development. For example, Davies and Cummings (1994) found that level of parental agreement was related to symptoms of childhood depression and anxiety, as well as to aggressive and delinquent behavior.

Although the cycle has commonalities between families, differences in symptoms and family structures can change the cycle.

Emily and Craig had been finding PEP to be interesting and helpful, but when the discussion about negative family cycles started, they both seemed to get a little more involved in the discussion. Their son, Dan, was 12. He had volatile episodes that were often triggered by simple requests, typically from his mother. Emily recognized that life was hard for Dan: There was not much that he enjoyed, and he was often irritable. Dan was also easily overstimulated and went through periods of being very agitated. Emily bent over backward to avoid creating stress for Dan, but she needed to make minor requests of him on a daily basis (e.g., "Come to dinner," "Take a shower," "Turn off the TV"). In response to even small requests, Dan often got extremely upset. When Emily tried to coax him into doing what she needed him to do, or at least into calming down, his behavior escalated. Craig often entered the picture at this point and played the role of the "heavy." Emily then started feeling sorry for Dan, who would cry when his father yelled at him and sometimes needed to be physically restrained. Emily then pleaded with her husband to be easy on Dan, leading to the two of them having a disagreement. Everyone ended up feeling lousy!

In this situation, Emily and Craig would need to get on the same page in changing the pattern. The first step would be for them to recognize the pattern: Emily was playing a protective and coaxing role with Dan, while Craig was trying to fix the situations he walked into. Neither of them was stepping back to apply symptom management or problem solving. Instead of working together, they were ending up working against each other. An important first step in helping them work together could be distinguishing "can't" from "won't" behaviors. Were there uncontrolled symptoms that resulted in Dan's being unable to control himself, or was he just digging in his heels when he wanted his own way? Children like Dan who have become disengaged may need to feel rewarded to join in the problem-solving process. A helpful tool might be the Family Fix-It List: Is there a goal on the list that fits this situation? Should there be? In this case, maybe Emily and Craig could agree to come together when Dan was having a tough time, rather than taking sides against each other. Maybe they could team up, along with Dan, against the mood disorder!

Breaking the Cycle: Finding Positive Strategies

There is no single way to break negative cycles, but there are some general strategies parents can use. First and foremost, parents' awareness of how the cycle occurs within their family is critical. Second, parents need to work actively with the child to better manage his/her symptoms and to uncover the child's best characteristics. Having the child engaged in the process of seeing the mood disorder as "the Enemy" helps stop the negative cycle, too. However, in order to create real change in the family's interactions, parents need to become aware of and then change their own actions, thoughts, and (ultimately) feelings. The parent project for this session is aimed at helping parents to increase their own self-awareness. This is *not* to be confused with *blaming* parents for *causing* their child's symptoms. However, there are approaches they can take that will further fan the flames, or, alternatively, quench them. Instead of "walking on eggshells" or turning their lives inside out, parents are encouraged to make some strategic and specific changes that may help family interactions go more smoothly. As an example, let's return to the case of Emily, Craig, and their son Dan.

> Emily felt very strongly that Dan needed to do his homework before dinner, when she could help him and he was not too tired yet. A battle ensued over homework almost every day. The reality was that Dan was tired and very irritable after school. By the time Craig got home (around 6:30 P.M.), Dan and Emily were both feeling defeated, and very little homework was done.
>
> When Emily stepped back and really looked at her thoughts, feelings, and actions in relation to Dan's homework, she realized a few things. She noted that her feelings of anxiety about getting through Dan's homework started long before he got home each day. In response, she was having negative thoughts about Dan and his homework before he even walked in the door, such as "How are we going to get through his homework? We must start the homework right away." Her anxiety and these negative thoughts resulted in her approaching Dan immediately upon his arrival home and trying to coax him into doing his homework. As Emily began to recognize this pattern, she started working on changing her focus. At the same time, in talking about this situation during a therapy session, Craig pointed out that Dan was 12 and should be part of making a plan to manage his homework. Emily and Craig agreed that they would sit down with Dan during a calm moment and engage him in coming

up with a homework plan. For her part, Emily recognized that she needed to begin managing her own thoughts, feelings, and actions.

When they sat down as a family, Dan had some important points to add. He preferred doing math homework with Craig, and he also found it easier to do homework in the morning. In addition, his middle school had a work period built into each day. He had been staying in his rather large homeroom during that time and was having trouble getting much work done. Emily spoke with Dan's school counselor about how much trouble they were having with homework. The school counselor mentioned that he had work tables in his office, and that he opened his office during the work period for anyone who wanted a quieter/smaller setting to do homework. Armed with this information, Emily, Craig, and Dan made a plan. Dan and his dad would get his math homework done after dinner. If time and energy allowed, he might start some other homework after that, but they would plan for Dan to do the rest of his homework at the breakfast table. Dan also decided that he would start going to his school counselor's office during the work period at school, so that he wouldn't have so much work to do at home. Moreover, they planned to use Sunday afternoons to get ahead on projects and studying. Emily wouldn't mention homework on weekday afternoons, but would instead quietly take Dan's daily planner out of his backpack, review what he needed to do, and read any notes from his teachers.

By thus analyzing the negative cycle, when it occurred, and what seemed to trigger it, Emily and her family were able to break the cycle and significantly reduce family stress. Emily, however, first had to recognize her own anxiety and negative thinking about the homework battle. Getting Dan involved in finding a solution was also an important step. It allowed empathy toward Dan to play an important role in Emily's analysis. She recognized that Dan was really stressed out, and that his negative behavior escalated easily when he first came home from school. Her ability to look at things from his perspective helped her to recognize that she needed to take a different approach. Although Dan was fighting homework in the afternoon, he did need a structured environment and plan for after school. The challenge was to make this structure suitable to his need to relax and unwind. Freeing herself from afternoon homework duty meant that Emily and Dan could take the dog for long walks in the park in the afternoon or go on a bike ride. When Emily was focused on convincing him to do his homework, she was not able to be there to listen to him when he needed to talk. He needed her help to work through the social problems he brought home from school, his sibling conflicts, and his unpredictable mood swings.

It is important for parents to be ready to listen when kids are ready to talk. Really listening to children without imposing an adult agenda on them can help to eliminate triggers and reduce negative family interactions. When children are able to calm down, they will be able to communicate and solve problems more effectively, as will parents. It is important for parents of children with mood disorders to get in the habit of building extra time into the schedule to allow for challenges. It is not always possible to take a breather when the moment is stressful, but if building in "down time" becomes a family habit, it may be easier to push through the times when there is no buffer. This is a great time to review how the already completed child, parent, and family projects can help to change family cycles and can serve as the basis for moving ahead with problems identified on the Fix-It List.

When parents are constantly "walking on eggshells," they tend to be waiting for the "eggshells" to break, rather than appreciating when things are going well. This is an important cycle to break. Children need to hear praise. They need to know that parents are aware of when they are doing something right. It is equally important for parents to let kids know specifically why they are praising them, such as "You were really kind to your sister just now. I really liked seeing that." In addition to providing praise, parents can head off some problems by phrasing their commands in positive ways. Instead of saying, "Don't hit your brother!", parents might say, "Please keep your hands and feet to yourself." This is not only a more positive statement, but it is also more general. We want kids to eliminate physical aggression across all settings!

Take-Home Projects

New Project: Thinking, Feeling, Doing

For this session's take-home project, parents will complete Handout 62 (Thinking, Feeling, Doing) This same project will be introduced to the child during the next session; parents are getting a head start by applying it first to themselves. For simplicity's sake, we use the same blank handout for parents as we do for children. In introducing this project to parents, explain a fundamental principle of CBT: Thoughts, feelings, and actions are intertwined, and that when thoughts and actions are modified, feelings can change. The Thinking, Feeling, Doing handout contains a "Feeling" heart for recording emotions, a "Thinking" cloud for thoughts, and a "Doing" box for actions. The form is intended to help parents identify automatic negative thoughts that lead to, and are results of, unhelpful actions. These automatic negative thoughts and unhelpful actions emanate from and exacerbate difficult emotional states.

Parents start by identifying a trigger situation for a negative pattern and writing it in the oval under the light switch. They then reflect on how they would typically feel in response to that situation, as well as how they would rather feel. For example, they may feel angry and frustrated in a particular situation when they would rather feel calm. Negative feelings are written in the "Feelings" heart on the side with the minus sign. Positive feelings are entered on the side with the plus sign. The next step is to reflect on the actions that are typically carried out in the situation. In negative cycles, these are usually automatic and not very helpful. These are labeled "hurtful" in the child session. These are written in the "Doing" box under the minus sign. Automatic thoughts that typically accompany the unhelpful actions and feelings in the particular situation are written in the "Thinking" cloud. (Handout 61 is an example of how parents complete Handout 62.)

Once the automatic negative thoughts and actions have been recorded, the focus turns to more helpful actions in response to the situation, as well as more helpful ways to think about the situation. Through this process, the parents can develop a plan for how to handle the situation better. After you have reviewed Handouts 61 and 62 with the parents, instruct them to record several examples of Thinking, Feeling, Doing between now and their next session.

Ongoing Take-Home Projects

Parents should continue to monitor how their child is doing on the Mood–Medication Log (Handout 32) or Mood Record (Handout 20 or 21), and to review and update My Child's Treatment Team (Handout 52) and My Child's Educational Team (Handout 53) as necessary. In addition, although the selected healthy habit change and chart (Handout 40, 44, or 47) is the child's project, parents should be available to support their child's efforts, as requested by the child and discussed in the session.

Chapter 13

Thinking, Feeling, Doing with Children

IF-PEP Child Session 5
MF-PEP Child Session 4

Session Outline

Goals:	1. Teach the child the difference between helpful and hurtful thoughts, and the ways that thoughts can affect feelings.
	2. Teach the child how to use thoughts and actions to manage difficult feelings.
Beginning the Session:	Do a check-in and review Mood–Medication Log (Handout 32) or Mood Record (Handout 20 or 21).
	Have child identify and rate feelings (Handouts 1 and 2).
	Review selected healthy habits chart (for IF-PEP only) (Handout 40, 44, or 47).
	Review Taking Charge of Mad, Sad, Bad Feelings (Handout 60).
Lesson of the Day:	Using helpful actions and thoughts to manage hurtful feelings (Handouts 62, 63, and 64)
	• Reviewing triggers, hurtful feelings, and hurtful actions
	• Teaching the child to identify hurtful thoughts
	• Making connections among hurtful thoughts, feelings, and actions

   - Identifying helpful actions
   - Identifying helpful thoughts to manage hurtful feelings

Breathing Exercise: Child's choice (Belly, Bubble, Balloon Breathing)

Session Review with Parents

New Take-Home Project: Thinking, Feeling, Doing (Handouts 62, 63, and 64)

Ongoing Take-Home Projects: Selected healthy habits chart (for IF-PEP only)

New Handouts: 62. Thinking, Feeling, Doing (have multiple blank copies on hand)
                               63. Thinking, Feeling, Doing (Sample 1 for Children)
                               64. Thinking, Feeling, Doing (Sample 2 for Children)

Handouts to Review: 1. Feelings
                               2. Strength of Feelings
                               54. My Triggers for Mad, Sad, Bad Feelings
                               55. My Body Signals for Mad, Sad, Bad Feelings
                               56. My Actions When I Feel Mad, Sad, Bad
                               57. Building the Tool Kit (Sample)
                               58. Building the Tool Kit
                               59. Taking Charge of Mad, Sad, Bad Feelings (Sample)
                               60. Taking Charge of Mad, Sad, Bad Feelings
                               40. Sleep Chart *or*
                               44. Healthy Food Chart *or*
                               47. Exercise Chart (for IF-PEP only)

Session Overview

During the previous session, the child has started building a coping Tool Kit of activities to manage mad, sad, and bad feelings. This session expands to include a focus on hurtful and helpful thoughts and is based on a fundamental premise of CBT: namely, that emotional states can be managed or shifted by how an individual thinks and acts. This session teaches children to recognize their hurtful thought patterns, as well as how those hurtful thoughts increase their mad, sad, and bad feelings. It also helps children see the connections among thoughts, feelings, and actions. To engage in this session productively, children must be able to recognize triggers, and must have a clear understanding of feelings, actions, and thoughts. Younger children may need additional scaffolding of these concepts. (Refer to Chapter 1 for more on scaffolding.) The chapter culminates with a project that ties together thoughts, feelings, and actions, and helps children learn a critical set of skills to manage their moods. Leave enough time at the end of the session so the child can carefully explain (with your help) to the parents how Thinking, Feeling, Doing works.

Beginning the Session

Do a Check-In and Review Mood–Medication Log or Mood Record

By now, this check-in process has probably become routine. The session begins with a quick review of the week and, in IF-PEP, while parents are still in the room, a review of the Mood–Medication Log or Mood Record. When parents leave, check in with the child about his/her feelings (see below). Often by this point in the session, children no longer need a prompt to generate this information. You may determine that it is more beneficial to review projects with or without parents in the room, depending on the parent–child relationship and the child's level of maturity.

Review Selected Healthy Habits Chart

In IF-PEP, do a quick check-in with the child to see how the selected healthy habits plan is working, and review the appropriate healthy habits chart (Handout 40, 44, or 47). Spend some time on troubleshooting, as needed, to facilitate successful accomplishment of the child's goals.

Review Taking Charge of Mad, Sad, Bad Feelings

The Taking Charge of Mad, Sad, Bad Feelings project has two components: making a Tool Kit, and recording three uses of tools in it. Children are encouraged to bring in their actual Tool Kit. If a point system is being used, they should be awarded extra points for doing so. Check on whether the existing tools are sufficient to address the needs of various settings (e.g., at school, at home when others are sleeping, at home during the day, with peers) and for various feelings they often experience (e.g., sad, euphoric, anxious, angry).

For the second part of the project, children are asked to take three triggering events and use tools in the kit to cope with mad, sad, and bad feelings. While discussing the examples children provide, you can help them come up with ways to remember to use the Tool Kit, such as keeping it in a prominent location or having private signals with their parents. In some cases, you will see a need to prompt a child to add more activities to fit different situations, since by this point in PEP you will know each child and his/her challenges quite well. For example, a child may have come up with great tools to use at home, but may need to generate some tools that can be used on the playground.

Eli was 9 and struggled with sadness and self-doubt. Although he loved to play outside at home, he really struggled during recess. Most of the boys in his grade played sports like football, basketball, and soccer during recess. He preferred to play one of his own imaginary games, but it was hard for him to find someone else who wanted to play his game. It was a challenge for Eli to be flexible. When he couldn't find someone to join in his game, he became sad and then tended to wander around the playground, feeling left out. Knowing about this pattern, Eli's therapist suggested that they add some tools to help him deal with recess. When they started using the four Tool Kit categories (CARS) to talk about recess, Eli started to see that imaginary games were both creative and active. He explained to his therapist that there was a group of boys who always played some kind of imaginary game, but they usually didn't want to play *his* game. His therapist asked Eli whether it would feel worse to be flexible and play their game, or to walk around by himself. Eli thought about it and decided that being flexible would probably lead to his feeling better. As Eli and his therapist continued to review CARS options, Eli mentioned that he liked to play Four Square, which would count as an "active" tool. Eli described a group of kids who always played Four Square after lunch. Eli decided to add "Play Four Square" and "Join in whatever imaginary game is being played" to his Tool Kit.

Eli's therapist knew that recess was a trigger for him, so she was able to help him see that he had more tools available to him at recess than he had initially realized.

Sometimes a child has trouble applying the tools in his/her Tool Kit. In these situations, it is important for the therapist to help the child recognize ways the Tool Kit could make life better. It is important for the child to see that he/she has something to gain from using the tools.

Ally was 10 and had been having nightly tantrums while trying to complete her homework (see Chapter 10). She brought in a record of having used her Tool Kit when she was really frustrated about her math homework. Ally told her therapist about how she had been working for 30 minutes trying to figure out what she was supposed to do to solve some word problems. She started feeling frustrated and flung her math book and papers off the dining room table where she was working. She said that she had yelled really loud, which actually made her feel a little better at first—but it had probably bothered her brother, who was also working on his homework, because her mom scolded her later that day for yelling. Ally proceeded to tell her therapist that the Tool Kit didn't work.

THERAPIST: Wow, sounds like a rough afternoon. Which tools did you try?

ALLY: Oh. I don't really know.

THERAPIST: You described some hurtful actions when you were frustrated, but not any of the tools in your Tool Kit. Before we decide that your Tool Kit doesn't work, let's start from the beginning and see if we can figure out how it might work in that situation, Okay?

ALLY: Okay.

THERAPIST: Did you notice any signals?

ALLY: No, not really.

ERIC [Ally's father]: I noticed that her fists were clenched and that her face was red.

THERAPIST: Let's look at your Tool Kit. You were clearly pretty frustrated. What's a really quick tool to calm yourself down when you are frustrated? I'll give you a hint—it's one that we practice each week.

ALLY: Deep breaths. I could do some deep breathing.

THERAPIST: Great—you could do some Bubble, Balloon, or Belly Breathing. Now your dad was around while this was going on, right? Any tools in the social category that might help?

ALLY: I guess hugs help me a lot.

THERAPIST: Now you're getting it. You could ask your dad for a hug. Now let's do some more thinking. Your math has gotten you really frustrated. What else do you think you need to be ready to tackle the math?

ALLY: Maybe I could go outside for a little bit?

ERIC: You could take Dakota [the family dog] out and play with her for a little while—she's always game to play with her ball.

THERAPIST: After using those tools from your Tool Kit, do you think you might be better able to get through your math?

ALLY: Probably, especially if I asked my dad to help me with the hard ones.

Ally's case is a good example of using troubleshooting to get a child actually using the Tool Kit. Her trigger was the difficult math problems, which led to feelings of frustration. On her own, she had trouble applying her Tool Kit, but reviewing the situation with her therapist and father helped her recognize her signals and begin to see how some of her tools might really help. Her father was able to be helpful and supportive in helping her identify tools she could use to get through this challenging situation.

Have Child Identify and Rate Feelings

As in previous sessions, ask the child to identify his/her current feelings, to determine why he/she feels that way, and to rate the strongest feelings.

Lesson of the Day: Using Helpful Actions and Thoughts to Manage Hurtful Feelings

Reviewing Triggers, Hurtful Feelings, and Hurtful Actions

Much of what children need for this session has been taught and reinforced during previous sessions. Identification of feelings has been taught during the initial child session (Chapter 5) and has been reinforced during each child session since then. The role of helpful and hurtful actions in managing mad, sad, and bad feelings has been taught during the previous child session (Chapter 11). In that session, the focus has been on helping children to identify triggers for their mad, sad, and bad feelings, and then develop a Tool Kit of helpful actions. Thus, during prior sessions, children have practiced identifying feelings, recognizing triggers, and developing a list of actions that can be helpful in managing emotions. In this session, these components are tied together. Use the blank Thinking, Feeling, Doing worksheet (Handout 62) to go over the key components of a trigger, followed by hurtful feelings, followed by hurtful actions. The concepts of hurtful thoughts and their consequences are introduced in this context later in the chapter.

Identifying the Trigger

The first step is to ask the child to remember a situation when he/she felt mad, sad, or bad. Can the child identify what triggered the feelings? The trigger is recorded on Handout 62 in the oval below the light switch. Either you or the child can write down the child's responses. (Handouts 63 and 64 are examples of Handout 62 as completed by children).

> Ten-year old Carly (see Chapter 12) identified getting ready to go to the museum one day as an example of a trigger. She wrote down the trigger as "Feeling rushed to get ready to go to the museum with my family."

As described earlier in this chapter, 9-year-old Eli tended to struggle with sadness, get down on himself, and get easily frustrated. Through earlier sessions with him and through time with his parents, it became clear that Eli's thoughts were often hurtful. Some of the things he said out loud gave clues to how he was thinking. His parents reported that at home, Eli said says things like, "I'm such an idiot," "Nobody likes me," and "I'm not good at anything." One of Eli's most frustrating parts of the day was homework time. He made a lot of comments that reflected hurtful thoughts during that time. His therapist decided to use what she knew about Eli during homework time to help him understand helpful versus hurtful thoughts. He needed more scaffolding than an older child would.

> THERAPIST: Eli, I want to show you something. Let's look at this worksheet together [Handout 62, Thinking, Feeling, Doing]. Do you want me to do the writing, or do you want to do it?
>
> ELI: You do it!

Some children, especially older girls, like to fill in the handout themselves; other children, like Eli, find writing effortful and prefer to have the therapist do the writing.

> THERAPIST: See down here? This is a place where we can put one of your triggers that we talked about last time. How about homework time?
>
> ELI: Yeah, I hate doing homework.
>
> THERAPIST: (*Records "Homework time" in the oval below the light switch on Handout 62.*)

Identifying the Hurtful Feelings

After the trigger is recorded, the child's initial hurtful feelings are recorded in the bottom of the heart (on Handout 62). Minus signs are used to indicate where "hurtful" thoughts, feelings, and actions are to be recorded on the handout.

> In response to the trigger of getting ready for the museum, Carly was readily able to identify her hurtful feelings and write these down as "overwhelmed," "stressed," and "angry."
>
> Eli needed more help identifying relevant feelings.
>
> THERAPIST: What hurtful feelings do you have while you are doing homework?
>
> ELI: I get mad.
>
> THERAPIST: (*Writes "mad" in the bottom of the heart on Handout 62.*) So let's look at this sheet. I'm putting "mad" in the bottom part of this heart, because that shows the way you are feeling when you are doing homework. From what you told me before, it sounds like you get really frustrated, and like you also start feeling really bad about yourself. I'm also writing "frustrated" and "bad" in the bottom part of the heart. It must be really hard to do your homework when you are feeling frustrated and mad! How would you rather feel?
>
> ELI: Just normal.
>
> THERAPIST: So by "normal," you don't mean super-happy or wonderful, just calm. Is that right?
>
> ELI: Yeah.
>
> THERAPIST: How about if I write "calm" in the top part of the heart, because that would be a better way to feel?
>
> ELI: Okay.

Identifying the Hurtful Actions

The next step is for the child to identify the hurtful actions that followed from the trigger and the hurtful feeling. Working with the Tool Kit during the previous session and at home helps children to start thinking about their actions and the choices they can make about their actions.

> Carly talked about how she was trying to find a different pair of jeans and the right socks when she yelled at her sisters, who had come into her room and hopped on her bed. Usually she played with her sisters by piling clothes on top of them and pretending to look for them, but that morning, she just yelled at them to get out of the way and get out of her room.
>
> Eli's therapist asked him, "What hurtful things do you do when you are feeling frustrated?"

ELI: Sometimes I rip my paper or break my pencil.

THERAPIST: See this box at the bottom of the page [on Handout 62]? This box is for the things you do. I'm going to write "Rip my paper" and "Break my pencil" in the bottom part of the box where the minus sign is. I bet things get worse when you do those things.

ELI: Yeah, then I get upset that I won't be able to turn my homework in because it is ripped.

THERAPIST: So those are the hurtful things you do. We call those things hurtful because they make things worse.

Teaching the Child to Identify Hurtful Thoughts

As you progress through Handout 62, the next step is for the child to identify his/her hurtful thoughts. For some children, this will come easily; for others, it can be very challenging. Two questions that often help a child articulate these thoughts are "What were you telling yourself?" or "What were you saying to yourself in your head?" Recording thoughts in quotation marks can highlight that these are things children are saying in their heads.

Carly said that she was thinking, "I can't find anything to wear!", "I'm going to look stupid," "Why can't my sisters just leave me alone!", and "I hate my sisters."

When asked for thoughts, young children will often restate their feelings (e.g., "I think I'm really mad!") or action (e.g., "I think I'm gonna hit him!"). They may need additional queries to articulate their thinking. Previous sessions often provide clues regarding a child's negative thinking. For example, a child may have said, "Nobody likes me. I'm a loser," when generating the Fix-It List. It is important to question or make suggestions, but not to put words into the child's mouth during this exercise. Children's metacognitive skills are likely to dictate how much time is spent on this portion.

Again, Eli needed more support from the therapist. The following dialogue illustrates how he and his therapist worked through identifying thoughts and the consequences of negative thoughts.

THERAPIST: So now we have your hurtful feelings in the bottom of the heart, and the hurtful things you do in the bottom of the box. What do you think this cloud at the top of the page is for?

ELI: Maybe what I say?

THERAPIST: Sort of. It's for the things you say to yourself, which are your thoughts. Your mom said that you sometimes call yourself names while you are trying to do your homework.

ELI: I feel like an idiot when I can't figure things out, so I sometimes call myself an idiot.

THERAPIST: So I am going to write "I'm an idiot" in the bottom part of this cloud. How do you feel when you call yourself an idiot?

ELI: Bad.

THERAPIST: Do you say anything else to yourself or think anything else when you're trying to do homework?

ELI: Maybe that I can't do anything right or that I'm stupid.

THERAPIST: So when you think those things, does homework go better or worse?

ELI: Worse!

THERAPIST: Okay, so "I can't do anything right" and "I'm stupid" go in the bottom part of the cloud. This part has a minus sign, telling us that those are your hurtful thoughts. So now we know how you feel when you are doing homework. We know what some of your hurtful actions are, and we know what some of your hurtful thoughts are.

Once negative thoughts are identified, they should be recorded in the bottom of the thought cloud.

Making Connections among Hurtful Feelings, Actions, and Thoughts

After the hurtful sections of the "Feeling" heart, "Thinking" cloud, and "Doing" box are completed, children benefit from a review of the entire cycle—moving from the triggering event to feelings, actions, and thoughts, and focusing on the two-way arrows between the shapes. Children usually see how thinking and acting in hurtful ways can worsen their hurtful feelings.

For example, yelling at her sisters made Carly feel angry at herself and more stressed—not only because she hurt their feelings, but because it could also get her in trouble.

In the previous session, children have been given three questions to help them identify hurtful actions: (1) "Does it hurt me?" (2) "Does it hurt someone or something else?" and (3) "Does it get anyone in trouble?" They can use these same questions to consider the connections among hurtful feelings, actions, and thoughts.

Usually, with help, children can see the connections. Hurtful actions intensify hurtful feelings. Hurtful thoughts also intensify hurtful feelings, as well as encourage hurtful actions (and vice versa).

Carly's thought that she would look stupid made her feel more stressed, and her thought that she hated her sisters made her feel even more angry.

As the child grasps the connections, you can return to feelings with the query "How would you rather feel? Calm? Relaxed? Content?" Often children with mood disorders hope for "calm."

When asked how she would have preferred to feel, Carly thought for a moment and then said, "It would have been better to feel excited about going to the museum. Or it would have been okay to feel calm."

These more pleasant or neutral emotions should be recorded in the top of the heart on Handout 62. Distinguishing among thoughts, actions, and feelings can be difficult for children, but when they are able to do so, and to see the connections among all three, they are ready to learn how altering actions and thoughts can influence feelings.

Identifying Helpful Actions

Up to this point, children have talked about the cycle of Thinking, Feeling, and Doing as if the three elements were bound together and could not be changed. The focus now shifts to the idea that a child can make choices about thoughts and actions. Those choices can change the impact of the child's feelings and the outcomes of situations. The PEP motto—"It's not your fault, but it's your challenge!"—can help children understand.

> "We can't keep all triggers from happening; nor can we automatically change our feelings. Those things aren't our fault. But we can change our thoughts and actions in response to triggers and feelings—that's the challenge. For example, sometimes we're not sure what to wear, and we can't always get good grades on projects. Those things aren't always our fault. The challenge is to respond by acting and thinking in more helpful ways."

The next step is to identify helpful actions. In general, actions are easier for children to recognize than thoughts. This builds directly on the Tool Kit exercise from the previous session. You might probe with "What might be more helpful actions in that situation?"

> Carly thought for a moment. "I could have put some music on, and if I picked something with a fast beat, I might have even been able to get ready faster. I also could have asked my sisters to help me find some socks."

> Eli's therapist asked, "What are some helpful things you could do from your Tool Kit that you made last time that might help you calm down when you are frustrated?" The therapist then pulled out Eli's Building the Tool Kit worksheet (Handout 58) from his folder, and they looked at it for ideas.

> ELI: I could take a break and pet my cat. I could ask my mom for help, and I could take some deep breaths.
>
> THERAPIST: Great. I'll write those down.

The new, more helpful actions get listed in the top part of the "Doing" box.

Identifying Helpful Thoughts to Manage Hurtful Feelings

The final step of generating alternative thoughts will vary, depending on the child's age and verbal reasoning abilities. Some children will be able to grasp the idea of helpful thoughts quickly, whereas others will need more coaching. The question "What kinds of things could you tell yourself that would help you?" can make it easier, especially for younger children, to generate helpful thoughts.

> Carly was able to generate the following helpful thoughts: "My sisters are just try-ing to play like we usually do," "None of my friends are going to see me there, any-way," "Maybe my sisters can help," and "I don't need to look perfect to go to the museum."

Next, the child considers the impact of these helpful thoughts and actions on his/her feelings. Often children will note that the intensity of the hurtful feeling will decrease, so helpful feelings can emerge.

> When her therapist asked Carly whether she would have felt less overwhelmed and angry if she had done those things or had those thoughts, Carly said that she would have a felt a little more calm, and then maybe she would have been able to enjoy being with her family.

> Once again, Eli needed more support from his therapist to generate helpful thoughts, as well as to understand the positive impact they could have.

>> THERAPIST: Now let's talk about your thoughts. We know what your hurtful thoughts are, but we need to figure out some helpful thoughts. Can you think of more helpful things to tell yourself when you are working on your homework, maybe to encourage yourself?
>>
>> ELI: I could tell myself, "Just do your best," or "Ask for help if you need it."
>>
>> THERAPIST: Yes, those are helpful thoughts. When you say things to yourself that help you feel better or encourage you, those are thoughts that help. So your helpful thoughts could be things like "I just need to do my best," and "If I get my mom to explain it to me, I bet I can do this without any problems," and "I have always figured my homework out before, so I bet I can figure this out too!" So, Eli, what happens to your feelings when you have hurtful thoughts like "I can't do anything right" and "I'm such an idiot"? (*Points to arrows between sections of Handout 62 to emphasize connections.*)
>>
>> ELI: Huh?
>>
>> THERAPIST: Do you feel better or worse when your thoughts are hurtful?
>>
>> ELI: Oh, worse.
>>
>> THERAPIST: And what about when your actions are hurtful, like ripping your paper? Do you feel better or worse?
>>
>> ELI: Definitely worse.
>>
>> THERAPIST: You are really getting it! When your thoughts are hurtful, like "I'm such an idiot," do you think your actions are more likely to be helpful or hurtful?

ELI: Hurtful!

THERAPIST: Exactly. Hurtful thoughts make you feel worse and lead to more hurtful actions, and hurtful actions make you feel worse and encourage hurtful thoughts. So what about your helpful actions? What do you think they would do to your feelings? (*Points to the top part of the "Doing" box on Handout 62.*)

ELI: If I take a break and pet my cat, I'll probably feel a little better.

THERAPIST: Good point. And what might happen with your thoughts if you took a break?

ELI: Maybe I could start thinking some more helpful thoughts.

THERAPIST: Exactly! Helpful actions help you feel better and encourage more helpful thoughts, and helpful thoughts make you feel better and lead to more helpful actions.

Children usually need to work through several examples of the Thinking, Feeling, Doing exercise to understand the connection between thoughts, feelings, and actions. Again, two examples are provided in Handouts 63 and 64. You can also use events noted as triggers in last session's Tool Kit project to start another example; these situations are usually fresh in the child's mind, and since they have come up previously, you might be able to provide some helpful prompts to get the example flowing. The goal is to help the child understand that he/she can make choices to think and act in helpful ways to improve the outcome. Actively choosing helpful thoughts and actions is part of the challenge of managing a mood disorder.

One problem that many children have is identifying the potential effects of their feelings; it can help children to label their feelings as "helpful" or "hurtful." In some cases, the child may focus on anger as the primary hurtful emotion, because angry responses have often led to getting in trouble. In such a case, it is important for the child to recognize that sadness or worry often precedes feelings of anger. Recognizing and managing sad feelings are also important, as Mario needed to learn.

Mario reported that when he got his math test back, it had a lot of problems marked wrong. He had gotten really sad, and although he didn't actually cry, he felt like crying. Mario thought that feeling sad was a helpful feeling in response to not doing well on his math test. If he had felt angry, he probably would have ripped up his paper. His therapist praised Mario for identifying anger as a hurtful feeling that could cause problems for him. He asked Mario what had happened after he got his math test back, since he felt so sad. Mario said that he just sat in his chair staring at the wall and thinking about his math test. The therapist asked whether it was hard for him to do his work when he was feeling so sad. Mario said that he didn't finish his social studies assignment that afternoon and then had to take it home for homework. Mario's therapist pointed out that feeling down on himself and having a hard time concentrating on his other work had hurt him, and that the sad feeling, although different from anger, could be hurtful too. His therapist continued by asking how he would rather feel at school, to which Mario answered, "Proud."

Breathing Exercise

Once again, review the three breathing exercises—Belly, Bubble, and Balloon Breathing. Ask the child to choose one, and then practice it together.

Session Review with Parents

The end-of-session review with parents is particularly important in this session and often takes more time to complete than in other sessions. Ideally, the child will lead the parent(s) through Handout 62, and thus teach and reinforce the skill just learned during the session. The Thinking, Feeling, Doing handout and exercise have been presented to parents during their previous session (or in this session, for parents in MF-PEP), and so they are in a position to support and encourage the child's efforts. Any questions that parents have about Thinking, Feeling, Doing should be answered during this session review. Make sure that both child and parent understand the different parts of Handout 62. Also make sure both realize that the skills used in completing this handout are new and will need practice before they will become a solution the family members can use readily. If the child and/or parents seem to struggle with the concepts and skills of this exercise, it may make sense to use an in-the-bank session to review and reinforce the skills and concepts.

The core concepts taught and reinforced during this session are critical components of PEP. Children with mood disorders experience frequent unpleasant mood states that can be easily escalated by hurtful thinking and hurtful actions. Children can significantly diminish the impact of these moods when they learn how to work through difficult situations without escalating them.

Take-Home Projects

New Project: Thinking, Feeling, Doing

For this session's project, children are asked to use Handout 62 (Thinking, Feeling, Doing) to manage one or more difficult situations during the interval between sessions. Children identify a triggering event; the hurtful thoughts, feelings, and actions they had; and then the helpful thoughts, feelings, and actions they did take or could have taken in the situation.

Ongoing Project: Selected Healthy Habits Chart

For children in IF-PEP, encourage them to continue charting their selected healthy habit on Handout 40, 44, or 47.

Chapter 14

Problem-Solving and Basic Coping Skills for Parents

IF-PEP Parent Session 5
MF-PEP Parent Session 5

Session Outline

Goals:	1. Develop parents' problem-solving skills.
	2. Enhance parents' coping skills.
Beginning the Session:	Do a check-in and review Mood–Medication Log (Handout 32) or Mood Record (Handout 20 or 21).
	Review Thinking, Feeling, Doing (Handout 62).
Lesson of the Day:	Problem-solving and coping skills Handout 65)

- Problem-solving steps
  - What is the problem?
  - Who needs to know about it?
  - What are the possible solutions?
  - What are the pros and cons?
  - Pick one solution and try it
  - Evaluate how it worked
  - Do it again or try another solution
  - Wrapping up problem solving

- Coping skills
  - Hold the child's feelings; avoid rapid reassurance.
  - Listen for the underlying message; don't take negative comments literally.
  - Take breaks; don't try to be constantly available and positive.
  - Move beyond guilt.
  - Create balance; recognize imbalance
  - Break big decisions into smaller ones during acute episodes.
  - Adjust expectations to the child's symptoms.
  - Practice self care and self-preservation.

New Take-Home Project: Problem Solving: Symptoms and Family Conflicts (Handout 65)

Ongoing Take-Home Projects: My Child's Treatment Team (Handout 52)
My Child's Educational Team (Handout 53)
Mood–Medication Log (Handout 32) or Mood Record (Handout 20 or 21)

New Handouts: 65. Problem Solving: Symptoms and Family Conflicts

Handouts to Review: 62. Thinking, Feeling, Doing

Session Overview

During the previous session, parents have learned what negative family cycles are and how to recognize them. This session focuses on specific problem-solving and coping skills that parents can use to change negative family cycles, reduce family conflict, and improve symptom management. Healthy coping depends on the ability to recognize problems and address them as they arise. This session also covers some important dos and don'ts of responding to children, such as holding the child's bad feelings rather than trying to reassure him/her too quickly, and listening for the underlying message of inflammatory comments. Parents should leave this session with a firm understanding of how to incorporate problem solving into their day-to-day lives for symptom management, improved quality of family life, and personal stress management.

In teaching problem solving, use examples that parents bring to sessions. From this point forward, role playing is increasingly used.

Beginning the Session

Do a Check-In and Review Mood–Medication Log or Mood Record

By now, the session check-in and review of whichever mood chart the parents are keeping should have become a well-practiced routine.

Review Thinking, Feeling, Doing

Begin the session by reviewing the Thinking, Feeling, Doing project from the previous parent session. Parents often gain significant insight about their automatic negative responses to their child through completing this exercise. As discussed in the case of Emily and Dan in Chapter 12, for example, a mother may realize that she begins getting stressed out about getting through homework before the child even gets home.

In some cases, parents will come to this session having recognized the hurtful patterns in which they are stuck, but will still be at a loss for how to change these maladaptive patterns. Reviewing their project provides an opportunity for additional coaching. You can help parents work through the second half of the exercise on developing helpful responses. So, to replace hurtful thoughts about homework, a parent might be encouraged to think in a more helpful and strategic way; "I like to unwind after a long day, Alyssa does too," or "I'm glad we're finally tackling these problems Jack has been having." These more helpful thoughts can lead to more helpful actions, such as letting Alyssa have some "down time" first to relax, or having an upbeat conversation with Jack instead of immediately quizzing him about his homework load for the evening. These issues lead right into the Lesson of the Day, which focuses on problem solving.

Lesson of the Day: Problem-Solving and Coping Skills

Problem-Solving Skills

Problem solving is a particularly important set of skills for families facing the challenges of a child with a mood disorder. Encourage parents to think of symptoms, as well as family conflicts, as problems to be solved. The key steps of problem solving are recognizing the problem, identifying possible solutions, choosing a plan of action, executing it, and evaluating the outcome (see Box 14.1 for the complete list). Working through problem solving within a family may require significant flexibility, since finding an adequate solution to a problem may involve multiple perspectives. In some cases, the problem is one that only adults can solve (e.g., how to schedule transportation so that all children in the family can make it to their individual activities on a given day). In other cases, involving the child and siblings in the solution will make success much more likely. Families encounter many different kinds of problems—some related to very concrete or logistical situations (e.g., how to get everyone where they need to go), and some more relational

---

BOX 14.1. Problem-Solving Steps

- Step 1: What is the problem?
- Step 2: Who needs to know about it? (Parents, child, siblings, treatment/school team members?)
- Step 3: What are the possible solutions?
- Step 4: What are the pros and cons? (considering everyone's needs)
- Step 5: Together, pick one solution and try it.
- Step 6: Together, evaluate how it worked.
- Step 7: Do it again if it worked, *or* try something else next time if it didn't work.

---

and emotional (e.g., how to manage after-school stress related to homework). When the situation involves the child, it is particularly important to include the child in the process. Similarly, siblings are often both part of the problem and part of the solution, so they need to be included as well. See Box 14.2 for tips on how to involve children successfully in problem solving. Discuss this issue with parents, and point out that problem solving will be the topic of the next child session (or, for MF-PEP, this session).

What Is the Problem

Problem solving starts with defining the problem. This means not only establishing *what* the problem is, but also defining *who* is involved in the situation and needs to know about

---

BOX 14.2. Including Children in Problem Solving: Dos and Don'ts

---

DO:

1. Approach the child (and any siblings) at a calm time.
2. Ask each child for his/her perspective.
3. Empathize with the child.
4. Ask whether the child would like suggestions before offering your ideas.

DON'T:

1. Assign blame.
2. Insist on coming up with a solution during highly emotional times.
3. Jump to choosing one of your ideas before hearing your child's ideas.

---

the problem. Ask parents for examples of problems they face, and use those for the discussion. Using frequently occurring or particularly distressing problems will make the discussion especially helpful for families.

> Jane and Peter, parents of 8-year-old Mark, received his diagnosis of BD about 1 year ago. Their biggest problem was that Mark had meltdowns at bedtime almost every night. The therapist asked Jane to describe their typical evening. She reported that after dinner (which they usually finished by 6:30), she focused on getting the kitchen cleaned up, while Peter often went to the computer to finish up emails for work. They typically sent Mark and his 10-year-old sister, Becky, off to play and sometimes to watch TV. Jane described how she and Peter often got caught up in doing other things around the house and only turned their attention back to Mark about 7:30 P.M., when it was time for him to get ready for bed. By this time, Mark was often totally revved up and very difficult to manage. Trying to get Mark ready for bed was a long process that typically resulted in his getting to bed later than he should and having a meltdown. As Jane and Peter described how their evenings typically went, they looked at each other. Until talking through an evening during PEP, they hadn't really noticed how established the pattern had become and how uncomfortable it was.

At first blush, the problem seemed simply defined as Mark's having meltdowns at bedtime. A closer look revealed that Mark spent the hour or so beforehand getting wound up instead of beginning to settle down. Moreover, during the critical period for Mark (6:30 to 7:30), his parents were busy with household or work activities. If the problem had been defined as "Mark has meltdowns at bedtime," then it would seem that the solution should involve Mark's doing something differently. However, as the therapist and parents delved further into problem definition, they learned that Mark's being without close parental attention during the last hour or so before bedtime resulted in his getting wound up and having a very difficult time settling down for bedtime. Jane and Peter might respond to this discussion by deciding to leave emailing and kitchen cleaning until after the children go to bed. If that worked, and having a parent with him helped Mark to get to bed in a calm and timely manner, the problem would be solved.

Who Needs to Know about It?

What if Jane and Peter tried spending one-on-one time with Mark before bedtime, and he still got wound up and had a very difficult time getting to sleep? Now we have begun to define a symptom—sleep disturbance. Difficulty settling down to sleep is a common problem for children with BD. Now an important step in problem solving needs to be activated: Relevant members of the team need to be made aware of the problem. If a child is getting revved up at bedtime every night, as Mark was, it is a really good idea to make sure that the child's prescribing doctor is aware of the problem. A shift in medication timing might be part of the solution. The treatment team might be able to add potential solutions or help with the definition of the problem.

What Are the Possible Solutions?

Once the problem is defined, the next step is to consider possible solutions. Creativity and flexibility are very helpful in this process. It is tempting to evaluate and dismiss potential solutions before listing them or fully considering them. We strongly encourage recording all possible solutions and saving evaluation for later in the process. As Jane, Peter, and the therapist contemplated the family's evening "ritual," a number of strategies seemed to have potential. It seemed that sending Mark off to play without an adult with him at that time of the day was just leading to problems. One solution was for Jane and Peter to take turns doing activities with Mark after dinner while the other cleaned up the kitchen. Another possibility was to leave the kitchen for after the kids were in bed and to focus on both the kids between dinner and bedtime. Another possibility was to vary the routine: Sometimes they could have family time after dinner, and then Jane and Peter could clean up the kitchen together after the kids were in bed. It was also possible that shifting the timing of Mark's medications could reduce the intensity of the evening problems.

What Are the Pros and Cons?

When problems are evaluated, differences in priorities can become apparent. For instance, when Mark's parents evaluated the solutions, Jane felt strongly about cleaning up the kitchen before the kids went to bed. This strategy allowed time for her and Peter to relax and talk together later in the evening. For this reason, Jane was less comfortable with leaving the kitchen until later and wanted to see whether other solutions could help before trying it. Mark seemed to need one-on-one support from a parent, so that he could slowly wind down. Becky, his sister, didn't need one-on-one support but might need some guidance from the person working in the kitchen, who could stop and help her when needed. Adjusting the timing of Mark's medication also seemed like a good possibility to consider. They could talk to Mark's psychiatrist. Possibly dividing one dose of Mark's medication (which would not change his total dose for the day) could lead to better evenings.

Pick One Solution and Try It

Jane and Peter decided that one parent would stick with Mark between dinner and bedtime, while the other parent would clean the kitchen and have Becky hang out nearby, to address any concerns that might arise with her. At the same time, they would explore with Mark's psychiatrist possibilities related to his medication.

Evaluate How It Worked

At the child session a week later, Jane and Peter reported that things were going much better during the evening for everyone. Mark was really enjoying the time he was spending with his parents; Becky was appreciating the much quieter evening atmosphere; and Jane and Peter were feeling significantly less stressed. With Mark's psychiatrist, they had decided to divide the dose of one of his medications, which seemed to contribute further to calmer evenings.

Do It Again or Try Another Solution

In the case of Jane and Peter's family, the first solution they tried worked well, and they continued with it. However, problem solving often does not go so smoothly. In many cases, the first attempt is met with partial success at best. When this happens, it is important that you help coach families through the "try another solution" step of problem solving. Encourage them to go back to another one of the potential solutions they had identified and keep trying solutions methodically until they find one that works for their situation.

Wrapping up Problem Solving

Encourage parents to adopt the perspective that the many challenges of raising a child with a mood disorder all represent problems to be solved. Parents often find that defining the problem is the most challenging step; it is often not as straightforward as it first appears. In your session, encourage parents to look at problems from different perspectives and to really *talk* through possible solutions, so that new, more effective means of coping can be developed.

Coping Skills

Parents of children with mood disorders also need a significant number of coping skills, to help them navigate the complicated situations they will encounter. First, we focus on how parents can prevent some problems by replacing common interaction patterns with better alternatives.

Hold the Child's Feelings; Avoid Rapid Reassurance

It is easy for parents to fall into the trap of providing reassurance too rapidly. Telling a child who feels miserable that everything will be okay automatically invalidates what the child has said. It is important for parents to acknowledge the bad feelings and be able to "hold" those feelings for and with their child, rather than immediately try to make them go away. If parents can learn to accept a child's painful feelings, they gain the opportunity to hear more of their child's thinking. This is a key step in helping their child begin to feel better.

We help parents understanding this point by using visual imagery and role play. We encourage parents to imagine themselves as a "feelings container"; this might be a plastic bowl with a tightly sealing lid, a big garbage can to hold the "slop" of emotions from their child, a handmade pottery bowl, or a coffee can. Ask parents to shut their eyes in the session and picture their "container." Then we advise parents to take a moment during an interaction with a child to shut their eyes and picture their "container" instead of offering a too-rapid reassurance. This gives parents a little interruption in the interchange, which can help them remain calm when their child is not. The two scenarios can also be role-played with parents, as in the following sample dialogues:

REASSURING TOO QUICKLY

CHILD: I hate my life. Nothing ever works out!

PARENT: Oh, it's not that bad. Everything will work out fine.

CHILD: I wish I was dead! (*Storms away, and parent–child interaction ends on a negative note.*)

HOLDING THE FEELINGS

CHILD: I hate my life. Nothing ever works out!

PARENT: (*Momentarily shuts eyes, takes a deep belly breath, imagines her "container."*) Sounds like it was a rough day.

CHILD: Yeah, my teacher blames me for everything!

PARENT: She does?

CHILD: Yeah, like today. She yelled at me when I wasn't even doing anything!

PARENT: Really? What happened?

CHILD: Bobby was throwing pieces of eraser at Mark. I told Bobby to stop, and then Mark yelled at me because he thought I was throwing things at him. Mrs. Smith didn't even give me a chance to tell her what happened. She just sent me out in the hall. It's not fair.

PARENT: No, that doesn't sound fair. Wow, it's hard when something unfair happens to remember that everything isn't bad, isn't it? Do you want to do anything about this situation?

CHILD: Maybe … yeah. Can we send Mrs. Smith an email?

PARENT: Sure. Right now?

CHILD: No. Will you shoot baskets with me first?

PARENT: Sure, that sounds like fun!

Listen for the Underlying Message; Don't Take Negative Comments Literally

In the heat of the moment, children often make inflammatory comments such as "I hate you," "You wish I was never born," or "I wish I was never born." If parents take these comments literally, the first instinct is to argue the point, become very hurt or angry, or fall back into the reassurance trap. Instead, parents should listen to these sorts of comments for their underlying message. "I hate you" probably means something like "I am incredibly angry at you and frustrated, because you aren't doing what I want or need you to do." The underlying message of "You wish I was never born" or "I wish I was never born" may be "I'm really annoyed because I keep making mistakes, and I'm afraid that you will give up on me," or "I feel inadequate." Parents should be encouraged to hear these comments and listen for the underlying message. This is an important part of being able to accept and "hold" a child's feelings.

Take Breaks; Don't Try to Be Constantly Available and Positive

Parenting is a 24-hour, 7-day-a-week job. Children with mood disorders need even more than nondisordered children do from their parents. The burden can be tremendous. Help parents to recognize that they cannot do everything and that they will not be able to be constantly positive. A parent who tries to be constantly available will eventually burn out. This burnout may occur at a critical moment, so the best strategy is for parents to recognize up front the impossibility of being able to do everything all the time. Once parents recognize that they need breaks, they can start to work toward a plan. This may mean "tag-teaming" with a spouse or seeking respite care from friends, family, or agencies. This PEP session may be the first time that the idea of a respite plan has been raised. Parents are often relieved to hear this is a healthy option rather than a "cop-out." Talking about the importance of respite gives parents genuine permission to seek breaks.

Move beyond Guilt

We often feel that parents see the word "guilt" in flashing neon lights. Moving past guilt is one of the toughest tasks for parents. In particular, parents can start to feel guilty about not being able to meet their child's every need or for being the "genetic link" that caused their child's disorder. In the former case, it can be helpful to discuss with parents that they will ultimately be of more benefit to their children if they approach caretaking as a marathon, not a sprint, and pace themselves. In the latter case, it is useful to point out that parents don't choose the genes they get or the genes they pass on to their children. These are nearly always relevant topics for discussion. Some parents will admit for the first time in this session that they sometimes do not like their children; being able to articulate this in a safe, confidential setting can relieve considerable pressure. When this occurs, parents can begin to differentiate the symptoms they dislike from the children themselves. Refer back to the Naming the Enemy exercise to facilitate this discussion. Other parents simply find themselves feeling guilty about everything. Being able to discuss this with someone who really understands can help parents begin to let go of some of those guilty feelings.

Guilt is also forced on parents by society, by family members, and even sometimes by mental health professionals. Many parents of children with mood disorders have been told in one way or another by treatment providers that their parenting is partially or even completely to blame for their child's problems. No one would wish a mood disorder on anyone, least of all their own child.

Nicky is 8, and his parents, Evelyn and Mike, each have an older child from a previous relationship. Nicky's half-brother and half-sister are 16 and 17, respectively. Between their older children and their relatives, Evelyn and Mike get more parenting suggestions than they know what to do with. Nicky has always been challenging, but over the past 2 years his mood symptoms and his challenging behaviors have escalated. Nicky was recently diagnosed with depression, and Mike and Evelyn are in the process of finding a medication regimen that will provide significant symptom relief. In the meantime, Nicky's older siblings frequently point out how different the expectations were for them at the same age, and Nicky's grandparents, in an attempt to be helpful, offer "guidance" as well. Mike and Evelyn dread taking Nicky out to restaurants or stores, because his behavior is unpredictable and volatile. When he melts down, they get looks from people that range from pity to disgust and are mortifying for them. Mike and Evelyn are trying to find ways to help Nicky feel better and be more successful, but they also second-guess their approaches to Nicky and feel guilty that they aren't better able to help him. Sometimes they give in and try to take a hard line with him, as their relatives have advised. This typically catapults Nicky into a meltdown and leads to more guilt. In response, they drop expectations and ignore behaviors that they would not normally let go. Evelyn and Mike are becoming immobilized by guilt and blame.

Guilt is inherently unhelpful and can lead parents to respond in counterproductive ways. As parents begin to let go of guilt, they often discover that they now have the energy to move in constructive directions. It is important for parents to let go of guilt and move forward.

Create Balance; Recognize Imbalance

Parents will acknowledge that they "give in" to avoid a fight with their child. Once the disorder has "taken over," it is hard work for a family to regain balance, but it is possible. The first step is to help parents recognize the need to find balance. Your perspective as both a therapist and a family outsider is useful in this regard, and initial PEP sessions typically help parents gain insight, if needed. Parents then need to make sure that all of the necessary treatment components are in place (this is discussed in the sessions focused on treatment and educational teams; see Chapters 10 and 16). By this session, parents are usually ready to admit how the disorder has taken over their family, and they can begin to generate ideas about how to begin getting life back in balance.

Chris and Barb were referred to PEP by their psychiatrist when they admitted to her that their son with BD, Brian, had been hitting and kicking them for months. They had become so afraid to set him off that they had not been addressing his aggressive behavior. They had dropped almost all expectations for him, and the whole family had been walking on eggshells. Their PEP therapist brought up his aggression toward them and the degree to which Brian had taken control of the household. Barb seemed immensely relieved to be identifying the problem and beginning to think about potential solutions.

Raising children with mood disorders is a complicated balancing act. One of the most challenging problems for parents is how to create balance. In some cases, parents need to step back and look at the bigger picture of their family life.

Bob and Kathy's son Matt (age 10) was diagnosed with BD at age 7. The last 3 years had been challenging for the whole family. At times Matt was very aggressive toward his 8-year-old sister, Amanda (i.e., chasing her, threatening to hurt her). Amanda had learned to steer clear, or at least if she saw a problem developing, to run and lock herself in her room. Matt needed a great deal of parental help to get through homework and other daily routines. He was very sensitive to household tension and tended to get agitated if the household routines were disturbed. Matt's therapist and psychiatrist worked well with the family but were a 30-minute drive from their home. Kathy was working on her master's degree in social work, and Bob put in long hours as a civil engineer. They were financially stretched, and their days were very full. Amanda took dance and piano lessons, and Matt played at least one sport each season. To help ease the financial stress, Kathy took a part-time position offered through her graduate program: supervising a group home. The position was supposed to be flexible and to require only 20 hours per week. Not only did it turn out to take more time, but, even worse, Kathy was getting many calls at night and on the weekends. Kathy had a history of recurrent depression, and when her sleep was disturbed, she tended to get depressed again. As Kathy and Bob participated in the group discussion about creating balance, they realized they had become a prime example of losing balance.

Finding balance can be very challenging and may involve sacrifices. Kathy and Bob ultimately decided to sell their home and downsize, in order to reduce their expenses and eliminate some financial stress. This would allow Kathy to finish graduate school without taking a job at the same time. Once she was finished with graduate school, the downsizing would allow her to work part-time.

Break Big Decisions into Smaller Ones during Acute Episodes

Crises often lead families to choice points, such as the need for hospitalization. However, permanent or family-altering decisions (e.g., a divorce, a family move) usually should not be made during acute episodes. Giving parents a two-step process for problem solving can be useful: (1) What is the immediate problem that needs to be resolved? and (2) Is there an underlying issue that needs to be addressed over the long term? An episode may bring to light an underlying issue such as custody arrangements, but thinking will be clearer when the child's acute episode has resolved.

Over the 3 years since their divorce, Laura and Burt had had multiple disagreements over the custody and visitation arrangements for their son, Chase. The situation was compounded recently, after Chase made a suicide attempt and was briefly hospitalized. The inpatient social worker, well versed in PEP, helped Laura and Burt conceptualize a two-step process for their decision making. Immediately after Chase's hospitalization, they agreed that Chase should spend time with his father on days when his younger stepbrothers would not also be at his father's house. Chase had always found them to be pesty, and he was generally better behaved and in a better mood when they weren't around. Laura and Burt further agreed that the long-term goal should be for Chase to spend more time at his father's house; however, they would reevaluate how and when to do this after Chase's symptoms subsided.

Adjust Expectations to the Child's Symptoms

One of the greatest challenges for parents of a child with a mood disorder is adjusting expectations up or down, depending on the child's functioning at a given point in time. Sometimes it is very difficult for parents to determine whether a child's behavior is willful. During the previous session, the idea of "can't" versus "won't" has been introduced. In a phase when a child is very agitated, irritable, and prone to escalating his/her behavior, the focus should be on finding stability, not on completing household chores. Problem solving is an important part of this process. Given that the first step in problem solving is to define the problem, doing so might help to identify agitation or mood instability rather than a specific behavioral issue as the problem. By the same token, as mood stability improves, expectations of being courteous to family members and making a reasonable contribution to the household become tenable again. Parents are engaged in the intricate dance of figuring out how much and when to push; you, as the therapist and as an outsider looking in, can provide valuable perspective to parents in this process.

Practice Self-Care and Self-Preservation

If a parent isn't healthy, a child has a very hard time becoming healthy. As parents learn to let go of guilt, it is important to encourage them to take care of themselves. This may mean making the time for a 30-minute walk each morning or evening, or sleeping in on a Saturday morning. Everything parents and children have been learning about healthy habits applies to parents as much as it does to children! Make the following suggestions, as needed:

> Maintain a healthy sleep schedule.
> Eat well.
> Exercise regularly.
> Take time to socialize with:
>> Spouse.
>> Friends.
>> Relatives.
>> Community organizations.
> Spend time with pets.
> Read a book.
> Listen to or make music.
> Pray or meditate, alone or in a congregation.
> Maintain a sense of humor.
> Pursue a hobby.

In some cases, parents also need to seek their own professional treatment. Self-preservation includes stress management. Parents need to recognize sources of stress and to engage in problem solving as necessary to manage that stress. Some common sources of stress and potential solutions are outlined in Box 14.3.

BOX 14.3. Becoming a Good Stress Manager

1. Explore changes to your and/or your spouse's work schedule. Can you:
   a. Reduce your hours?
   b. Work flexible hours?
2. Delegate household tasks.
3. Set up carpools to reduce driving time for kids' activities.
4. Examine your children's schedules—are they too full?
5. Prioritize your "to-do" list. Can some items at the bottom of the list be eliminated?

Take-Home Projects

New Project: Problem Solving: Symptoms and Family Conflicts

The new take-home project for this session is to identify a problem in the family related to the child's symptoms (e.g., "Matt has meltdowns almost every evening") and use the problem-solving steps to solve it. On Handout 65 (Problem Solving: Symptoms and Family Conflicts), parents should record how they identified and defined the problem, engaged the relevant family members, brainstormed potential solutions, picked a solution, tried it, evaluated how it worked, and decided what (if anything) to do differently next time.

Ideally, parents will pick a problem that does not require extensive child involvement. However, using the tips provided in Box 14.2, parents can include the child's perspective. Although children in IF-PEP will not learn the steps of problem solving on their own until their next session, they can certainly participate in the process with parental guidance.

Ongoing Take-Home Projects

Children have now added using helpful thoughts and actions to manage challenging emotional states. Parents should encourage the children to use their new strategies, and parents should record on the Mood–Medication Log (Handout 32) or Mood Record (Handout 20 or 21) whether or not a particular strategy was helpful.

The next scheduled parent session reviews and troubleshoots any issues with the child's school team, so it may be useful for parents to review Handout 53 (My Child's Educational Team). Handout 52 (My Child's Treatment Team) should also be reviewed as necessary.

Chapter 15

Problem-Solving Skills for Children

IF-PEP Child Session 6
MF-PEP Child Session 5

Session Outline

Goal:	Teach the child the steps of problem solving and ways these can be used to navigate daily challenges.
Beginning the Session:	Do a check-in with parents. Review selected healthy habits chart (for IF-PEP only) (Handout 40, 44, or 47). Review Thinking, Feeling, Doing (Handout 62). Have child Identify and rate feelings (Handouts 1 and 2).
Lesson of the Day:	Introducing problem solving • Stop: Take a moment to calm down. • Think: Define the problem and brainstorm strategies. • Plan: Decide which strategy to use. • Do: Carry out the strategy. • Check: Evaluate the outcome.

Breathing Exercise:	Child's choice (Belly, Bubble, Balloon Breathing)
Session Review with Parents	
New Take-Home Project:	Problem Solving (Handout 67)
Ongoing Take-Home Project:	Selected healthy habits chart (for IF-PEP only) (Handout 40, 44, or 47)
New Handouts:	66. Problem Solving (Sample) 67. Problem Solving
Handout to Review:	62. Thinking, Feeling, Doing

Session Overview

At the beginning of the session, allow time to review and troubleshoot the child's previous take-home project, the Thinking, Feeling, Doing exercise. This session then introduces problem-solving skills to the child. Five steps are taught: "Stop," "Think," "Plan," "Do," and "Check." Make sure that the child leaves with a clear understanding of the five steps. Our ultimate goal is for children to experience challenges they face as problems that can be solved. Teaching the problem-solving steps helps move children in the right direction. The take-home project asks a child to apply the steps to at least one trigger, and more practice is encouraged.

Beginning the Session

Do a Check-In with Parents

By now, the check-in with parents should be a very quick process. Parents may still find it helpful to bring in their Mood–Medication Log or Mood Record, or they may simply give a quick run-down of how things have been since the child's last session.

Review Selected Healthy Habits Chart

The healthy habits review is only for children in IF-PEP. Review while the parents are still in the room, and troubleshoot as necessary to address issues that may be impeding progress toward the child's goals. As appropriate, spend more time after the parents leave the room addressing concerns the child may have about accomplishing healthy habit goals. Remind the child that at the next child session, he/she will pick a second healthy habit to address.

Review Thinking, Feeling, Doing

During the review, you can also correct any misunderstandings and help the child fill in any incomplete sections of Handout 62 (Thinking, Feeling, Doing). This project is the most complex task children complete in PEP. They may come in with only parts of the handout completed and need help thinking about how the exercise could have been more helpful.

> Marta, a 10-year-old with BD-II, completed her Thinking, Feeling, Doing project about an incident with her mom, Christine. Marta explained that on Sunday afternoon, she was struggling with her book report. Her mom was sitting with her, helping her summarize the book, when the phone rang. Marta's dad answered the phone and told her mom that it was someone from work calling for her. Marta's hurtful feelings were "angry" and "frustrated." Her thoughts were "She's ignoring me again for that stupid job," and "If it's not important enough to Mom to stay and help me, it's not important enough for me to do." She threw down her pencil, slammed her book shut, and went to play computer games.
>
> At that point, Marta had gotten stuck and had not filled in anything else on the handout. Her mother reported talking on the phone for about 15 minutes. When she went to get Marta to start up again, Marta was caught up in her computer game and responded angrily to her mother's prompt to restart her school assignment. The interaction escalated into a big argument.

THERAPIST: From what you described, you did a great job of identifying the trigger: Mom getting that call from work when you were in the middle of working on your summary.

MARTA: Yeah, I got really mad and frustrated when Mom went to answer the phone.

THERAPIST: (*turning to Christine, Marta's mother*) How did you feel?

CHRISTINE: I was really frustrated as well. Marta was working really hard, and that call really threw her off track. I guess I have a problem I need to solve, because I have really been getting too many calls at home on the weekend!

THERAPIST: So you were both frustrated. Marta, did you know that your mother was upset that her phone call was so frustrating for you?

MARTA: I guess I didn't really think about it. I was just really mad.

THERAPIST: Well, I also noticed that you did a great job of identifying your hurtful thoughts! (*Points to the part of Handout 62 Marta has filled in.*) Those thoughts really summed it up. Your thoughts that your mother cares more about work than you, and that your book report isn't important, really turned your mother's phone call into something awful.

MARTA: Yeah, I got really upset.

THERAPIST: I see that you put "Throwing down my pencil" and "Slamming my book shut" under hurtful actions, but that you didn't put "Playing computer games" in either the helpful or hurtful category. Where do you think "Playing computer games" should go?

MARTA: Probably in the hurtful box, because playing computer games made it hard to get back to my book report.

THERAPIST: That makes sense. Now let's think about filling in the helpful boxes. Frustrated and angry are probably feelings that are going to interfere with getting your book report done. How would you rather feel?

MARTA: Calm? Or maybe patient?

THERAPIST: Okay. Do you want to write, or do you want me to?

MARTA: I'll do it. (*Adds "calm" and "patient" to the "Feelings" heart.*)

THERAPIST: Now how about actions? What actions might have been better?

MARTA: I could have started by taking some deep breaths.

THERAPIST: Great idea. What else?

MARTA: Well, my dad was around. I guess I could have asked him to sit with me while my mom was on the phone. Or I could have worked on the picture I need to draw while I waited for her. I like to draw anyway.

THERAPIST: Great. What about some helpful thoughts?

MARTA: I could have thought about how much I had done already, and how if I just kept working on it, I would still have time to play outside later in the afternoon. (*Writes, "Wow, it's going fast. Maybe I can still ride my bike later if I keep going."*)

THERAPIST: Super! You were able to think of something positive about the book report, and you could look forward to more fun later in the afternoon. How might that make you feel?

MARTA: Pretty good—way better than I expected when I started working on the book report.

THERAPIST: Are there any other helpful thoughts you might have?

MARTA: I also could have thought about how my mom is also probably getting sick of the calls from work. (*Writes, "Mom's sick of work calls, too."*)

THERAPIST: You got it. If you took some of those helpful actions and thought those helpful thoughts, it would have been a lot easier to be patient and get more of the book report done. The situation wouldn't have seemed so awful, like your mom was trying to do something mean to you.

Marta knew what her hurtful thoughts, feelings, and actions were, but in the moment and immediately afterward, she hadn't been able to activate more helpful thoughts or choices. However, in the context of the session, she showed that she really understood the concept. With continued practice, children can begin to generalize the skills and use them to navigate more easily through difficult situations. It is important to remind children periodically to keep practicing all of the skills they have learned!

Have Child Identify and Rate Feelings

After the project review, the parents leave the session. At this point, do a quick check-in with the child. Reviewing children's current feelings, the reasons why they feel that way, and the strength of their feelings on Handouts 1 and 2 reinforces their foundation skills. They need to be aware of their feelings in order to manage them.

Lesson of the Day: Introducing Problem Solving

Today's lesson again builds on the therapeutic content of previous sessions. At this point in PEP, children should be well acquainted with the idea that "triggers" set off challenging situations. They have previously worked on developing helpful actions and thoughts in response to triggers. Now we want them to take things one step further and look at triggers as problems they can solve. We want children to recognize how easy it is to react to a trigger without thinking, and how those unthinking reactions can make the situation worse for them and/or those around them. A key point to make is that when hurtful feelings are triggered by a distressing event, a child can learn to make better decisions. In PEP, children learn the following five steps of problem solving:

1. Stop. Take a moment to calm down.
2. Think. Define the problem and brainstorm strategies.
3. Plan. Decide which strategy to use.
4. Do. Carry out the strategy.
5. Check. Evaluate the outcome.

This session teaches children what is meant by each step and coaches them in how to carry them out. As you work with a child to illustrate the steps of problem solving, use triggers or problems relevant to this particular child. Any event that resulted in hurtful feelings or behaviors can be used. If the child has trouble coming up with a relevant example from his/her own life, review the example provided in Handout 66, Problem Solving (Sample). Once a problem has been selected for solving, children tend to jump in at the Do step. They may need help to backtrack and consider Stop, Think, and Plan, as in the following example.

> Dr. Burk asked 9-year-old Joey whether there was a problem he was having that they could use as an example for problem solving. Joey quickly came up with fights between him and his younger brother about what to watch on TV.
>
> JOEY: My brother and I could take turns deciding who gets to pick! Like on Mondays, Wednesday, and Fridays I could pick, and on Tuesdays, Thursdays, and Saturdays, he could pick!
>
> THERAPIST: That's a great idea, but we missed some important steps in problem solving. Like, I don't really understand exactly what the problem is, because we didn't stop and define the problem. So, let's really go through the steps, okay?
>
> JOEY: Okay.
>
> THERAPIST: When do you and your brother fight about the TV?

JOEY: Mostly we fight about the TV in the morning. My brother gets downstairs first, and he always puts stuff on that I don't like to watch—baby shows.

THERAPIST: Does anyone else get involved in the problem?

JOEY: Well, my mom is always yelling at me about getting ready in the morning.

THERAPIST: That sounds like something important. Is it hard for you to get ready in the morning?

JOEY: Well, it's really hard for me to get up in the morning, and I guess I get distracted a lot, so yeah, I guess getting ready is kind of hard. My mom has to remind me a lot, and I almost miss the bus a lot of days.

THERAPIST: So does the TV distract you from getting ready?

JOEY: Yeah, I want to watch when my brother is watching, but I don't like to watch his stupid baby shows, so then we get in fights about it.

THERAPIST: Does your brother need to get ready for school?

JOEY: No, because he goes to afternoon kindergarten.

THERAPIST: So it sounds like the problem isn't just the TV in the morning. Are there other times you fight with your brother about what to watch?

JOEY: Not really. After school we both like to watch cartoons.

THERAPIST: So how do you think we should define the problem?

JOEY: Maybe that getting ready in the morning is hard, and seeing the TV makes me want to watch one of my shows instead of my brother's baby shows.

THERAPIST: Great job! So now that we know what the problem really is, would alternating days for picking shows in the morning solve the problem?

JOEY: I guess not.

THERAPIST: Right. We needed to define the problem before we could do the "Think" step and come up with ideas. What ideas do you have?

Joey's case is a great example of how children can want to jump in and start coming up with solutions before defining the problem. As demonstrated above, it's helpful to talk a child carefully through the problem definition step and show him/her how much it can change the potential solutions. Joey was calm as he engaged in problem solving within the session, away from his younger brother and the stress of getting ready in the morning. Typically, when problematic situations arise, strong emotions come along with the problem. This leads into a discussion of the first step.

Stop: Take a Moment to Calm Down

The Stop step asks children to recognize the point in a stressful situation when their feelings are in the "Danger Zone" on the mood thermometer of Handout 2 (Strength of Feelings). Children should be reminded that strong feelings are a Danger Zone, because they keep us from thinking straight and making positive choices. The Stop step means "Don't act; don't react; take a minute to calm down by using a strategy from the Tool Kit." Stopping is often the most difficult step for children to learn. You can explain by using an analogy like riding a bike: Going fast and not slowing down before a sharp turn usually result in losing control of the bike and crashing. If children "speed" or rush into a difficult situation, their emotions can get out of control, and a hurtful outcome is often the result.

After explaining the meaning of the Stop step, ask the child to identify at least two coping strategies he/she could have used in the sample situation to calm down. Children should learn that having at least two options is a good idea, because one may not work or they may not be able to do it. For example, if Joey wanted to watch TV for 10 minutes as a way of calming down, he would be unlikely to get approval from his mother for that particular calming strategy in this situation. Taking some deep breaths or getting a hug from his mother might be better ways to calm himself down during the morning.

Think: Define the Problem and Brainstorm Strategies

In the Think step, children first define the problem and then generate a list of actions they could take next. As illustrated by Joey's example, you may need to provide some prompting to help a child get at the underlying or actual problem. For some children, this step might also involve talking to another grownup to help define the problem. During the discussion, it might be helpful for the child to identify adults who could help with this step (parents, grandparents, teachers, guidance counselors, etc.).

Another challenge for children is generating several options for solving the problem. This may take some coaxing from you or another adult. The list should contain at least two helpful options, but not all have to be equally useful. Sometimes children can identify the hurtful behaviors they might engage in if the triggering event were to happen to them and they did not use the problem-solving steps. It can be useful to include those actions on the list and evaluate them as part of the Plan step.

Plan: Decide Which Strategy to Use

In the Plan step, pros and cons of each possible outcome are considered, and a specific action is chosen as the one to try. Again, you and the child can discuss what might happen if the child chose each option. In addition, remind the child of the three questions used earlier to determine whether outcomes are helpful or hurtful ("Does it hurt me?", "Does it hurt someone or something else?", and "Does it get anyone in trouble?"). Children may have difficulty anticipating the consequences of their actions, so you may need to provide assistance. At the end of this step, the child should choose one option to try.

Do: Carry Out the Strategy

The Do step is straightforward: The child carries out the option chosen during the Plan step.

Check: Evaluate the Outcome

The Check step is easily overlooked, but it is critical to helping children make better choices about their future behavior. In this step, children examine whether the outcome is helpful or hurtful, and consider whether they would use that strategy again. When you are teaching the steps, the Check step often reiterates the expected outcome generated in the Plan step. When children use the steps, the Check step helps them see whether they correctly anticipated the outcome. It also helps to improve their Plan skills in predicting what might happen.

Children should work through as many additional examples as session time permits.

Breathing Exercise

Review the three breathing techniques with the child, and then practice the one chosen by the child.

Session Review with Parents

Problem solving is a fundamental skill set for all families, but it is particularly critical for families of children with mood disorders, who face frequent and complicated problems. As the child summarizes the session content for the parents, make sure that everyone understands the steps and their relationship to the problem-solving steps taught in the previous IF-PEP parent session (or this MF-PEP parent session).

Take-Home Projects

New Project: Problem Solving

The new take-home project for this session (Handout 67, the blank version of Problem Solving) requires children to apply the problem-solving steps to a trigger that led to a hurtful outcome. Children should be encouraged to complete additional examples and bring them to the next session also. As with many skills, practice makes perfect; the more often children use the strategy, the more likely they are to use it when stressful events occur.

Ongoing Project: Selected Healthy Habits Chart

By this point, the child should have made some progress on the first healthy habit selected for change. The next IF-PEP child session (Session 7) takes up a second habit for change. (This session is not covered in a separate chapter; refer to Chapter 9 for instructions on conducting the session.) Healthy habits are not covered in discrete MF-PEP sessions, although, as noted in Chapter 9, their content may be incorporated into other sessions.

Chapter 16

Addressing School Issues with the School Team

IF-PEP Parent Session 6
Not a session in MF-PEP

Session Outline

Goals:	1. Improve communication between parents and school personnel. 2. Develop or enhance school accommodations and/or services.
Planning the Meeting:	When to schedule? Who will attend? Where should the meeting be held? Parental comfort with disclosures to the school Agenda planning
At The Meeting:	Your role as the therapist Handling difficult situations
New Take-Home Project:	No new project
New Handouts:	None
Handouts to Review:	52. My Child's Educational Team

Sesion Overview

This chapter covers arranging and participating in a meeting with parents and the school personnel who are members of the child's educational team. This is not a standard parent session, and so it does not follow the standard session format. In Chapter 10, we have addressed in general how parents can create an effective educational team. However, many families of children with mood disorders still struggle with how to work effectively with staff members at their children's schools. Therefore, as part of IF-PEP, the therapist, parents, and school professionals meet as a team to work on the nuts and bolts of the child's particular school issues. The school team meeting is generally scheduled after parents have been taught problem solving. Parents are encouraged to use the problem-solving skills before and during the meeting, and to attend in the spirit of collaboration and team building. Parents have the responsibility of coordinating the logistical arrangements with school personnel and the IF-PEP therapist. Regardless of when in IF-PEP this session is scheduled, a preceding session should address the meeting-planning information described below. This may be done during the parents' third session, where they focus on treatment teams; during the parents' sixth session, when school issues are revisited; or during an in-the-bank session. Preparing for a school meeting makes an ideal problem-solving goal, so it can also be discussed at the end of the parents' fifth session on problem solving. If a child is not having any particular problems at school, this session can be skipped.

Planning the Meeting

When to Schedule?

This meeting is usually scheduled during the latter portion of IF-PEP, but in some cases a child's needs will dictate that it be scheduled sooner rather than later. This is where our mantra of "flexibility with fidelity" becomes relevant. In some cases, a regularly scheduled IEP meeting will appear on the school calendar, and this can become the occasion for the parents and you to meet with the school professionals. In other cases, there will be a critical need for this meeting to take place as soon as possible. Although it makes sense for the meeting to occur after the foundations of PEP have been covered, you do have the flexibility to hold the meeting sooner. In some cases, as noted above, this session is not necessary if the child is functioning well at school.

Who Should Attend?

This meeting includes parents, you (the IF-PEP therapist), and some or all of the professionals who are members of the child's school team. If the child has an existing IEP or 504 plan (see Chapter 10 for a discussion of these plans), a meeting can be requested with the existing IEP or 504 team from the school. If there is no preexisting 504 Plan or IEP, the personnel to invite to a meeting will vary. The classroom teacher should be included in most cases. Other possible attendees include the school counselor, school psychologist, the instructional support teacher, and school administrators.

Where Should the Meeting Be Held?

School professionals often have time for meetings built into the school day. Therefore, the most successful method for getting the whole school team together is usually for you and the parents to join the school staff at school. Most school personnel's schedules are not compatible with traveling to a therapist's office. (This may be a little different for specialized schools, where more time is built into staff schedules for meetings.)

Ideally, everyone should be physically present in the same place, but if this proves impossible, an audio or video conference call can be arranged. The parents may be at school with the school personnel while you join them via speakerphone or video. Alternatively (but less preferably), the parents could join you in your office, and you could all communicate with the school representatives by speakerphone or video. However, since one goal of this session is to build the relationship between parents and the school staff, it's best if they are in the same room as the school personnel. If an audio or video conference is held, it is especially important that any documents to be reviewed during the meeting be provided in advance to all parties. This should include any written information you would like to share with the other members of the educational team. Even when planned carefully, phone or video conferences are challenging, especially if many people are in the room. Box 16.1 offers tips for participating in phone or video conferences and avoiding some common communication problems.

Parental Comfort with Disclosures to the School

A meeting with you and the school personnel gives parents a valuable opportunity: They will have school personnel available, as well as a professional who knows their family and situation to clarify issues and facilitate planning. Yet, if the child has not had problems at school, parents are sometimes reluctant about disclosing the child's diagnosis and other issues to the school staff. Parents may fear that their child will be stigmatized. This issue has probably been explored in the earlier session where the school team was discussed,

---

BOX 16.1. Tips for Participating in Phone or Video Conferences

- Have all parties clearly state their names and roles at the beginning of the meeting.
- Don't be afraid to ask people to repeat themselves or to speak louder.
- Have all parties say their names prior to speaking each time.
- Place the speakerphone in the middle of the table, or have people move as necessary to be closer to the video conferencing microphone.
- Be sure that papers are not rustled near the speakerphone or microphone.
- Let people know right away if you cannot hear them.
- If you are joining a meeting by phone, no one can see your nonverbal signals that you want to add something. You may need to jump into the conversation.

but if the parents still have concerns, those should be addressed before the meeting. Parents may not realize that working with the school professionals may help to prevent problems or catch them while they are still small, as in the following example.

Christina was 9 and in the middle of third grade. Two years earlier, she had been diagnosed with a mood disorder, and she had been taking the same mood-stabilizing medication for the past year. At routine parent–school conferences, teachers talked about how much they enjoyed Christina in class, as she had lots of ideas to share and was an enthusiastic learner. During the IF-PEP session on systems of care, her parents talked about how much the teachers loved having Christina in school, but how hard it was to get her through homework and the afternoon/evening routines. Christina often had major meltdowns after school. Due to the history of stressful afternoons, the parents had cut out most of her extracurricular activities. Homework completion often stretched into the late evening, which led to difficult mornings. Christina had gone to school late twice during the past month. When Christina's parents suggested writing a note to her teacher explaining why she hadn't completed all her homework, Christina became distraught.

Christina's parents were hesitant to bring these issues up with the school staff. Mike, their IF-PEP therapist, talked about the cycle they were living with—difficult afternoons leading into late nights and increasingly difficult mornings. Without intervention, this cycle was likely to worsen and lead to escalating mood symptoms. Mike thus convinced Christina's parents to share what was happening at home with the school personnel. In the meeting, Christina's classroom teacher and the school counselor listened carefully to what her parents were describing. When they had finished, her teacher said, "I am so glad you told me this. Christina is quite a perfectionist about her work, and while I appreciate the work she does, she probably spends more time than necessary on some of her assignments." Mike joined in and asked how much time they expected a typical third grader to spend on homework. Christina's parents were surprised to hear that the school district expected third graders to spend 30–45 minutes on homework each evening. Christina was often spending 2–3 hours on homework each night. Given how intense Christina's issues were at home and how they interacted with homework, Mike suggested that a 504 plan would be appropriate. The school counselor and the teacher agreed. The school counselor was the 504 plan coordinator for Christina's school. She began to draft a plan in which Christina would check in briefly with the teacher each afternoon to preview homework, estimate the amount of time each assignment should take, and prioritize so that Christina would do her most challenging assignments when she was feeling the most relaxed. They also included a weekly 30-minute meeting with the school counselor in the plan, so that Christina could work on some stress management skills. Christina's parents, teacher, and school counselor agreed to stay in close communication and to meet again in the near future, so that they could touch base on how things were going.

If school professionals are not aware of problems at home, they will be unable to provide sufficient support. Although they may not always have answers for how to help with homework or other issues, they may have ideas for what to try.

Agenda Planning

It is important to guide the parents on planning their agenda prior to their meeting with the school staff, so that time is used efficiently and productively. If the school personnel and the parents see eye to eye, the meeting can be used to initiate assessment requests, obtain a progress update, or fine-tune the program that is currently in place. The meeting may also serve as an opportunity for the school professionals to ask questions of you, the IF-PEP therapist, and to benefit from your expertise. In addition, this meeting may provide a chance to plan ahead—for example, if a child will be transitioning from elementary to middle school in the coming year.

If there is no current IEP or 504 plan, but the parents have concerns related to school, this meeting can serve as an opportunity to clarify issues for the school personnel. The school staff may then decide to either seek a 504 plan or to initiate an MFE (see Chapter 10) and consider whether an IEP would be appropriate. Sometimes teachers feel they can handle issues at school, but when they see the whole picture of how a child is doing across domains, they begin to realize that accommodations and services are necessary.

> Jalen was in fourth grade and had BD and ADHD. Every year, his mother, Karen, requested that he be assigned to a very structured teacher who would establish clear expectations. This year she made the same request, and Jalen was placed in class with the most seasoned teacher on the fourth-grade team—one who had a reputation for being tough but fair. Karen also always wrote the teacher a note at the beginning of the year explaining how hard it was for Jalen to stay focused, and that it would help him to sit close to the teacher and away from distractions. Aside from getting distracted, Jalen had never previously had any behavior problems at school. This year, however, he seemed to be struggling more with peers. He had gotten into a couple of arguments on the playground, and the recess aides had intervened, but no further action had been taken. He was also coming home extremely irritable and really struggling with his homework. When Karen and her husband, Dennis, scheduled the school meeting with their IF-PEP therapist, they saw it as an opportunity to share their observations of Jalen this year and enlist the school's help.

Jalen was struggling but did not have a formal plan. In the past, close communication with the classroom teacher had been enough to provide Jalen with the added support he needed to succeed in school. Now his symptoms were beginning to creep through. In a situation like this, a meeting can be very helpful. It provides an opportunity for the parents and the teacher to share what they have been seeing, and ideally to get the whole team on the same page. When everyone on the team is aware of the same issues, there can be more productive educational planning, whether through Section 504 or IDEA mechanisms.

If there is an IEP (or 504 plan) in place, but either the parents or the school personnel still have concerns about how things are going, this meeting is particularly important. Children with mood disorders can be "moving targets." Accommodation needs can change, depending on several factors: the season (e.g., worse depressive symptoms during the winter months or more manic symptoms during the spring); a child's development (i.e., challenges can change as the child gets older); curriculum changes in higher grades (a child with a mood disorder may have trouble dealing with these); or episodic changes (i.e., a child in a depressive or manic episode may need increased or different supports).

> Caroline, a third grader, had been diagnosed with DD and ADHD. Over the past couple of months (January and February), she had experienced a worsening of her depressive symptoms, which included fatigue, agitation, and declining attention. Although she described sadness at home and her parents observed an increase in her irritability, she worked hard to hide these symptoms at school. However, her teachers were starting to send notes home expressing concern about Caroline's difficulty completing work. Caroline had a 504 plan, but it mostly addressed her ADHD symptoms (preferential seating, communication notebook between parents and teacher, check-ins about comprehension of assignments, etc.). At the meeting, Caroline's parents described their concerns. Her teacher also had concerns, but had been seeing the problem as distractibility and poor organization. Caroline's IF-PEP therapist helped bridge the two perspectives. He raised the possibility that this worsening could be seasonal, and he made a note to himself to check in with Caroline's parents at their next session about possibilities for symptom management (e.g., a light box). The team collaborated to add some accommodations to the 504 plan and agreed that if things did not improve over the next month, they would meet again and consider initiating an MFE. A plan for increased communication was put in place for the next month.

Caroline's situation is not uncommon: Her mood symptoms were manifesting differently at school than at home, and her school dysfunction (i.e., not finishing her work) was being interpreted as a behavioral issue. The team meeting provided a bridge between the parents' and school's perspectives, which enabled a plan to be put in place.

At the Meeting

Your Role as the Therapist

Part of your role as the IF-PEP therapist at this meeting is to help the school begin to focus on symptom management with a problem-solving approach, rather than focusing solely on behavior management. Problem solving and symptom management are particularly important in regard to children with mood disorders. Most important of all, your role is to encourage school staffers to think of themselves as part of a team that includes the parents and, when possible, the mental health team. Box 16.2 outlines the varying roles of a therapist and school personnel at a school meeting.

School professionals will vary in their openness, as will parents. Often school staff members will be receptive and willing to be creative in their educational planning for a child with a mood disorder, but they may lack the trained personnel or resources to follow through. They may also find themselves feeling overwhelmed; at times, their best efforts at behavior management may not work in the face of escalating mood symptoms. The school staff may be grateful to have access to the resources and knowledge that you bring to the meeting.

BOX 16.2. Roles of Therapist and School Personnel during Meeting with Parents

---

ROLE OF THE THERAPIST

- Provide information about mood disorders to the school personnel.
- Collaborate with the school personnel to develop interventions.
- Bridge the parents' and the school's perspectives.
- Provide increased understanding of the child's needs.

ROLE OF SCHOOL PERSONNEL

- Share the school's perspective on the child.
- Know what resources the district has and how they can be accessed.
- Help differentiate the child's needs—cognitive? emotional? behavioral?

Julio was 8 and in second grade. In kindergarten and first grade, he loved school and was a strong student who was well liked by peers. During the summer prior to second grade, however, Julio began exhibiting some symptoms of depression, such as sadness and frequent meltdowns. As his depression got worse, he began having an extremely hard time controlling himself in almost any setting. His parents sought a consultation with a psychiatrist and began working with her to find effective medication for Julio. He started the school year in a regular classroom, with close communication between his teacher and parents. After some meltdowns and episodes of Julio's running away from school staffers, the school began to work with his parents to establish a setting at school that would work for him until he could begin to recover. Both his parents and the school staff were optimistic that Julio would return to his previous level of functioning and that intervention would be temporary. When Julio and his parents began IF-PEP, he was doing one-on-one work with an aide in a spare classroom. Before the school meeting, the parents and his IF-PEP therapist talked about options. At this point, 3 months of the school year had gone by. Julio was not participating in any special-area classes (i.e., art, gym, music, library) and was really missing them. Although he was doing some schoolwork, each day was a struggle. One option they talked about was establishing an IEP for Julio and then possibly transferring him to another school in the district where there was an emotional support classroom. In the actual meeting, it became clear that all parties had independently come to the same conclusion. The focus then shifted to how to help Julio with the transition, rather than whether the transition was necessary.

Sometimes everyone agrees, and this makes for a very productive meeting. On other occasions, you'll be asked to attend or facilitate a meeting that involves considerable tension and disagreement. In some cases, you'll be able to help the parents focus on their most significant concerns and agree on a bridge-building strategy for working with the school. The knowledge and skill you bring to the table may help refocus all team members on the child's needs.

Handling Difficult Situations

In some cases, you will come into a situation in which the level of discord is beyond what you can resolve in a meeting. When tension is very high, it is best to treat the school meeting as a chance to gather information and share concerns, with less emphasis on obtaining results. This is a good opportunity to model team building and problem solving. If you feel that the family and the school are too far apart in their perspectives, one question to raise is whether another team member is needed—perhaps someone else from the school district, such as the supervisor of special education or another administrator. Sometimes it is a matter of getting the right school team members on board. For example, if a 504 plan coordinator has denied a request for an MFE to determine the need for an IEP, it may then be helpful for the family to reach out to a school administrator. If the school meeting does not go well, this is probably a good time for an in-the-bank session, during which you can redefine the problem and begin to brainstorm solutions. If necessary, an independent professional such as an educational advocate or an educational lawyer may help facilitate progress.

If the situation is becoming overly contentious, and this is a school district you are likely to work with for other clients, you should consider what role you are comfortable playing. Sometimes the relationship between the family and the school becomes highly conflictual and is not easily repaired through bridge building and sharing information. You need to have a positive working relationship with the school district for the long term, but must also be in a position to support your clients. If the situation becomes too conflictual, it may be helpful to suggest that the family hire an educational advocate (or, in extreme situations, an educational attorney). Above all else, be sure that you do not get pulled into the role of giving legal advice or becoming part of the conflict. As in all other clinical and ethical dilemmas, be sure to consult with a colleague or mentor if the situation becomes difficult to navigate.

School meetings can be both challenging and rewarding. When bridges can be built and creative problem solving facilitated, these meetings can be valuable to the family and enjoyable for the clinician. At other times, the meetings can be frustrating and unproductive. It is important for you as an IF-PEP therapist to keep in mind that this meeting is an important step in building a collaborative relationship among members of the child's educational team. In some cases, it is a first positive step; in others, it is one of several productive steps; and in still others, it is a step in the right direction.

Chapter 17

The Communication Cycle and Nonverbal Communication Skills for Children

IF-PEP Child Session 8
MF-PEP Child Session 6

Session Outline

Goals:	1. Define "communication" for the child, and introduce the four steps of the communication cycle.
	2. Increase the child's awareness of his/her own nonverbal communication.
	3. Increase the child's awareness of nonverbal communication in others.
Beginning the Session:	Do a check-in with parents.
	Review second healthy habit chart (for IF-PEP only) (Handout 40, 44, or 47).
	Review Problem Solving (Handout 68).
	Have child identify and rate feelings.
Lesson of the Day:	The communication cycle and nonverbal communication skills
	• What is communication?
	• Two ways to communicate
	• The communication cycle
	• Types of nonverbal communication
	• Introducing the Paying Attention to Feelings project

Breathing Exercise:	Child's choice (Belly, Bubble, Balloon Breathing)

Session Review with Parents

New Take-Home Project: Paying Attention to Feelings (Handout 71)

New Handouts:
68. Communication
69. The Communication Cycle
70. Nonverbal Communication
71. Paying Attention to Feelings

Handouts to Review:
40. Sleep Chart *or*
44. Healthy Foods Chart *or*
46. Exercise Chart (for IF-PEP only)
67. Problem Solving

Session Overview

The most recent child sessions have been focused on problem solving and (for IF-PEP) on healthy habits. The associated take-home projects are reviewed at the start of this session. This session is the first of two devoted to communication skills. This first session introduces the two types of communication (nonverbal and verbal), describes the communication cycle, and then focuses on nonverbal communication skills. The next child session will focus on verbal skills. As mentioned previously, children with mood disorders often have difficulty reading and interpreting social cues. Improving their nonverbal communication skills can help them improve family and peer relationships. It is helpful to have a mirror on hand in this session, so that children can check their own facial expressions.

Beginning the Session

Do a Check-In with Parents

Begin the session with parents and children together for a quick check-in on how the week has gone. Mention briefly the Lesson of the Day.

Review Second Healthy Habit Chart

Children in IF-PEP should have been working on their second healthy habits topic (sleep, diet, or exercise) since their last session. For most children, check in on their progress and review the appropriate healthy habits chart (Handout 40, 44, or 47) while the parents are still in the session. An older child will want more autonomy in this review; in those instances, wait to complete the review until you are alone with the child. If a child has encountered problems, prompt him/her to use problem-solving skills to find solutions. See Chapter 9 for more on healthy habits.

Review Problem Solving Project

Review the completed Handout 67 (Problem Solving) with the child. Ask the child to explain the challenging situation he/she encountered and how the child handled it. If the child has recorded more than one scenario, and if time permits, review these additional scenarios. You may need to clarify the problem-solving steps or simply talk with the child about how the plans worked and what he/she will do the next time. If the problem was outside the home, reviewing Handout 67 with the parents can help the parents gain insight into the child's struggles. If the problem was at home, you may be able to guide both the parents and child in ways they could fine-tune their problem solving in the future, or simply highlight their newfound success. The child should be encouraged to continue using problem solving and to ask for help from the parents in the future as needed. As the parents have also been working on problem solving, they are also welcome to bring up issues that have arisen while completing the parent problem-solving project.

DR. SANCHEZ [therapist]: So, Lindsay, did you come up with a problem to solve this past week?

LINDSAY: Yeah, I picked a problem with my friend Rosa at school.

DR. SANCHEZ: Can you tell your dad and me what was going on?

LINDSAY: Sure. I was walking in the hallway before classes started. I saw Rosa across the hall by her locker. I waved to her and called her name. Usually we hang out before the bell rings and walk to our first period class together. By the time I got across the hall, Rosa was gone. Then at lunch, I saved her a seat, but she sat way down at the end of the lunch table. She even was sitting next to girls we aren't really good friends with. I couldn't figure out what was wrong. Then I started worrying about how soccer practice would go later in the afternoon, 'cuz Rosa is my only real friend on the team.

DR. SANCHEZ: Wow, sounds like you were getting pretty concerned about this. What would you say the problem was?

LINDSAY: Well, I guess I thought Rosa was being mean to me, and I was afraid she wasn't going to be my friend any more.

DR. SANCHEZ: That's a tough problem to have. You did a nice job defining it. What did you do?

LINDSAY: I remembered I was supposed to do my problem solving, so I started making a list in my head of all the things I could do.

DR. SANCHEZ: Good for you! What kind of ideas did you come up with?

LINDSAY: Well, I thought I could ignore Rosa until she said something to me, and then I could ask her what was going on. Or I could bring it up when I had a chance to talk to her alone. She and I usually get dressed for soccer before the other girls do, or I could ask her on the ride home from practice. Or I thought I could just skip practice; then she would have to find me to ask me what was going on, and I could ask her then.

DR. SANCHEZ: Good. You came up with a pretty long list of options. Which one did you choose?

LINDSAY: I couldn't stand not knowing. I asked Rosa what was going on while we were changing in the locker room. She told me I hadn't done anything wrong, and she didn't mean to ignore me. She still looked pretty upset, so I asked her if something else was wrong. She told me that her grandmother went to the hospital by ambulance that morning. Rosa is really close to her grandmother—they live together. Rosa was super-worried about how she was doing. I was so glad I asked, because then I was able to give her a hug and tell her I was sorry about her news.

DR. SANCHEZ: Wow, solving the problem this way really turned things around, didn't it?

LINDSAY: It sure did. I went from thinking that Rosa was mad at me and maybe didn't want to be my friend any more, to being really glad I could be there for her because she was worried about her grandmother.

DR. SANCHEZ: Good for you, Lindsay. You are using your new skills to manage your own feelings and to be a really good friend. I'm proud of you.

BRUCE [Lindsay's dad]: Hey, Lindsay, I'm proud of you, too. Mom told me you made a card for Rosa and for her grandma the other night. That was so thoughtful of you.

Have Child Identify and Rate Feelings

After the parents leave the session, do a quick check-in with the child to identify his/her feelings and rate their strength.

Lesson of the Day: The Communication Cycle and Nonverbal Communication Skills

What Is Communication?

One way to begin a discussion about communication is by asking a child whether he/she sometimes gets in trouble for not listening or not following directions at home or at school. Most children can provide examples of times they have gotten into trouble for not listening. From there, you can go on to explain that listening is one part of communication. Using Handout 68 (Communication), discuss with the child what "communication" is. Important points to cove include these:

- Communication is an exchange between two or more people.
- It includes sharing ideas and feelings.
- It is a process of give and take.

This flows into a discussion of why communication is important: (1) It lets other people know what you need, how you are feeling, and what you expect; *and* (2) it lets you know what others need, how they are feeling, and what they expect.

Two Ways to Communicate

Next, children need to understand the two ways to communicate—verbal and nonverbal—and the differences between them. In verbal communication, people use words to exchange information. In nonverbal communication, people exchange information without using words. Both kinds of communication are important. Explain that you will be discussing nonverbal communication today and verbal communication at the next session.

The Communication Cycle

Then, using Handout 69 (The Communication Cycle), introduce the communication cycle to the child. Children need to understand clearly that there are four important steps where communication can be effective or go awry: (1) in the sending, (2) in the receiving, (3) in the response, and (4) in how the response is understood. If a child clearly grasps this, you can move on quickly to the next stage. However, many children benefit from a more thorough discussion of this topic. Using humor can keep this from sounding "preachy."

For example, one way to show that communication doesn't happen unless the message is received is for you to make a request to an inanimate object. For instance, you might face the wall and politely ask for a pencil or piece of paper. Despite your doing this repeatedly, the wall will not respond because it cannot receive a message. Next, ask the child, "Close your eyes, cover your ears, and pretend to be in a different room." Then make a request the child can fulfill (e.g., "Hand me a pencil"). The child will not fulfill the request. Next, tap the child's shoulder and make the request again when the child's eyes are open and ears are uncovered. If the child complies, thank him/her for letting you know that the child received the message. Although these quick activities may seem elementary, they can help remind children about the importance of eye contact, proximity, and letting someone know you have received a message.

Alternatively, you can generate examples with a child of times when each step of the communication cycle has gone amiss for him/her.

> THERAPIST: Let's think about an example of the communication cycle. For instance, your mom is in the kitchen and asks you, while you're in the living room, to turn off the TV and come to dinner. You may or may not receive this message. What could keep you from receiving the message from your mom?

JOSÉ: If the TV is too loud, I might not hear her.

THERAPIST: Right, the TV might be too loud and drown her out. What else could keep you from getting the message?

JOSÉ: I'm so involved in the show that I tune her out.

THERAPIST: Right, being focused on the TV might keep you from hearing her. What would help you get the message from your mom?

JOSÉ: I hate it when people yell from the other room to ask me to do something. I usually just ignore them. She should come in the room and tell me.

THERAPIST: Sure, it would help if your mom came into the room. You would see her and focus your attention on her instead of the TV. She can make sure she has eye contact with you before she says what she wants. This is also more effective because you can see her nonverbal communication, too. Like if she says it with her hands on her hips and a stern voice, or if she smiles because she cooked one of your favorite meals. But your mom might not be able to come into the room if she can't leave what she's cooking, or if she's busy setting the table. What else might help you get the message?

JOSÉ: My mom won't let me turn up the TV past a certain level. That means I am more likely to hear her calling me.

THERAPIST: Good point. So keeping the TV volume lower makes it more likely that you will hear her when she calls from the other room. How would your mother know if you had received the message?

JOSÉ: I would be at the dinner table if I had.

THERAPIST: Okay, you could follow the direction, and then she would know you received the message. What other ways could you let her know you received the message?

JOSÉ: I would usually yell back, "The show's over in 5 more minutes."

THERAPIST: Okay, José, you would say something in response. That is the part of the picture where the person sends a message.

JOSÉ: She usually just yells at me to turn the TV off.

THERAPIST: So your mom receives the message and sends you another one telling you what she wants you to do. You know she heard you because of the message she sent back.

JOSÉ: Yeah, I guess. I'd rather just finish the show.

THERAPIST: So, we've gone through all of the steps in the communication cycle. Your mom sends a message; you receive the message; you send a message acknowledging the first message; then your mom receives that second message and sends you another one. Communication doesn't really happen unless the person reacts to the message by saying or doing something.

Wrap up this discussion of the communication cycle by having the child explain the four steps involved in the cycle.

Types of Nonverbal Communication

Explain to the child that the rest of the session will focus on nonverbal communication. Five types of nonverbal communication should be presented: facial expressions, body gestures, body posture, tone of voice, and personal space. You can each these most easily by sending a nonverbal message to the child, followed by a discussion of whether the child has read the nonverbal cues correctly or incorrectly and what the result is. When you are role-playing, use several types of nonverbal communication simultaneously, just as people naturally combine them in everyday situations.

> DR. SANCHEZ [therapist]: Lindsay, do you remember how you described misunderstanding Rosa? You thought she was angry with you, when really she was sad. Now that we've talked about the different types of nonverbal communication, what do you think you were noticing about her that you "misread"? Let's go through each of the five types of nonverbal communication and think this one through.
>
> LINDSAY: Well, her facial expression was "bleah." Usually she gives me a big smile when she sees me in the morning. Her body gestures were that she walked away from me. Her body posture—I'm not sure there. She didn't have a tone of voice, because she wasn't talking to me! And personal space—way too much!
>
> DR. SANCHEZ: And now that you know what her situation was, how do you rethink what you saw?
>
> LINDSAY: Well, her facial expression was just blank—like she was numb, not ignoring me. Same kind of thing with her walking away and personal space: It wasn't on purpose, it was like she was really spaced out.
>
> DR. SANCHEZ: Okay, that's a really good lesson in how to carefully check out nonverbals before you act on them. Great job, Lindsay.

Facial Expressions

Children can usually identify facial expressions depicting surprise, sadness, anger, and happiness. Using as a prompt the various emotions shown on Handout 71 (Paying Attention to Feelings), have the child guess what feeling you are portraying. Next, switch sides, and guess what emotion the child is portraying. Having a mirror nearby so that a child can see his/her own face can be helpful for children whose demonstrable emotions can be hard to detect.

Body Gestures

Gestures can be exaggerated for teaching purposes, and most children can identify several common gestures (e.g., waving "hello," "goodbye," or "come here"; shrugging your shoulders; looking at your watch; shaking your head "no"; nodding your head "yes").

Body Posture

Ask the child to identify the meaning of various body postures (e.g., crossing your arms to indicate that you are not listening or you are angry; turning your back to indicate that you are not interested; or slouching in your chair to indicate that you are bored or tired).

Tone of Voice

Tone of voice can be demonstrated by saying the same words while delivering different messages via tone of voice. For instance, you can say, "Yeah, sure," in agreement (with a positive tone) or in disagreement (with a sarcastic tone). Messages can be delivered in a whisper, a loud voice, a high-pitched tone, or sarcastically. Several phrases can be used to demonstrate (e.g., "I like you," "No, thanks," "What do you need/want?"). The same sentence can also be used to communicate several messages, depending on which word is emphasized. For example, say the sentence "I am going with her to the store," and ask the child to interpret what you mean when each word is emphasized in turn as follows:

Word(s) to Be Emphasized	*Associated Meaning*
I	*I* am going, not you or somebody else.
Am	I *am* going to go, and nothing is going to stop me.
Going	I haven't already gone; I am about to *go.*
With	I am taking her *with* me, not leaving her behind.
Her	I am going with *her,* not with someone else or you.
To [the]	I am starting my errand here, not at the store.
Store	I am going to the *store,* not someplace else.

Personal Space

The final type of nonverbal communication to be discussed is personal space. Demonstrate the use of personal space by asking, "How are you?" from various distances (e.g., across the room, at several arms' length, and close to the child). Base your choice of the closest distance on the child's comfort level; some children become distressed when they are very close to another person. Children are usually able to state that the physical distance relates to how much the person seems to care about the answer to the inquiry "How are you?"

Although close proximity can signal relational closeness, failure to maintain appropriate personal space can cause significant social issues. Children with BSD can especially lose track of boundaries and personal space in their expansiveness. Some children may need work on concrete rules for what constitutes appropriate personal space in different situations. A child may follow personal space "rules" at school and in structured situations, but may get too close to other children and family members at home and in less structured situations. Role playing is a useful way to demonstrate appropriate and inappropriate personal space for different situations.

Integrating Nonverbal Cues

Wrap up your review of nonverbal cues by an integrated presentation of all five nonverbal components as you communicate different emotions. For example, state the following sentences twice; each time, nonverbally convey one of the two emotions in parentheses. Have the child guess the emotion you mean to convey.

> "I have a test tomorrow." (scared, confused)
> "I won second place." (sad, proud)
> "Are we there yet?" (annoyed, bored)
> "I don't want to get up." (angry, relaxed)

Introducing the Paying Attention to Feelings Project

This session's take-home project emphasizes correctly reading nonverbal communication within the family. As many family members as desired can join in, using Handout 71 (Paying Attention to Feelings). The child begins by randomly selecting a feeling from the left-hand column of the handout and demonstrating it nonverbally. When parents correctly guess the feeling, a check mark is put in the box next to that feeling. A question mark is put next to feelings they cannot guess. Then roles are reversed, and parents nonverbally act out the feelings (in a mixed-up order) while the child guesses which feeling the parents are showing. There is an extra line at the bottom of the handout for the family to add another feeling to the list. Explain that no words can be used, but they can say "blah, blah, blah" if they want to show tone of voice, and they can use props from the room they are in if they wish. This project provides more practice in understanding nonverbal communication, as well as an opportunity for family members to discuss how to communicate more effectively within the family.

> Corey (age 10) and his mother, Belinda, were working on their project together. When it was Corey's turn, his first nonverbal cue was to put his hands on his hips. Belinda immediately laughed and guessed that he was acting out "angry." When it was Belinda's turn to act, Corey interpreted her nonverbal communication of "confused" as "angry." This helped Belinda see why Corey became defensive when she was asking him about his homework or activities.

In addition to the project in Handout 71, tell the child to pay attention to the nonverbal communication signals of the people around him/her (family members and kids at school), as well as to his/her own nonverbal cues.

Breathing Exercise

Review the three breathing techniques with the child, and then practice the one chosen by the child. Encourage the child to continue to practice at home between sessions.

Session Review with Parents

This session covers an exceedingly important aspect of communication, especially for children with weaknesses in reading the nonverbal cues of those around them. Make sure the child and parents understand the session's key points, which are the four steps of the communication cycle and the five types of nonverbal communication.

Take-Home Projects

New Project: Paying Attention to Feelings

Nonverbal communication skills are typically learned through modeling and observation. Encourage the child and parents to practice Paying Attention to Feelings multiple times, in order to strengthen an often weak area.

Chapter 18

Communication Skills for Parents

IF-PEP Parent Session 8
MF-PEP Parent Session 6

Session Outline

Goals:	1. Improve communication within the family.
	2. Help parents identify hurtful communications and replace these with more helpful communication strategies.
Beginning the Session:	Do a check-in and review Mood–Medication Log (Handout 32) or Mood Record (Handout 20 or 21).
	Review Problem Solving: Symptoms and Family Conflicts (Handout 65).
Lesson of the Day:	Improving communication skills

- The communication cycle
- General communication traps to avoid
- Communication traps specific to mood disorders
- How to communicate effectively with moody children

New Take-Home Project:	Out with the Old Communication, In with the New (Handout 73)
New Handouts:	72. Out with the Old Communication, In with the New (Sample)
	73. Out with the Old Communication, In with the New
Handouts to Review:	53. My Child's Educational Team (for IF-PEP only)
	65. Problem Solving: Symptoms and Family Conflicts

Session Overview

In this session for parents, the focus on coping skills continues. This time, the emphasis is on communication within the family. Communication can be a particular challenge for families coping with mood disorders. During times of transition or crisis, communication can sometimes lapse and intensify problems. An important goal of this session is to help parents identify hurtful communication patterns and styles within their own family, so they can begin to replace them with more helpful strategies.

Beginning the Session

Do a Check-In and Review Mood–Medication Log or Mood Record

Check on how the child and family have been doing since your last session. In IF-PEP, if the previous session was with school professionals, review the parents' perceptions of how the meeting went, as well as any remaining questions, concerns, or follow-up issues pertinent to the child's school situation. If there are still many issues to resolve, an in-the-bank session may be needed to address them.

Review Problem Solving: Symptoms and Family Conflicts

Next, turn your attention to the parents' Problem Solving: Symptoms and Family Conflicts project (Handout 65). The goal is for parents to begin approaching symptoms, as well as other situations related to their child's mood disorder, as problems that can be solved. Having a clear definition is half the battle; with a well-defined problem, parents are likely to be much more successful with a solution. If parents have defined the problem well and the solution they tried still did not work, they should be encouraged to keep trying. Sometimes problems cannot be definitively solved, but situations can be improved through problem solving.

Lesson of the Day: Improving Communication Skills

Although PEP emphasizes to parents that the cause of mood disorders is largely biological, remind them now that the course of illness is significantly affected by the stresses of daily life. Eliminating stress from day-to-day interactions may help to reduce the frequency or severity of symptoms. Improving communication within the family makes interactions less stressful and more productive, and can significantly improve both child and family functioning.

The Communication Cycle

In IF-PEP, parents may already be familiar with the communication cycle through hearing about their child's previous session. In reviewing the cycle for parents, emphasize the role of interpretation and misinterpretation.

Each time one family member communicates, either verbally or nonverbally, the receiver (another family member) makes an interpretation of what was meant. The receiving family member then communicates back, and this is then interpreted by the original sender. Communication is not perfect in any family, and most families have room for improvement, but the need for effective communication carries extra weight for families of children with mood disorders.

As the therapist talked about the communication cycle, Randee and Steve listened intently. Their 12-year-old daughter, Lydia, tended to be very irritable. They were becoming increasingly frustrated at how poor communication was within their family. Randee described a typical interaction: Often Lydia walked into the house looking annoyed. Randee, worried about how the afternoon and evening would go, hesitated to say anything and then asked, "Do you have a lot of homework?" Lydia generally screamed back something like "Stop yelling at me!", followed by a couple of choice curse words. Randee described feeling furious at Lydia for being so disrespectful to her. She typically resorted to threatening Lydia with a consequence for cursing at her. According to Randee, they almost never had positive communication after school.

THERAPIST: If we think about the communication cycle, how do you think Lydia might be interpreting your question about whether she has a lot of homework?

RANDEE: Well, I'm just trying to help her plan if she has a lot ...

THERAPIST: Your intentions are coming from the right place, but how do you think Lydia might be hearing the question?

RANDEE: Well, I guess if she has had a hard day and is already feeling stressed about her homework, she might feel stressed out when I ask about homework. I guess when I'm having a stressful day and the kids come in, and the kids jump right in with "What's for dinner, Mom?" instead of "How was your day?", I get annoyed.

THERAPIST: Now you are seeing the communication from Lydia's perspective. She's had a tough day, she is stressed about having to do homework, and then you ask her about homework.

Many 12-year-olds would roll their eyes and then stalk off to their bedroom in response to a parent's asking about homework. Parents who often experience extreme mood episodes with their children can often feel "on edge"—worrying about when the next episode is coming, while feeling helpless because nothing they say ever seems right. Lydia probably sensed Randee's anxiety about homework, which only added to her own anxiety. She also may have been hearing Randee's question as a criticism: "I know you aren't going to be able to handle your homework, so lay it on me: How much is there tonight?" By paying attention to her own nonverbal and verbal communication, Randee could probably significantly change the interaction.

THERAPIST: How could you change the communication cycle in this case?

RANDEE: I guess I could start by offering her a snack. She doesn't like it when I ask her how school was, either.

THERAPIST: That's a great thought—you could offer her a snack. How do you think that would sound?

RANDEE: Something like "Hey, I went to the grocery store and they had really great-looking pears. Want to share one with me?"

THERAPIST: That sounds like a great idea. What other communication strategies might work with Lydia?

RANDEE: She seems to relax the most and talk more when I'm not asking her questions. She likes to hear stories about my day, and things always go better when I can get her laughing.

THERAPIST: Those are good ideas. Don't forget about the power of being quiet. It might work for you to greet Lydia, offer her a snack, and then let things be quiet, which would give her the opportunity to steer the conversation.

STEVE: It seems like we should bring Lydia into this discussion, since she is a big part of the cycle we get into each night.

Randee and Steve decided to discuss with Lydia how the afternoons could go better if they changed their communication patterns. It became clear to Randee that although she had initially felt helpless, there were ways she could shift the cycle by changing her own verbal and nonverbal communication, and also by applying the problem-solving skills they had been working on.

General Communication Traps to Avoid

Some communication missteps are subtle, whereas others feel wrong as soon as they leave the lips. Some clear examples of hurtful communication are worth reviewing during this session. Often parents are able to recognize mistakes they are prone to making; knowing how common these mistakes are can help the parents let go of guilt and move on. The idea is to leave hurtful communication strategies behind, not to feel bad about them. As parents begin to recognize traps, they can start to find new ways to communicate. Some strategies are more obviously hurtful than others. For example, most parents know that calling names or swearing should be avoided. However, well-meaning parents easily fall into other hurtful communication strategies.

Offering Advice and Lecturing

Parents often offer advice and end up lecturing their kids. As adults, they badly want to share their experience and knowledge with their children. Kids, however, just tend to hear "Blah blah blah blah blah" and feel resentful and annoyed. If instead, parents listen carefully—asking open-ended, reflective questions, while waiting for kids to ask for assistance—the communication door opens. If parents then follow up those questions with a question such as "What ideas do you already have?", the communication cycle is well on its way to working smoothly!

Denying

Children are more prone to fall into certain traps, while parents tend to "own" others. For example, kids often make comments such as "I don't know" or "I don't care." These comments can be used to deflect attention from missteps or from something that is particularly upsetting. When children (or parents) deny, the parents (or children) can fall into the trap of arguing about the topic that is being denied.

> Randee brought up another pattern that often occurred in her communication with Lydia. In her best dramatic preteen voice, Lydia would say, "It's no big deal, Mom!" Randee talked about how frustrating it was to know that a social situation or a problem at school must be very stressful for Lydia, yet to hear Lydia dismiss the problem. Frequently, attempts at conversations about a situation that Randee saw as a "big deal" and Lydia saw as "no big deal" erupted into arguments.
>
> > THERAPIST: So how could you respond when you think something is a big deal and Lydia is in "leave me alone" mode?
> >
> > RANDEE: I guess I could try giving her some space rather than arguing with her. I do find that if I sit down near her or lay down next to her at night, she often just starts talking. I guess for me, the challenge is to avoid the trap of arguing with her. If we argue, she definitely won't talk! If it's important to her, she'll eventually start talking.

Mind Reading

Mind reading is a trap that both parents and children fall into. Kids assume what parents are thinking ("You think I'm stupid!"), and parents sometimes assume what kids are thinking. Either way, the assumptions involved in mind reading tend to shut conversation down and create significant frustration.

Trash Collecting

Both parents and kids fall into the trap of "trash collecting." That is, they bring old conflicts into the current situation (e.g., "Here we go again. Are you going to start throwing things again, like you did last time you had a meltdown?!") One of the greatest struggles for parents of a child with a mood disorder is that 5 minutes after a major meltdown, the child may behave as though the meltdown never occurred. Unfortunately for parents, memories of meltdowns tend to linger and sometimes grow bigger over time. It is critical that parents have ways to cope with their own feelings about their child's mood and behavior, other than venting their frustration onto their child.

Box 18.1 lists other hurtful communication approaches to avoid, along with examples. These include blaming, giving up, changing the subject, "ventriloquism" (speaking for others), and more.

While the focus is on communication, it is important to get parents thinking about the communication between adults in the household/extended family. The same communication strategies that are hurtful in parent–child communication can have a negative impact on adult relationships. Trash collecting, for instance, is a problem within many adult relationships.

BOX 18.1. Hurtful Communications to Avoid

Name calling/swearing:	*You *#@! idiot!*
Blaming:	*It's your fault!* Or *It's not my fault!*
Denying:	*It's not a big deal!*
Giving up:	*What's the use?*
Mind reading:	*You think my idea is stupid!*
Trash collecting (bringing up old conflicts):	*You're just like your mother!* *You never help me!* *You always work late!* *You ought to be more like Karen's husband*
Changing the subject:	*Well, how about when you . . .*
Not listening—tuning out, focusing on your own thoughts/responses:	
Interrupting:	*Wait, that's not the way it went!*
Ventriloquism (speaking for others):	*Benny really wants me to help him.*
Lecturing/giving advice before asking whether suggestions are wanted:	*How many times have I told you? Just walk away like I do.*

Communication Traps Specific to Mood Disorders

There are some "hot-button" words and phrases for children with mood disorders. These kids are often thought of as "having a bad attitude," "being lazy," "not trying hard enough," "doing things on purpose," and "acting crazy," among other things. The behaviors that evoke these hot-button phrases are often symptoms of depression, mania, or comorbid disorders. Parents need to find and use alternatives. Here are some general rules for them to follow:

- *Don't guess intent; describe behavior.* It is impossible to judge another person's effort or motivation; it is only possible to observe behavior.
- *Avoid the word "lazy."* "Lazy" is inflammatory and aggravates a situation. Lack of energy is a common symptom of depression.
- *Avoid the word "crazy."* This is name calling at its worst, and speaks to many children's inner fears that they indeed *are* crazy.
- *Avoid "You know better than that."* Comments like this serve no useful purpose. Remember the symptoms your child is struggling with. Many children with mood disorders struggle, for example, with impulsivity.

In addition, the sentences in italics in the following list are some specific alternatives to common inflammatory ones:

- Instead of "You're never going to get anywhere with an attitude like that!"
  - *"You seem really annoyed. What do you think would make the situation better right now?"*
- Instead of "You're just being lazy."
  - *"You don't seem to have much energy right now. What could help rev your engine a bit?"*
- Instead of "You're not trying hard enough."
  - *"I'm concerned that the evening is almost over and you haven't started your homework. How do you want to structure this next hour to get your work done?"*
- Instead of "You did that on purpose just to irritate me!"
  - *"I'm really frustrated because you missed the bus, and now I need to drive you to school before going to work. After school today, let's work on a better morning plan."*
- Instead of "You're acting crazy."
  - *"You look really upset to me. What would help you calm down right now?"*
- Instead of "Why did you just do that? You know better than that!"
  - *"I need you to put the markers down now. We'll discuss after dinner how to make amends with your brother for scribbling on his homework."*

How to Communicate Effectively with Moody Children

So if parents shouldn't call names, blame, give up, read minds, interrupt, or lecture ... what should they do? We give parents the following recommendations.

Be Empathic

The first thing parents need to do is be empathic. If parents can stop and consider what their child is feeling before responding, many opportunities for communication will go better. When Randee put herself in Lydia's shoes (what a challenge it was for Lydia to get through the school day, how much she needed a break before homework), she immediately thought of several better ways to approach Lydia after school instead of bringing up homework.

Remember That Timing Is Everything

Often parents and children do need to communicate about challenging topics such as homework completion and household chores. *When* a topic is broached can be almost as important as *how*. Again, Randee found that just when Lydia had gotten off the school bus and before she had had a snack was not a great time for Randee to bring up a difficult topic. Also, if a child is in the midst of a "can't" time, when anything a parent says is likely to lead to a blow-up, the parent should let the topic go. No chore or piece of homework is worth a rage. If the parent lets it go, there is a reasonable chance that an improved mood is around the corner and that things will work out better than if dealt with in the "can't" moment.

Be Aware of Your Own—and Your Child's—Nonverbal Cues

Children read every nonverbal as well as verbal communication that parents make. Sometimes they read in more than what was intended, or understand a communication to mean something different from what the parent intended. As discussed in Chapter 17, nonverbal cues include facial expression, body gestures, posture, tone of voice, and personal space. Noticing a child's nonverbal communication may help parents understand what he/she is trying to say, as well as how intensely their child feels about an issue.

Hold and Acknowledge the Child's Feelings

One of the extra challenges for parents is being ready to hold and acknowledge the child's feelings. Acknowledging a child's feelings can be a very helpful communication tool and can lead to productive conversations.

> After discussing holding and acknowledging feelings during the session, Melissa said, "I think I know what you are talking about." She went on to describe an interaction she had had with her 8-year-old son, Brandon, after his first day of third grade. He had come off the bus looking miserable. A couple of kids from the street were hollering at Brandon to come play, but Melissa had just gotten the sense that he needed a little break. She called out to him, "Brandon, I have something to show you inside. Come in for a few minutes to see it, and then you can join your friends." Brandon yelled to his friends that he would be out in a few minutes and walked home with his mother. Once they were inside, she showed him a funny card she had gotten in the

mail that day and gave him a snack. She also asked whether he would like his back scratched (something he tended to like when feeling upset). As she scratched his back, she said, "You seem upset today." That one comment opened the floodgates. Everything that had bothered him about the day came flooding out.

In this example, Melissa got a number of things right. She was empathic; her timing was good; and she read her son's verbal and especially his nonverbal communication very well. She also gave him a face-saving way of leaving his friends: The lure of something she wanted to show him made him more likely to follow her suggestion without protest or humiliation. Finally, her timing for addressing his feelings was very good—she waited until he was inside and she had provided some initial comfort before commenting that something seemed wrong.

Make Sure Positives Outweigh Negatives

It is often easier for parents to criticize than it is to find something positive to emphasize. However, people respond better to positive comments than they do to negative comments. This leaves parents with a significant challenge—how to address behavior problems and simultaneously motivate change. The secret lies in the balance. Parents need to find a way to make at least one, and preferably two, positive comments for each negative comment. Alternatively, negative comments can be rephrased positively. For example, "You left the door open again. You have to close the doors!" can be restated in a more positive way, such as "Please close the door. I know you care about keeping our pets safe." The habit of making negative comments can be a tough one for parents to break, especially when a child is exhibiting challenging behavior throughout the day. One little strategy parents can use is to start the day with a number of pennies or paper clips in one pocket and then shift them one by one to the other pocket for each positive comment. This system not only reminds parents, but keeps track of the number of positive comments a parent has made, and so it can help build the positive comment habit.

Be Direct

We all need to vent sometimes to a good friend, but it is also important to address problems directly with the other person involved, especially issues that occur regularly.

As the discussion about direct communication progressed, Belinda (see Chapter 17) got very quiet. She said very little during most of the session.

THERAPIST: You seem very quiet, Belinda. Are you okay?

BELINDA: I'm feeling kind of bad about something. When you were talking about direct communication, I started to wonder if I have been falling into that trap a lot.

MAC [Belinda's husband]: What do you mean?

BELINDA: Well, I talk to my sister Molly a lot, and I sometimes vent to her, but I don't think that really helps communication at home.

THERAPIST: You're right. Although venting can feel good at the time, it doesn't tend to change things. What specifically has been bothering you that you haven't been communicating about?

BELINDA: Well, I sometimes don't feel like we're working as a team in raising Corey. I have been silently wishing that you would be more involved in Corey's treatment, except, of course, for when I complain to Molly.

MAC: I guess I'm surprised to hear this, since Belinda has never mentioned any of this to me before.

THERAPIST: The good news is that you are both here now. This can be the beginning of more direct communication and more collaboration.

Belinda probably experienced a lot of relief after having this discussion, while Mac, as he noted, probably felt taken by surprise. Most people are poor at mind reading. Clear, positive, direct communication is much more effective at getting needs met than wishful thinking is!

Take Ownership

If one person in a dyad owns his/her part of an issue, it is easier for the other half of the dyad to accept and follow through at his/her end. Using what we refer to as "*XYZ talk*" can be helpful. *XYZ talk* sounds like this: "When you do *X*, I feel *Y*. I would like you to do *Z*." In the real world, it sounds like this example: "When you come home right in the middle of bedtime, the kids get all wound up, and I feel resentful and frustrated. I would like you to come home in time to help with bedtime, or, if you absolutely have to work late, come home after bedtime." This strategy works best when the *XYZ* statement is delivered without a lot of emotion.

Ask Questions First

Questions, when used judiciously, are an incredibly important communication tool. Questions should be used by the listener to make sure that he/she understands (e.g., "Do you mean you don't want to go to soccer?"), as well as by the speaker to ensure that he/she is being understood (e.g., "Am I making sense?"). Questions are particularly critical with kids who may shut down unless they feel understood. In addition to parents' needing to use questions to keep the conversation going, children tend to skip parts of stories, so that questions become especially important.

Apply the Golden Rule

The "golden rule" that many of us learned in kindergarten certainly holds true in family communication: It is important for parents to remember to speak in both words and actions (nonverbal communication) in the same way they would like their children to address them. Children tend to be particularly sensitive to tone, and parents are often accused of "yelling." Children will sometimes use the word "yelling" to describe anything they perceive as an angry tone. Given that parents often find angry tones to be disrespectful, it is important for parents to model a pleasant tone, so that children will also learn to use a pleasant (or at least neutral) tone when communicating with others.

Take Turns

The give and take of conversation with kids is different from that between two adults. It is easy for adults to fall into the trap of talking too much. It is really important for parents to take turns talking and listening. Listening to kids can involve being quiet, a lot!

Keep Cool

In the midst of communication, it is critical for parents to "keep their cool." This means watching their tone of voice and body language throughout an interaction. If parents find that they cannot stay calm during a particular interaction, their best bet is to find a way to take a break, then resume the conversation once they are calm again. In some situations, and with some children, this can be used as an opportunity to model respectful communication strategies (e.g., "I am so frustrated right now that I need to take a break before we finish talking about this"). In other situations, particularly if a child would escalate his/her behavior upon sensing a parent's high emotional level, it is better to use a neutral excuse to take a break (e.g., "I've got to go to the bathroom—I'll be right back").

Use Humor, but Avoid Sarcasm

Using humor means saying and doing things that parents and child can laugh about together. A silly comment or slapstick maneuver can often significantly reduce tension and possibly facilitate communication.

However, biting sarcasm is likely to worsen rather than facilitate communication, for several reasons. It is difficult for children, for many teens, and sometimes even for adults to interpret, and a person in a heightened emotional state will have a difficult time reading it. Children with learning disabilities (verbal or nonverbal) may have particular difficulty interpreting sarcasm. Moreover, sarcasm can be a form of verbal aggression that is thinly veiled as humor. Sarcasm is often delivered without awareness of its negative impact; parents need to be self-aware about their use of it. It can escalate a situation. Children often respond to sarcasm with comments like "Stop yelling at me" or "You're being mean."

> Belinda could feel her frustration building as she tried to get Corey to start on his homework. Having just talked about communication the night before in her PEP session, she thought about her nonverbal communication. She realized that her hands had gravitated to her hips, and that her body language probably looked pretty threatening and tense. Corey had complained before about how she put her hands on her hips and looked "angry" when she "yelled" at him. She decided to make fun of herself and said, "Corey, will you look at this? My hands just jumped to my hips against my will! Help me get them off!" After a friendly wrestling match and a good laugh, Corey was able to settle down to work on his homework.

Deal with Issues When They're Small

Parents should strive to address issues when they are small, rather than waiting until a crisis builds. In general, communication and problem solving are much more effective when the issue being addressed has not become a crisis.

Be Brief and Clear

Communication needs to be concise and clear—for example, "Please move your back-pack from the floor to your bedroom now." Parents should avoid including extraneous information in their requests for action. Lots of reasoning or justification hides the request in too many words.

Take-Home Project

New Project: Out with the Old Communication, In with the New

The new parent project for this session focuses on improving verbal and nonverbal communication. It is easy for parents to fall into the trap of using hurtful communication strategies. Out with the Old Communication, In with the New (Handouts 72 and 73) encourages parents to become more aware of their own communication and begin to replace hurtful strategies with more helpful ones. Parents are asked to record one time each day when they lapsed into an old or hurtful communication pattern, when they caught themselves, and what new or helpful communication pattern they could use instead. Handout 72 is a sample completed version that can be used to explain the project. Handout 73 is the blank form for parent completion.

Chapter 19

Verbal Communication Skills for Children

IF-PEP Child Session 9
MF-PEP Child Session 7

Session Outline

Goal:	Help the child recognize components of effective verbal communication.
Beginning the Session:	Do a check-in with parents. Review Paying Attention to Feelings (Handout 71). Have child identify and rate feelings.
Lesson of the Day:	Effective verbal communication • Review of communication cycle and nonverbal components • Helpful versus hurtful words • "I" statements • Misleading slang
Breathing Exercise:	Child's choice (Belly, Bubble, Balloon Breathing)
Session Review with Parents	
New Take-Home Project:	Let's Talk (Handouts 75 and 76)

Ongoing Take-Home Project: Selected healthy habits chart (for IF-PEP
                                only) (Handout 40, 44, or 47)

New Handouts: 74. Verbal Communication
                             75. Let's Talk (Sample)
                             76. Let's Talk

Handouts to Review: 68. Communication
                             69. The Communication Cycle
                             70. Nonverbal Communication
                             76. Paying Attention to Feelings

Session Overview

The previous child session has covered general issues related to communication, as well as specific nonverbal communication skills. The key points from that previous session are reviewed, and then this session covers verbal communication. The focus is on how to stop hurtful words and phrases and to replace them with more helpful verbal expressions, including "I" statements. Most of the therapy content has now been taught to the child, and you should use opportunities as they arise in the session to refer back to previously learned concepts (Thinking, Feeling, Doing; problem solving; the Tool Kit; etc.) to reinforce learning and generalization of new skills.

Beginning the Session

Do a Check-In with Parents

Check in with the child and parents about the child's week at the start of this session. Also ask whether they have any questions related to their last session on communication skills. This leads into a review of the project from the previous child session.

Review Paying Attention to Feelings

Next, review the Paying Attention to Feelings project (Handout 71) from the previous child session. Reviewing this with the parents and child together allows the family to discuss which feelings were challenging to demonstrate and interpret, and how misperceptions can interfere with everyday life.

THERAPIST: (*looking toward Ranjit*) During our last session, we talked about nonverbal communication, and your project was to really pay attention to your own nonverbal communication, as well as other people's nonverbal communication. Do you remember the different types of nonverbal communication?

RANJIT: I remember facial expressions and gestures and tone of voice. I can't remember the other ones.

THERAPIST: Body posture and personal space.

RANJIT: Oh, yeah. I paid attention to tone of voice a lot, because I'm sometimes not sure if people are mad at me.

LAKSHMI [Ranjit's mother]: Ranjit has asked me, and even his teacher a couple of times, whether I am mad at him. It really helps when he asks instead of assuming and getting angry back.

THERAPIST: Good work. I'm glad you are paying attention. It's definitely better to ask if you aren't sure! The times you asked, did your mom or your teacher ever say they were angry?

RANJIT: No.

THERAPIST: Hmmm … they could sound angry and not realize it, or maybe you are extra sensitive and worried about people being angry. What do you think?

RANJIT: I think maybe I am extra sensitive, but when my mom is busy, sometimes she sounds angry.

THERAPIST: So you learned about yourself, and also about your mom. What can you do if your mom looks busy?

RANJIT: I could offer to help her, and I could remind myself that she is busy.

THERAPIST: Those are great ideas. It's important to understand things about yourself, but also about the people around you, so keep practicing. Maybe practicing will help you be a little less sensitive and worried, and will remind you to pay attention to what is going on with the people around you. How did your practice games go?

LAKSHMI: We had a good time playing the games as a family. We made cards and played charades all together.

THERAPIST: I'm so glad you had a good experience. It sounds like Ranjit learned some things. I really encourage you to keep practicing paying attention to non-verbal communication—both your own and other people's.

This project tends to be enjoyable for families and easily incorporates siblings. The review of this exercise is likely to be brief. Families should be encouraged to continue to attend to how nonverbal communication is perceived, and to be mindful of what they express nonverbally.

Have Child Identify and Rate Feelings

After the parents leave the session, do a quick check-in with the child to identify and rate the strength of his/her feelings. If needed, use Handouts 1 (Feelings) and 2 (Strength of Feelings) to prompt the child to provide this information.

Lesson of the Day: Effective Verbal Communication

Review of Communication Cycle and Nonverbal Components

This session begins with a brief review of (1) the reasons why communication is important (i.e., to let others know what we are thinking and feeling, to learn what others are thinking and feeling, to build relationships, and to solve problems); (2) the four steps in the communication cycle; and (3) components of nonverbal communication. Explain that whereas the previous session focused on understanding nonverbal communication, this session will focus on verbal communication.

Helpful versus Hurtful Communication

Next, engage children in a discussion of helpful versus hurtful verbal communication. Ask children to provide examples of times when they have said things that they did not mean or later regretted. Add these examples to the column of hurtful verbal statements in Handout 74 (Verbal Communication). Then ask children how they felt after the hurtful communication happened. Children need to recognize the consequences of hurtful communication. By this session, children are used to thinking in terms of "helpful" and "hurtful," so this is usually an easy concept to convey. It also reinforces learning in previous sessions (e.g., Thinking, Feeling, Doing).

> DR. SANDY [therapist]: Lisa, can you think of any times when you used hurtful words with someone?
>
> LISA: Yes (*looks down at the floor*) The other day I was really mad, and I yelled at David [her little brother]. I told him I hated him and I wished he was dead.
>
> DR. SANDY: Wow, those are pretty strong words. What did David do when he heard them?
>
> LISA: He started to cry, and he hasn't played with me since then.
>
> DR. SANDY: So that's a pretty good sign that those words were really hurtful, because you've told me before how much David likes to play with you. It is extra hard to hear hurtful words from someone who is important to you. We're going to work today on coming up with more helpful words that still let you communicate what you are thinking and feeling, but in a way that doesn't hurt other people.

Children need to understand how to express their thoughts and feelings in ways that honestly convey what they are thinking and feeling, yet that do not violate the rules they have learned for evaluating actions: (1) "Does it hurt me?" (2) "Does it hurt someone or something else?" (3) "Does it get anyone in trouble?" Discuss with children how people who are upset or have strong feelings often say hurtful things to others. Because it can be quite difficult to communicate in a helpful way while feeling very strongly, remind children to use an idea from their Tool Kit to calm themselves down before communicating.

DR. SANDY: Lisa, can you think of certain times or situations when you have been more likely to use hurtful words?

LISA: Not really. They just pop out sometimes.

DR. SANDY: Hmmm … let me think. You've given me a couple of examples of using hurtful words when you've either been really tired or feeling pretty stressed. Do you think being tired or stressed makes it more likely that you would use hurtful words?

LISA: Yeah, I guess. I hadn't really thought about that before.

DR. SANDY: Well, I know you've been working really hard on getting your sleep schedule back on track, and from all the stuff you've been telling me, I think that is working pretty well. So maybe today we could focus on what you can do when you're feeling stressed.

LISA: Okay.

DR. SANDY: For example, when you said those words to David, it was right after your mom got a call from your teacher and then asked you about the trouble you had gotten into at school. How were you feeling then?

LISA: Pretty embarrassed and mad at myself for getting into a fight at school.

DR. SANDY: I bet you were. And good for you that you can recognize your hurtful feelings and how they are connected to the hurtful words you spoke. After your mom talked to you, what might you have been able to do to help yourself calm down?

LISA: I probably should have gone to my room. That's one of my best tools for calming down.

DR. SANDY: Okay, it's good you could think of a tool from your Tool Kit. Would it be useful for your mom to suggest in a nice way that you go to your room if she sees you are upset?

LISA: Yeah, as long as she said it nicely and not like it was a punishment.

DR. SANDY: That's a really good point. If your mom can prompt you nicely, it will help you make good choices. Let's make sure we talk with her about that at the end of the session. But now let's think about how your conversation with David could have gone differently.

LISA: Well, if I had gone to my room and started to cool down, then David came and asked me to play a game, I might have just told him that I would play with him later, that I wasn't in the mood to play right then.

DR. SANDY: How do you think David would have responded to those words, instead?

LISA: Well (*laughs a little*), he still would have wanted to play right away, but he's usually pretty good about waiting if I tell him I'll play with him later.

DR. SANDY: Excellent. Words like "I'm not in the mood to play right now, David" are very helpful. They communicate how you are honestly thinking and feeling, but in a very helpful way.

"I" Statements

In learning how to replace hurtful words with helpful ones, children need to learn specific communication strategies. "I" statements are among these important strategies. Using "I" statements can convey thoughts and feelings without hurting someone else. "I" statements allow children to express themselves without placing blame on others who might become defensive or fail to receive the message; take responsibility or ownership of their thoughts and feelings; and communicate their thoughts and feelings about a specific situation. The formula for an "I" statement is "I feel _____ when _____." Provide some examples of situations where "I" statements could be helpful.

LETICIA [therapist]: D'Shaun, let's think about how things went when you were the last kid to be picked up after play practice at school. Do you remember what you said to your dad and what happened next?

D'SHAUN: Boy, do I ever—I was grounded for a week! And my drama teacher was super-annoyed that I wasn't allowed to come to the next rehearsal.

LETICIA: So let's do the play-by-play. When your dad came 30 minutes late, you said …

D'SHAUN: (*in an angry voice*) Didn't I tell you when you were supposed to be here? How come you had to make me wait so long? I'm the last one to get picked up, and it's freezing outside!

LETICIA: And then your dad said …

D'SHAUN: (*imitating his father*) Son, you can just be glad you're getting a ride at all. And if it's such a problem to come home from play practice, you can just skip it for the rest of the week!

LETICIA: Ouch! Now let's think about how that whole scene could have gone differently. Try using an "I" statement, like we were just talking about. Your dad comes 30 minutes late to pick you up, and you *could* say …

D'SHAUN: I feel worried when all the other kids have been picked up and you aren't at school yet. I tried calling you on your cell phone, but you didn't answer. I didn't know if you wanted me to just wait for you, call Mom, or start walking home.

LETICIA: What do you think your father might have said?

D'SHAUN: He might have said something like "I'm so sorry! My cell phone died, and I hit a lot of traffic. Next time something like that happens, you should call Mom."

LETICIA: Wow, things can really turn out differently when you use those "I" statements!

Review several examples of how communication can be transformed from hurtful to helpful when "I" statements are used.

Misleading Slang

A final, common issue in verbal communication is the ubiquitous use of slang expressions by children. Phrases such as "I could just die!" or "I could kill him for saying that!" are common playground talk. However, for parents of a child with a mood disorder, these otherwise insignificant phrases can strike terror in the heart ("What if he really means it?"). To help children recognize more clear and direct ways to communicate their feelings, calmly point out to them that although these phrases may be commonly used by other children their age, their literal meanings are very alarming. Finish this discussion by having children replace the hurtful statements in Handout 74 (Verbal Communication) with helpful ones.

Introducing the Let's Talk Exercise

Next, turn the discussion to how communication can go poorly or well within the family. Using Handouts 75 and 76 (the completed-sample and blank version of Let's Talk), ask children what steps could be taken within their own families to improve communication. Children often need a concrete example from which to work, such as a topic over which children and parents often argue. Help children to list three things they wish their parents could do differently to communicate better about this topic, and three things the children themselves could do differently. Often children can generate a list of how their parents could behave differently, but struggle to find their own ways to contribute constructively. Help children, as needed, to convert negative (e.g., "They don't listen") or absolute (e.g., "Let me do all the talking") terms into more positive, less black-and-white terms. For example, "They don't listen" can be replaced with "Allow me time to talk." "Let me do the talking" can be changed to "Let me share my side." Completing both arrows in Handout 76 (what children can do and what parents can do) reiterates the importance of give and take in communication about a contentious topic, and of reaching a compromise through problem solving.

Breathing Exercise

Do a quick check-in with a child on the whens and wheres of ongoing breathing practice, and share a couple of deep breaths with the child in session. This allows you to check on the child's correct diaphragmatic breathing, as well as the mastery of slow, measured breathing in and out.

Session Review with Parents

Have the child "teach" the Lesson of the Day to the parents: helpful versus hurtful words, using Tool Kit strategies to calm down, using "I" statements, and avoiding misleading slang.

Take-Home Projects

New Project: Let's Talk

Have the child show parents Handouts 75 and 76 (the Let's Talk sample and the blank version you and the child have filled in). Give the family a second blank copy, and ask them to work on completing it together.

Ongoing Project: Selected Healthy Habits Chart

In IF-PEP only, the child should continue working toward changing the second habit selected in the previous healthy habits sessions (and on maintaining change in the first habit).

Chapter 20

Planning for Symptom and Crisis Management with Parents

IF-PEP Parent Session 9
MF-PEP Parent Session 7

Session Outline

Goals:

1. Help parents develop strategies to manage mood symptoms and plan for crises.
2. Help parents develop stress management strategies for themselves.
3. Prepare for sibling session (for IF-PEP only).
4. (for IF-PEP only) plan any additional in-the-bank sessions.

Beginning the Session:

Do a check-in and review Mood–Medication Log (Handout 32) or Mood Record (Handout 20 or 21).

Review Out with the Old Communication, In with the New (Handout 73).

Lesson of the Day:

Planning for symptom and crisis management
- Managing mania
- Managing depression

- Creating a safety plan
- Managing suicidality
- Hospitalization: When it's necessary and how it works
- Managing parental stress
- Preparing for the IF-PEP sibling session

Take-Home Projects: Preparing the child in treatment and siblings for the IF-PEP sibling session
Let's Talk (for MF-PEP) (Handouts 75 and 76)

New Handouts: 75. Let's Talk (Sample) (previously distributed to child)
76. Let's Talk (previously distributed to child)

Handouts to Review: 72. Out with the Old Communication, In with the New (Sample)
73. Out with the Old Communication, In with the New

Session Overview

This is the last regularly scheduled parent-only session. It is designed to address the unique challenges of raising a child with a mood disorder, and it helps parents apply the skills learned in previous sessions to the specific aspects of their child's mood disorder. Parents should come away from this session with a commitment to planning ahead to prevent, or at least to deescalate, future crises. Content to cover includes the following: strategies for managing manic and depressive symptoms; the importance of having a safety plan, and the elements that this plan should include; managing suicidal concerns; learning about hospitalization; and managing parental stress. In MF-PEP, cover all these issues, as they will apply immediately to at least some group members and may apply to others in the future. In IF-PEP, it is important to prepare for this session with the child's symptoms and the family's needs in mind. For example, if the child is young and symptoms have been mild, focus on those topics most relevant to the family; although knowledge is empowering, too much information about symptoms that have not been encountered can be anxiety-provoking. The next scheduled session in IF-PEP is for siblings, so take time in this session to plan how best to structure that session. Parents also typically use this session to review concerns about unresolved family and school issues. Decisions about the need for additional in-the-bank sessions should be made before the end of this session.

Beginning the Session

Do a Check-In and Review Mood–Mediation Log or Mood Record

Complete a brief review of how the child and family have been doing since the last session.

Review Out with the Old Communication, In with the New

In the previous session, parents were assigned to use Handout 73 (Out with the Old Communication, In with the New) to notice and record their "old, hurtful" language and write "new, helpful" language that could replace it. We have been impressed with how honest parents are in admitting to the use of hurtful language. Many parents are surprised to see how pervasive a pattern this can be within their homes. It can be a powerful intervention to review this exercise empathically with parents, acknowledging how easy it is to fall into a rut with negative language. At the same time, emphasize the importance of getting out of this rut and adopting healthy communication patterns with, and for, their children. If parents themselves experience mood symptoms (most notably irritability), changing communication patterns in the family can be very significant; it can improve much more than the child's symptoms. We have seen "ripple effects" in improved communication and relationships between spouses and other parent–child dyads within the family when this exercise is actively utilized.

> DR. JACKSON [therapist]: So, Marlene and Todd, how did you do with monitoring your communication with Benjamin this past week?
>
> TODD: To tell you the truth, it was pretty embarrassing. Marlene has told me before that I'm too hard on Benjamin, but I didn't really realize it until we started recording after last session.
>
> MARLENE: Yes, and I'm not innocent, either. My mom used to get on my case all the time when I was growing up—and when we filled out our worksheet after last session, I realized I was saying the same kind of negative stuff that drove me crazy listening to her when I was a kid.
>
> DR. JACKSON: Wow. Sounds like this exercise was a pretty important one to do in your family. How long would it take after you said the unhelpful words for you to catch yourself?
>
> TODD: The more I started to pay attention, the quicker I got. By this past weekend, I even was able to stop myself before saying some things I probably would have regretted, and reworded what I wanted to tell Benjamin.
>
> MARLENE: Once I caught on to how much I was sounding like my mom, I got a lot quicker at catching myself as well.
>
> DR. JACKSON: Excellent—and how did you do with coming up with more helpful, constructive communication to replace your hurtful words?
>
> MARLENE: That took some work, but I think I'm getting there.

TODD: Same with me.

DR. JACKSON: Well, we don't have an "official" project at the end of this session, other than to plan for next week's session, when Melissa and Rachel [Benjamin's older and younger sisters] attend. So maybe you could keep recording your communication between now and then, to make even more progress and really solidify the new habits you are developing. I think you'll notice that as your communication with Benjamin becomes more positive and constructive, you'll see the same kind of changes coming from him.

TODD: Makes sense to me!

In this example, Todd and Marlene each experienced an "aha" moment in response to doing their project. In other cases, however, the level of parental stress and/or severity of parental mood symptoms (irritability in particular) can make it difficult for parents to consistently replace unhelpful communication with more helpful ways of talking to their child. As you review this project with parents, assess how successful the parents have been. If they are catching on and making some progress, encourage them to continue working on it. If you sense that high stress or parental mood symptoms are impeding progress, you may need to address these issues specifically—possibly through suggesting the use of an in-the-bank session—in order for family communication to improve substantively.

Lesson of the Day:
Planning for Symptom and Crisis Management

Explain to parents that unique skills are needed to parent a child with a mood disorder. Parents need to know what to do when their child exhibits symptoms of depression or mania, particularly when suicidal or other dangerous behavior is involved. The information in this session can help parents become more effective in maximizing their child's health and well-being.

Managing Mania

Children with BSD periodically exhibit some very challenging symptoms. Parents need to be aware of these symptoms and what they can look like in the early stages. When symptoms are recognized early and problems are treated while still small, the course of illness can be significantly improved.

THERAPIST: Tracy, Keely has been diagnosed with bipolar disorder for a couple of years now. It seems like you are getting really good at monitoring where she's at with her mood. What do you notice as she is starting to cycle?

TRACY: Well, just after starting to work with you a few months ago, I noticed that Keely's sleep was changing. She was having trouble falling asleep, but she was also getting up 30 to 40 minutes before she needed to, in order to get to school on time. This made me really nervous, as we had just gotten her settled down the month before.

THERAPIST: So what did you do when you noticed this?

TRACY: I called Keely's psychiatrist's office. They were really good about it and got me in for an appointment right away. We decided to slightly increase the evening dose of one of Keely's medications. Once we did this, Keely began falling asleep easier, and her morning routine began to shift back to normal. I felt like we "dodged a bullet."

THERAPIST: Good for you! You have really gotten good at monitoring Keely and problem solving when you see worrisome signs.

When the early stages of a manic episode are noticed and caught, medication adjustments are often easier. However, it can be difficult to pick up the early stages of mania if the child has been depressed and uninterested in anything for a long period of time. The beginnings of a "high" mood may initially seem pleasant, especially in contrast with the irritability and anhedonia that depression can bring. This is a good time to remind parents how important it is to keep records on a child's moods.

During the early stages of mania, it is important to avoid highly stimulating situations such as large gatherings or sleep-disrupting activities (e.g., sleepovers). Parents should focus on maintaining structure and sticking as close to the sleep routine as possible. During a manic episode, it is helpful to avoid arguing and carefully pick which battles are important to fight for health and safety reasons. If mood symptoms raise any safety concerns (e.g., reckless behavior, suicidality, or aggression toward others), parents will need to plan accordingly. Safety planning is discussed in more detail later in this chapter.

Diego had been quiet for much of the discussion about managing mania, but when the therapist raised the issue of avoiding arguments, he began to share his thoughts. His 9-year-old son, Miguel, had been diagnosed with BD-NOS 1½ years ago. Diego talked about how long it had taken him to learn to avoid arguing with Miguel. He talked about how frustrating it was to listen to Miguel talk on and on about some unrealistic plan that was doomed to failure and likely to cause profound disappointment. Diego described how strong the urge was to argue with him, set him on a more realistic path, and ultimately protect him from the disappointment of the plan's failure. He shook his head. "I have finally learned to just quietly nod my head, then to be there to support Miguel when his unrealistic plan fails. At least then Miguel feels supported by me."

With mania come grandiosity and lack of insight. Problem-solving skills are clearly affected by this! If a child feels that he/she is able to accomplish some unrealistic feat, it is not useful to argue about whether or not the feat is possible for the child. It may be important, however, to forbid the activity if it is dangerous, is too expensive, or requires time or participation from someone who is not available. For example, parents are not available at dinnertime on a school night for a special trip to the office supply store. An important topic to discuss in this session is how to say "no" in these situations without arguing and, ideally, without triggering meltdowns. Helpful strategies to suggest include starting out with empathy (e.g., "Wow, it's really important to you to do this project, isn't it?"), and engaging the child in a joint problem-solving process so that the actual project or its timing can be made more feasible (and often can be scaled down). If the child is already too high in the mania, a calm, quiet response focusing on bringing the child's mood back down will be necessary before other problem solving can occur.

Manic episodes often do not end abruptly. Full remission may take weeks or even months to accomplish. As symptoms wane, expectations should gradually increase, so that the child and family can get back to "business as usual." Behavior during manic episodes can be embarrassing, so a child should not be reminded of how he/she acted during an episode. The exception to this rule occurs when a child is either unaware of the symptoms or denies that there is a problem. In this case, it may be important to review symptoms (preferably in a therapy session), to help the child increase his/her awareness and become a part of managing the illness. Readiness for being an active participant in symptom management varies from child to child.

Managing Depression

Just like mania, depression can sneak up on families. Gradually increasing irritability can seem situational until it reaches a critical point. However, when family members regularly monitor a child's mood and check in with each other, the early signs of depression can be caught. These may include sleep changes, critical or negative thinking, loss of interest in activities, social isolation, decreased concentration, and increased problems at school. So, in addition to bringing accurate information about symptoms to their treatment teams, what else can parents do to help their child manage?

A return to the Tool Kit and Thinking, Feeling, Doing is a good first step. Both children and parents need to choose helpful actions and focus on helpful thoughts. Communication strategies become even more important, as do healthy habits (i.e., eating well, maintaining good sleep hygiene, and exercising regularly). As we have noted throughout this book, healthy habits are "free treatment"; they have no side effects and typically no financial cost. They are tremendously beneficial in the face of depression. Unfortunately, depression can make it difficult to maintain these habits, and it may take some creativity to sustain them. Children may say that playing video games or increasing "screen time" helps them when they are depressed, but these are often short-term fixes. Other innovative ways to keep a child engaged in pursuing healthy habits include these:

- Help others in need (e.g., animals, the elderly, persons with intellectual deficiencies)
- Write in a journal
- Spend time with a special person
- Exercise:
  - Stretching (relieves tension)
  - Aerobics (lets off steam, energizes)
  - Strengthening (builds stamina)

- Engaging in an activity that the child usually enjoys
- Doing something creative (art, music, building)

As with managing mania, children vary in their self-awareness and ability to take an active role in managing their depressive symptoms.

Creating a Safety Plan

Families with children whose mood symptoms are mild may only need a very brief mention of this section's resources. However, families with children whose symptoms are moderate to severe often benefit from a more detailed discussion of safety issues. Parents' advance preparation can shift a difficult situation from dangerous to manageable. As with childbirth, having a plan reduces anxiety and provides focus for family members who might otherwise panic!

First, parents need to think about how their child's crises have manifested themselves in the past. They can then begin to think ahead about how to plan for safety. If a child's mood shifts have been associated with violence, siblings may need to be able to lock their bedroom doors so that they have someplace safe to go. Locks on doors provide physical and emotional safety for siblings during outbursts and periods of aggression. If this strategy is employed, it is critical for the parents to have access to keys.

Parents also need to know how and when, or when not, to do a therapeutic hold with their child. If a mother is 5 feet 2 inches tall and weighs 120 pounds, and her son is 4 feet 10 inches tall and weighs 100 pounds, she probably cannot hold him safely in the midst of a crisis. Part of the plan should be identifying someone who is immediately available if the need for a therapeutic hold arises. If no one is available and anyone's safety is at risk (including that of the child in crisis), the police typically have the quickest response time. Part of a good safety plan includes knowing how and when to contact emergency services, such as the police. The idea of calling the police is extremely anxiety-provoking for many parents. Increasingly, however, community police are willing to meet with families prior to a crisis. This provides parents the opportunity to explain their child's condition, possible risks, and their preferred methods of deescalating emergency situations. As with all other aspects of crisis management, thinking things through and planning ahead will be immensely helpful.

A couple of months before Cindy started PEP with her 11-year-old son, Evan, they went through a very rough phase. Evan was having frequent meltdowns that often escalated into his throwing things and becoming aggressive with Cindy. During these episodes, Cindy would send her 8-year-old daughter to her room so that she would be safe—but then Cindy would struggle with Evan, trying to prevent him from destroying things or hurting her. At one point, she was covered with bruises and felt that she was at the end of her rope. Evan's adjustment to his medication had ended that episode, but Cindy was painfully aware that a similar episode could occur again. In session, she talked about how bad things had been.

Cindy and her therapist then worked together to identify triggers and ways to reduce the intensity and frequency of aggressive outbursts. They also worked on developing an emergency safety plan. Cindy was a single mother and could not think of anyone whom she could call to help her if Evan were to get aggressive again, so they talked about calling the police in such a situation. After that session, Cindy called her local police department and spoke with the sergeant in charge of juvenile affairs. She explained that her son had a brain illness, BD, and was getting treatment for it, but that sometimes crises arose. She asked the sergeant how a police officer would respond if she ever needed to call. He explained that the officer would attempt to talk with Evan and help him deescalate his behavior, and would only physically restrain him if talking was not working. The next time Evan started to get out of control, Cindy knew she had a plan. She calmly told Evan that hurting people and damaging property were not acceptable, and that he could find an appropriate choice (such as getting on the trampoline), or she would need to call the police to help him calm down. The first time she tried this, Evan did not respond, and she did call the police. As soon as he saw that his mother had called, Evan started crying and curled up on the kitchen floor. By the time the police had arrived, the aggression had stopped, and there was little for the police to do. The next time Cindy gave him the "find an appropriate way to manage yourself without hurting anyone or anything, or I will call the police to keep us all safe" talk, Evan stormed outside and spent the next 30 minutes jumping on the trampoline.

For Cindy and Evan, planning was everything. She knew the circumstances under which she would need to call. She had spoken to the police department in advance and knew, roughly speaking, how they would respond. She had explained the plan to Evan. She and Evan had also worked with his treatment team to find other ways to reduce his aggressive behavior (including an adjustment in the timing of his medication). Not everyone has such good success the first time. It is important for families to continue working as a team with their treatment providers to address problems and find increasingly better solutions.

Like Cindy, Wendy was a single mother of two children—David, age 6, and Lisa, age 10 (see Chapter 19). Lisa was recently diagnosed with BD after a couple of years of significant turmoil and, at times, major aggression. She often took her anger out on David; this was terrifying to Wendy, who felt helpless when Lisa got out of control. Recently, after multiple episodes during which Lisa had trashed the house, hit David with a broomstick, and left Wendy covered with bruises, Wendy called 911. Two police officers were dispatched to the house. Wendy found them to be very judgmental and blaming in the way they spoke to her. She was really upset when they put handcuffs on Lisa and put her in the back of a squad car. They insisted on taking her to the emergency room, from which she was discharged 10 hours later. Following that episode, Lisa was referred for case management, and Wendy and Lisa were referred to PEP.

Wendy's call to the police was a call of desperation and was the result of having no crisis management plan. The point of having such a plan is to prevent such acts of desperation.

THERAPIST: Wendy, it sounds like you had a really horrific experience the last time Lisa got out of control.

WENDY: Yes, it was so scary, and I was so upset with the police. They just made everything worse!

THERAPIST: Okay, so it seems we had better develop a different plan to handle Lisa if she gets so out of control again in the future. Am I correct in assuming you don't feel like you could adequately restrain her when she really gets activated?

WENDY: Correct. I'm still bigger than Lisa, although probably not for long, given how she's been putting on weight lately. But when she gets wound up, there is no stopping her! There's no way I could hold her down when she's like that.

THERAPIST: Do you have any relatives who live nearby?

WENDY: My sister and brother-in-law, Jenny and Steve, live about 5 minutes from me. Steve is not particularly close to Lisa, but he's a big guy. My sister would do anything for me; we've always been close. I bet she could talk him into helping out. I hadn't even thought of asking them before—it's pretty embarrassing how things get at our house, but Jenny knows the struggles we've been through.

THERAPIST: Excellent! Is Steve usually at home in the evenings?

WENDY: Yeah, he works the early shift, so he's usually home by 4 in the afternoon.

THERAPIST: That sounds really promising. You've had your biggest problems with Lisa in the after-school and early evening hours, so if Steve is available, that might make a really good resource for you. How about if you talk to Jenny and Steve after our session today? If Steve is willing to be a backup for you, then make sure Lisa knows that this is an option if needed. Sometimes when kids know parents have an outside resource like that, simply reminding them when using this resource is the next step helps them to deescalate their behavior.

WENDY: Okay, I'll do that.

THERAPIST: The other thing I'm going to ask you to do is to call or stop in at your local police precinct and ask to speak with the juvenile officer. Many families have better success working with the police if they do some preplanning. It might even be that if Lisa knows you are willing to call the police that she will pull herself together enough to avoid that outcome.

Parents should be coached to assemble necessary information for use during emergencies and keep it in a readily accessible location. Information about medication side effects is particularly important. Some side effects are serious, and it is important for parents to be able to have information about those side effects at their fingertips. Other vital information includes emergency phone numbers for treatment providers (including case managers, local inpatient units, crisis centers, police, etc.). It is also important to know how to get to the local emergency department or children's crisis center. Information about insurance coverage should also be easily accessible, including criteria for hospitalization and what is covered.

Managing Suicidality

Regardless of how serious a parent thinks a suicide threat might be, it is critical to take threats seriously. Parents need to remove any available methods, especially guns (see Chapter 6). Locking up guns within the house is insufficient—they need to be removed from the house. It is best to have this discussion with the gun owner. If Dad owns the gun, doesn't attend the session, and has a history of domestic violence and alcohol abuse, Mom should not be asked to go home and bring up this point; it sets Mom up for an unpleasant altercation. Kitchen knives may need to be temporarily locked up, and medications should be secured.

Hospitalization: When It's Necessary and How It Works

Parents need to understand when inpatient hospitalization is necessary and how it works. It should never be threatened as punishment or used to provide respite. It is used when a child is a risk to him/herself or is presenting a danger to others. Examples include suicidality or such reckless behavior that the child's safety cannot be maintained at home or the child is a danger to others (e.g., chasing a sibling with a knife). Inpatient stays are typically very brief (usually under a week) and are geared toward stabilization. Although medications may be adjusted during a hospitalization, stays are so brief that the process can only be started; it will then require outpatient follow-up. If treatment begins with inpatient care, it is critical that families are linked with ongoing outpatient care at discharge. For families already in outpatient care, it is important that parents understand how care will be coordinated between the inpatient and outpatient care providers. It is often helpful for parents to know where the local inpatient units are.

Managing Parental Stress

Spouses and partners also experience a range of emotions (e.g., resentment, anger, embarrassment, bitterness, jealousy, fear, isolation, loneliness) and should have their needs addressed. Parents benefit from having a collaborative relationship, sharing "heavy-duty" tasks, having access to respite, and sharing an understanding of the illness and its impact on each family member. Most importantly, parents need to preserve time for each other. The greatest danger for a couple is for the partners to get pushed apart by the child's illness rather than pulled closer together.

Remind parents of the coping skills for stress management covered earlier (Chapter 14), particularly the tips for self-care and self-preservation. Like healthy habits for the child, the following should be considered "free medicines" for the parents, with only helpful side effects:

- Get enough sleep.
- Eat well.
- Exercise.
- Plan fun activities.
- Keep a journal.

- Maintain a support system.
- Meditate/pray/do yoga.
- Keep your sense of humor!

As noted in Chapter 14, managing a child's mood disorder is a marathon, not a sprint. Therefore, resources of time, money, energy, and hope need to be carefully expended. Parents need to assess in a realistic manner how much stress they can handle and still remain physically and emotionally healthy. If their current set of stressors is beyond what they can handle, one option is to consider simplifying.

> Colin and Lynn were particularly engaged as the session turned to the topic of parental stress. It made them realize how very stressed they were feeling. Their 10-year-old son, Lucas, presented a lot of challenging behaviors on a regular basis. Colin had a demanding job that often required him to work long hours. Lynn worked during school hours, but often did not get home until 30–45 minutes after Lucas and his older sister, Marissa. The family was also under a lot of financial stress. During the session, Lynn looked at Colin and asked, "Could we change anything to reduce our stress?" Once that question had been raised, Colin and Lynn started to examine what they could do to make life easier. They asked a number of questions: Whom could they turn to for respite care? Could they simplify life in any way? What could they do to reduce their financial stress? Could they arrange their jobs so that one or both of them could work fewer hours and have more time and energy available for family needs?

Emphasize that parents need to take care of themselves. Worn-out, stressed-out parents are not able to contribute to their family, nor can they enjoy life. Participation in PEP should encourage creative problem solving. You can help family members to take a fresh look at their day-to-day lives, to ask these larger questions, and to make a transition into healthier, more balanced lifestyles.

As therapists, we have a unique ability to instill hope in families. On a bad day, parents may believe that all possible treatment options have been exhausted, but this is unlikely to be the case. You should know your local resources and help parents see what else can be tried next. This is best done in the context of supporting parents in taking care of themselves.

Preparing for the IF-PEP Sibling Session

The next IF-PEP session will focus on sibling relationships. A portion of this current session should be reserved to discuss which siblings will attend, what the goal of the session will be, and how to discuss this at home. In families where the mood-disordered child has no siblings, or in which this child's symptoms (usually mild) do not spill over excessively into family life, the sibling session can be skipped. However, in many families, this sibling session can be very beneficial if well managed. Who attends the sibling session will vary from family to family, based on the siblings' ages and concerns. Usually the child with the mood disorder does not attend this session. Parents attend only at the session's start and end.

Parents of a child with a mood disorder are often overwhelmed by this child's needs. When the issue of siblings' needs is brought up, parents can experience a new wave of guilt as they realize that needs of their other children have not been met. The challenge for you as a PEP therapist is to raise these issues while also making siblings' needs feel manageable. The reality is that small changes can significantly improve things for siblings.

Depending on family issues and composition, planning for this session may be more or less complex. It is important for the child in treatment to know what will (and won't) happen during this session. In particular, the child should be reassured about how confidentiality works in sibling sessions: The child's diagnosis is not a secret at home, but this does not mean that you will share thoughts or feelings the child has expressed in therapy.

Although this session is placed late in the sequence of sessions, it can be scheduled earlier, depending on family needs and clinical judgment. For example, if there has been physical aggression toward a sibling, addressing sibling issues may need to be scheduled sooner.

Heidi and Robert have four children. Their oldest, Karl, is 11 and was diagnosed with BD-II 6 months before they began PEP. His course of illness has been very difficult, and for the past several months, much of their time and the bulk of their emotional resources have been focused on Karl. Heidi and Robert have been very worried about the impact of Karl's illness on their other three children. Because of this, they have asked their therapist for a sibling early in treatment. Karl's sister, 10-year-old Michelle, seems resentful: She is aware of the amount of energy being dedicated to Karl and complains about not getting equal time, especially with her mother. Heidi and Robert have also begun to see a lot of anger exhibited by their two youngest—Jeremy, age 7, and Carrie, age 4. The little ones do not really understand what is going on, but are aware that something has changed and are responding negatively to the increased household tension. Michelle in particular has complained of being embarrassed because of Karl's behavior around her friends. Jeremy complains bitterly about how Karl treats him. For Carrie, the youngest, the past several months have been scary. With four kids in the house, there has always been significant commotion. However, major anger outbursts have recently been added to the household mix. Heidi is particularly worried about Carrie, who looks scared during Karl's outbursts. It has been hard to have play dates for the other children and to just allow the free flow of neighbors through the house, as they did in the past.

In this case, Carrie is too young to be able to verbalize how she feels about the situation, so Heidi and Robert have decided with their therapist to have Michelle and Jeremy attend the sibling session together. Their hope is that they can apply what they learn from Jeremy's and Michelle's input to help Carrie as well.

Issues to consider for the sibling session may include the need for siblings to have a safe place; the siblings' roles with younger children and/or the child with the mood disorder; and providing other adult support for the siblings, such as spending time with nearby relatives, seeing their own therapist, or meeting with a school counselor periodically.

Take-Home Projects

Preparing the Child in Treatment and Siblings for the IF-PEP Sibling Session

Parents in IF-PEP should leave knowing how to prepare their children for the upcoming sibling session. This should include telling the child with the mood disorder who will attend and what is anticipated to happen. In addition, before the session's end, determine whether additional in-the-bank sessions will be needed if parents are still struggling with any residual issues.

Let's Talk (for MF-PEP)

Parents and children will complete Handout 76 (Let's Talk), using Handout 75 (the completed sample) for guidance, as described in Chapter 19. There is no formal family project for IF-PEP, but parents should be reminded to continue working on using helpful communication strategies.

Chapter 21

Working with Siblings

IF-PEP Sibling Session 10
Not a session in MF-PEP

Session Outline

Goals:	1. Listen to and validate siblings' questions and concerns.
	2. Provide psychoeducation about mood disorders and mood symptoms.
	3. Identify concerns that can be addressed by parents.
Beginning the Session:	Introduction of clinician and siblings
Lesson of the Day:	Understanding and addressing siblings' perspectives
	• Elicit and validate sibling's concerns.
	• Provide information about mood disorders.
	• Explain the importance of a safe place.
	• Ask about family roles of siblings.
	• Raise sibling issues with parents and increase support.
Take-Home Project:	No formal project, but families may be asked to revisit problem-solving or communication skills to respond to sibling issues

New Handouts:	None
Handouts to Review:	None

Session Overview

In families of a child with a mood disorder, siblings can carry a significant burden, and parents often raise concerns about them. Siblings may experience a host of emotional reactions to the mood-disordered child and the situations that arise because of him/her. They often feel resentful, angry, sad, embarrassed, bitter, jealous, scared, isolated, lonely, and guilty. They often struggle with the direct impact of their brother's or sister's behavior, in addition to getting less parental attention. They are often frustrated by differences in parental expectations that feel unfair. The purpose of this session is to address some of these concerns and help the family cope better as a whole. This session is not meant to be a cure for all sibling issues, but it should establish sibling issues as an important part of managing a mood disorder within a family. Some families may choose to delve into sibling issues more deeply and add in-the-bank sessions.

Beginning the Session

Introduction of Clinician and Siblings

Like the school personnel session (see Chapter 16), this session does not begin with a review of the previous sessions' projects. Depending on the ages of the siblings attending this session, introductions may be brief and may take place in the waiting room, or the parents may accompany the siblings into the therapy room to set the agenda for the session. However, some things may be difficult for siblings to say in front of their parents, and for this reason, parents leave the room for a portion of the session. The parents may be quickly briefed at its end on topics to continue working on at home—or, depending on the issues raised and the developmental level of the siblings, it may be more beneficial for parents to rejoin the latter portion of the session to do some family problem solving with the aid of the therapist.

Lesson of the Day:
Understanding and Addressing Siblings' Perspectives

Elicit and Validate Siblings' Concerns

This session provides siblings with a chance to talk freely about what it is like growing up with a sister or brother who has a mood disorder. In many cases, siblings will recognize that their brother or sister does not have it easy, and will feel guilty about airing their own concerns. Therefore, the stage should be set at the start for siblings to talk freely.

Jay (age 11) and Kaitlyn (age 7) came into the session looking apprehensive. Their sister, Natalie (age 9), and their parents had been coming to sessions for a while, and they had been in the waiting room a few times when their grandparents hadn't been available to stay home with them. This time they had come with their parents, and Natalie had stayed home with their grandparents. They weren't sure what to expect. They had met the therapist, Louise, in the waiting room previously, and she had seemed nice. Louise started the session by asking them what it was like living with Natalie. When they both shrugged, she talked a little about some of the challenges she had heard about, such as Natalie's yelling a lot in the mornings and being demanding and loud at night. When Jay and Kaitlyn realized that Louise knew a little about what it was really like at home, they both started talking. Periodically, Louise had to ask them gently to take turns talking so she could hear both of them. After they had both vented for several minutes, she asked them whether they would like to make a list of things they would like to see change.

Once siblings realize that their concerns are valid and that the adults actually have a good idea of what is going on, they will often start talking openly. If siblings are a little more reticent, it can help to get them talking if you share some thoughts about how siblings of children with mood disorders often feel.

Episodes of aggression are upsetting to siblings, but they are often most bothered by chronic stressors, such as difficult mornings and stressful bedtimes.

After being invited to make a list of things that they would like to change, Jay and Kaitlyn both started rattling off changes faster than Louise could write. Louise asked them to come up with the two problems that bothered them the most. Without hesitating, Kaitlyn said, "All of the yelling in the morning and at bedtime." Together, they made those two problems into two manageable wishes: (1) having quieter mornings, which would include Jay's and Kaitlyn's being more cooperative and getting up slightly earlier so they could eat breakfast with their dad before he went to work; and (2) having at least 10 minutes of quiet time with Mom or Dad at bedtime.

As is common for siblings of children with mood disorders, Jay and Kaitlyn focused on disruptions to routines caused by their sister's mood symptoms. Routines are an important part of healthy development. Thus hearing these concerns from siblings should indicate areas that parents will need to address through problem solving. As the therapists, you should note such issues and make sure that they are raised with parents at the end of the session. Siblings may share some parental perspectives, but they often will have different perspectives about family situations. Some examples of how siblings tend to see situations include the following:

"He's so embarrassing! Every time we go somewhere, he has a meltdown."
"She's always in my space, and my parents never do anything about it."
"I lock my door and go in my closet when he's flipping out."
"I get in trouble for every little thing I do, but she never gets in trouble."
"I don't like to have friends over, because I never know what he's going to do. Once he grabbed my friend's butt!"

"She takes up all of my parents' time."

"I'm afraid he'll hurt my mom."

"I wish we went to different schools."

"I get yelled at when I try to help, but I'm afraid my parents won't be able to stop it."

Siblings get tremendous benefit from airing their concerns and having them validated. It is also beneficial for siblings to get a sense that the mood-disordered child's problems are being worked on in treatment. Siblings often worry that their parents cannot handle the needs of their brother or sister. Knowing that you, a well-trained professional, are helping their parents navigate the challenge can bring a much-needed sense of hope.

Provide Information about Mood Disorders

Some siblings will come to this session with very little knowledge about their sister's or brother's mood disorder. In an age-appropriate manner, give siblings information about the illness. This will help them understand that this is a no-fault illness—it isn't their fault, their parents' fault, or their sibling's fault. They may also need some education to understand why their parents' expectations for them are different from those for their sibling, and why their parents may differ in their responses to their sibling. It can be difficult for children to understand parents' decisions about which battles to pick.

Marcus, age 7, had a 9-year-old sister, Krystal, with BD-NOS. When he came to the sibling session with the family's PEP therapist, Jason, Marcus looked anxious. Jason started by talking about the basketball jersey Marcus was wearing, to put him at ease. Jason then shared with Marcus some of what he understood about what it was like to have Krystal as a sister. Marcus looked immensely relieved when he realized that Jason "knew the deal." Jason then gave Marcus an opportunity to talk about the biggest problems for him.

> JASON [therapist]: So, Marcus, what's one of the toughest times of the day for you?
>
> MARCUS: Dinner, definitely. At school, we've been talking about nutrition in health class, and my teacher keeps saying family mealtime is super-important. At our house, dinner is a nightmare! My sister usually yells at my mom before dinner because she wants dinner sooner. Then, once we start eating, she pitches a fit over some little thing my mom serves.
>
> JASON: Wow, that sounds pretty unpleasant—not at all like what your teacher described, huh?
>
> MARCUS: You got that right! Besides, we've always had a rule in our house that that we have to try everything Mom puts on our plate and eat our vegetables if we want dessert, but Krystal never follows those rules any more. She can eat whatever she wants and still gets dessert every night. It's not fair!
>
> JASON: Hmm ... why do you think it is that your mom is doing things so differently with Krystal these days?
>
> MARCUS: I don't know. I think she is just turning into a spoiled brat—every time she yells and screams, she gets more of what she wants.

JASON: Do you ever see your mom setting limits with Krystal?

MARCUS: Well, yeah, sometimes. Meals are probably the times Krystal gets away with the most stuff.

JASON: Lots of kids with bipolar disorder, like your sister, have certain times of day that are the most difficult for them. From what I know about Krystal, late afternoon seems to be her trouble spot. Do you think your mom might be cutting her some slack at that time of day just to make the day go better for everyone in the household, you included?

MARCUS: Hmm ... I hadn't thought about it that way before. (*Pause*) I guess I would rather know that Krystal can get dessert if I don't have to listen to her yell all the way through dinner! It does kinda wreck my appetite to see her being so mean to Mom.

JASON: I can tell you that Krystal isn't enjoying feeling out of control either, so you guys, believe it or not, are actually all in this together! Maybe you could talk as a family after this session, to make a plan to improve the atmosphere around the dinner hour. What do you think?

Children are both resilient and forgiving. It is reassuring for children such as Marcus to understand why their parents hold children in the family to different standards, and how they intentionally make choices to help all members of the family. Children do need to know that adults are in charge. It is also immensely reassuring to be able to turn family conflicts into problems that can be solved as a family.

Explain the Importance of a Safe Place

Ask whether the siblings have a safe place to go during crises, and if so, emphasize the importance of going to that safe place when necessary. Siblings sometimes mistakenly believe that they can or should help during a crisis, and thus they resist leaving the center of the conflict. In other cases, such resistance is driven by sheer curiosity and a desire to be in the thick of things. Either way, siblings need to leave during a crisis—both to protect themselves and to avoid inadvertently escalating the situation. If a sibling does not have a safe place or seems unclear about when to use it, make a note to discuss this with parents at the end of the session.

The safe place might be a sibling's own bedroom, which he/she is allowed to lock (parents should always also have a key to unlock the room); another room in the house; or, in some cases, a neighbor's or nearby relative's house. Having a parent create a special safe place in the house gives a clear message to siblings about their importance in the family.

Ask about Family Roles of Siblings

In many families, older siblings are relied on for help with younger siblings. In families of a child with a mood disorder, it is important for the clinician and parents to assess family members' roles carefully and ensure that the siblings are not carrying an undue burden. It may be fine for older siblings to help with younger siblings while parents manage crises. Older siblings may also be helpful in heading off crises by providing much-needed distractions at key moments. Regardless of a family's structure, you can check in with siblings—and later with parents—to make sure that current patterns are healthy for everyone.

Raise Sibling Issues with Parents and Increase Support

When parents return toward the end of this session, the siblings can be asked to summarize their main concerns, and you can add any problems that may be missed. Encourage parents and siblings to take a problem-solving approach, and remind parents that small changes can improve things significantly for siblings. For example, adding locks to siblings' bedroom doors may enhance a feeling of safety as well as protect personal space. Getting a sibling up 15 minutes earlier may provide the opportunity for a much-needed private morning check-in with a parent. Creative problem solving can go a long way.

Siblings often need more adult support than they are getting, but parents of children with a mood disorder may feel stretched completely thin already. Emphasize that not all support needs to come from parents. In some cases, siblings benefit from having their own therapist to meet with periodically. This may be a school counselor or a mental health professional in the community. In other cases, extra time with a relative who lives nearby can help. Setting aside some brief uninterrupted time for just a parent and a sibling can go a long way to convey to the sibling that parents understand and care about how he/she is doing. Emphasize that the needs of siblings do need to be addressed. Once parents start thinking about it, they are likely to have various creative ideas about how to address these needs.

Chapter 22

Wrapping Up with Parents and Children

IF-PEP Child and Parent Session 10
MF-PEP Child and Parent Session 8

Session Outline

Goals:
1. Address lingering questions and concerns.
2. Review important PEP lessons.

Beginning the Session:
Do a check-in with parents.
Review Let's Talk (Handout 76).
Have child identify and rate feelings.

Lesson of the Day:
Wrapping up PEP
- Address lingering questions and concerns.
- Follow up on continuing care.
- Review key PEP concepts.
- Celebrate.

Take-Home Project:
No assigned project

New Handouts:
77. PEP Take Home Messages for Parents
78. PEP Take-Home Messages for Children

Handouts to Review:
76. Let's Talk

277

Session Overview

By this final session, a family should have a treatment team in place to ensure ongoing care. If the family has an established treatment team to which it will return after PEP, be sure to plan for a summary of PEP to be provided to the team. If PEP has been the first step in treatment for the family, and the family will be starting with a new team, be sure to plan for some communication with the new team. If you will be continuing as part of the family's treatment team, then this session will focus on reviewing and planning next steps. In some cases—typically when the child's mood disorder was mild to moderate in severity when the family was referred, and now is in remission—this may be the termination session, with booster sessions available as needed in the future.

Take a few moments before this final session to identify any issues that may not have been adequately addressed, and review the significant "take-home messages" that have been the focus of the previous sessions. The session provides an opportunity to wrap up any lingering issues, to review important points, and to celebrate the completion of PEP.

In IF-PEP, depending on the dynamics of the family, this session can be conducted with the whole family together or divided so that there is some time alone with the child, some time alone with the parents, and some time all together. Review of PEP will take up much of this session, but some time at the end should be spent celebrating the family's accomplishments during PEP. If the family's treatment will be continuing with you, the focus can then shift to setting goals and priorities for further treatment.

In MF-PEP, parents and children separate as usual. Parents have a final chance to get remaining questions answered and concerns addressed. Children play a group game to test their knowledge of PEP, and then redeem their points for prizes. Finally, children rejoin their parents for a graduation ceremony in which certificates of completion are passed out, along with a brief speech from one of the child therapists about each child's most notable accomplishments during MF-PEP.

Beginning the Session

Do a Check-In with Parents

Begin the session with parents and children together as usual for a quick check-in on how the week has gone. Use the Mood–Medication Log (Handout 32) or Mood Record (Handout 20 or 21) as necessary.

Review Let's Talk

Families should arrive at this session with ideas generated by both parents and children for how to improve family communication. The more specific the ideas, the more likely a family will be to implement them effectively (e.g., "Use a calm, soft voice" is likely to be a more helpful suggestion than "Talk nicely"). It is also important for changes to be phrased positively rather than negatively (e.g., "Wait to talk until the other person is finished" instead of "Don't interrupt").

Anna came into session with her parents, excited to share their family project. She reported that they had worked on it the first night after their last session, and some of the ideas had really helped during the week. Anna eagerly showed her PEP therapist, Kate, their completed copy of Handout 76. Anna's to-do list was as follows:

1. Listen until the other person is finished.
2. Take a deep breath before talking, talk calmly, and use an inside voice.
3. Use kind words.

Her parents' to-do list included these things:

1. Say what you mean directly and without sarcasm.
2. Listen to Anna's ideas or thoughts.
3. Keep voice low and calm.

Anna reported that she had come home from school in a bad mood but with a lot of homework one day. She had remembered to take deep breaths before talking, which helped her to tell her mom how stressed and upset she felt without yelling or taking her mood out on her mom. Her mom had listened to her, but then had some ideas about how to break down the homework into chunks Anna could manage. After listening to Anna talk about her day, she had calmly asked Anna whether she wanted suggestions for how to handle the homework. Anna said yes, and then took some deep breaths while calmly listening to her mother's ideas. An afternoon that might have gone poorly turned out well.

Have Child Identify and Rate Feelings

If the session is structured for some time alone with a child, he/she can be asked to identify and rate current feelings when the parents leave. Otherwise, this task may be done immediately after the initial check-in and before review of the Let's Talk project.

Lesson of the Day: Wrapping Up PEP

Address Lingering Questions and Concerns

Any lingering questions or concerns of family members should be addressed. If family members do not raise any concerns, it may be helpful for you to prompt with some issues that you feel were left unfinished or that have been coming up repeatedly. Throughout this session, family members should be given ample opportunity to raise questions or concerns. However, it is helpful to try to identify and cover troublesome areas up front.

DR. PHILLIPS [therapist]: So, Tiffany and Mom, we've spent a lot of time together, and I think you've learned quite a few new skills to manage those pesky mood symptoms you've had to deal with. Can you tell me some of the most important things you've learned in our time together?

TIFFANY: Well, it is really nice to know that Mom and Dad don't blame me when I'm grumpy; they just try to help me get out of that mood. My Tool Kit is pretty good, but sometimes nothing seems to help.

DR. PHILLIPS: It's good you've got some steps you feel like you can take. But I agree that sometimes, your mood might stay stuck in grumpy. What can you do then?

DIANE [Tiffany's mother]: Tiffany has gotten pretty good at just going to bed early on those days. Usually when she gets up the next morning, she has a fresh new start, and her mood is better. My big question now is this: When should she go off her antidepressant? If we aren't seeing you any more, I'm not sure how I'll know if and when she's ready.

DR. PHILLIPS: That's an excellent question. You have several choices there. First, we talked about how it is smart to try tapering off medicine when Tiffany is in a low-stress time, like this coming summer. Second, you can always call me to reschedule a booster session or a consultation session if you'd like. Third, you've got a pretty good relationship with your pediatrician, and as he is prescribing Tiffany's medicine, that will be a really good question to ask at her next appointment.

Discussion about hot topics is likely to be spontaneous. Families often also find it helpful to talk about what they have learned, discuss how they plan to proceed, describe what they might do differently, and indicate what they have learned that they plan to continue doing.

Follow Up on Continued Care

Be sure to check with parents that ongoing care is in place. For some families, PEP becomes a lifeline. It is important that any questions about the ongoing treatment team be addressed before the close of PEP. If PEP is being provided to an individual family as a stand-alone intervention, it is important that transition to an already established treatment team should go smoothly. Families need to know how to access needed services as time goes on.

Review Key PEP Concepts

Once unfinished business has been covered and any spontaneous review has occurred, you can spur discussion by summarizing or restating important take-home messages from each topic area. Handouts 77 (PEP Take-Home Messages for Parents) and 78 (PEP Take-Home Messages for Children) can be used for this purpose. This review can also be tailored to the needs of specific families. In MF-PEP, the children play the PEP Review Game (Game Reproducible 21 in Part III; described in Chapter 3) and then redeem their points from all eight sessions. In IF-PEP, this last session may also be used to review material individually and then redeem the child's points for prizes.

Celebrate

For some families, PEP has been their first proactive step toward managing their children's mood disorders. For others, it will be one of many steps they have taken in becoming experts on their children and empowering themselves to move forward and help their children and their families be healthy. Parents and children should come away from PEP feeling empowered. They will have gained significant knowledge, learned new skills, and found support. As they go forward, we want them to remember to apply the knowledge, employ the skills, and always seek the support they need. For families who are continuing treatment with you, this session segues into maintenance treatment. For those who are returning to a new or previously established treatment team, this is a transition. Either way, families should enter the next phase of treatment with a new perspective and new skills—and a celebration is in order!

PART III

Child and Parent Handouts and Group Game Materials

Feelings

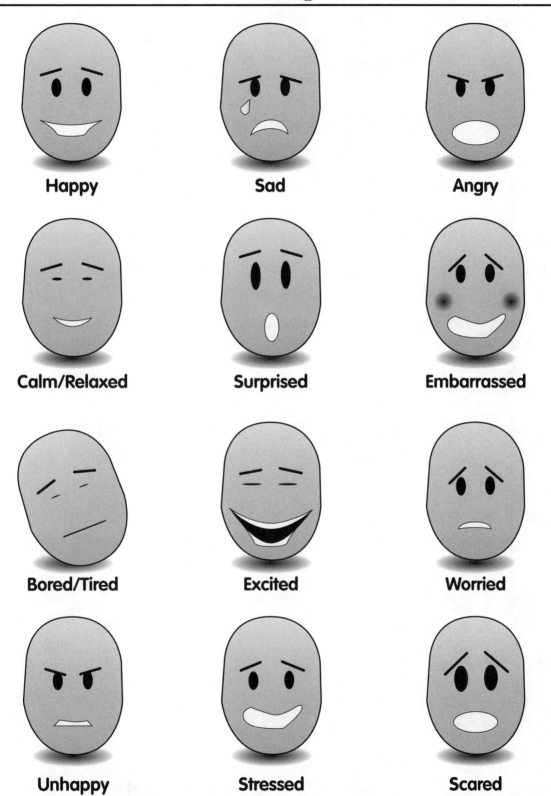

Strength of Feelings

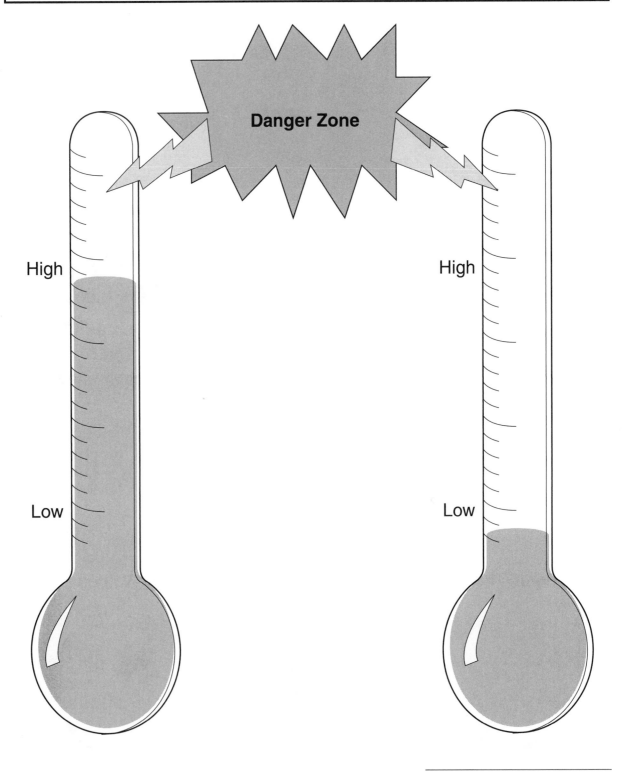

Feeling

Symptoms

Depression	Mania

What Is Depression?

➡ Mood: Very sad/worried

or very angry/irritable

➡ Feeling bored, as if nothing is fun

➡ Sleep and appetite: Up or down

➡ Trouble paying attention

➡ Feeling tired, no energy

➡ Wanting to move around a lot or not at all

➡ Feeling guilty or worthless

➡ Thinking about death/suicide

What is Mania?

➡ Mood: "Too happy" or "too angry"

➡ Feeling like you have special powers

➡ Getting distracted easily

➡ Not needing sleep

➡ Being a lot more active than usual

➡ Doing dangerous or really silly things

➡ Thoughts racing

➡ Talking fast and loud

➡ Doing or saying sexually inappropriate things

The Highs and Lows of Mania and Depression

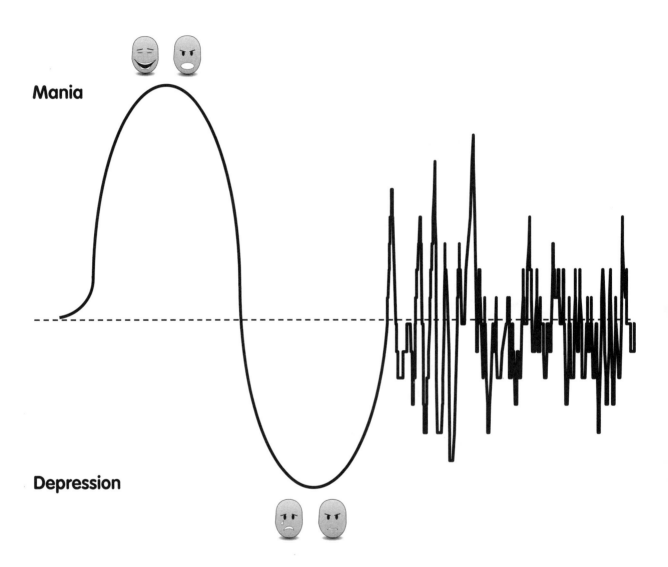

Mania

Depression

Other Symptoms That Cause Problems

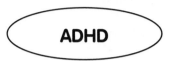

Trouble paying attention and staying on task
Feeling "hyper"
Acting without thinking

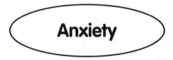

Feeling scared and worried a lot of the time

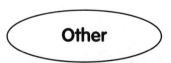

Hearing or seeing things that others don't see or hear
Having upsetting thoughts

PEP Motto

It's not your fault,
but it's your challenge!

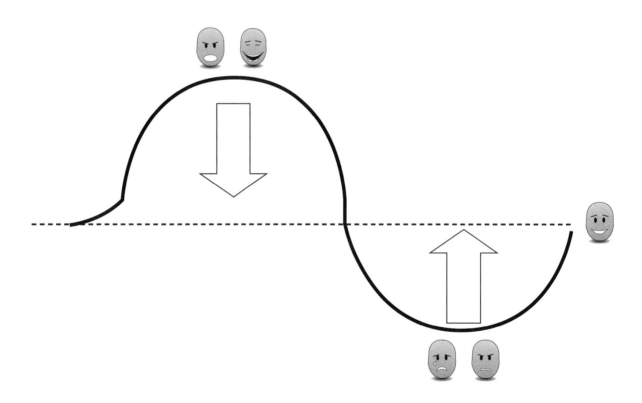

Fix-It List Areas (Sample)

Home

1. Arguing with my parents

2. Fighting with my brother and sister

3. Feeling bored

4. Not getting up on time

School

1. Can't finish work

2. In trouble for talking

3. Math is too hard

Friends

1. Can't find anything to play with friends

2. Friends never like my ideas

Fix-It List Areas

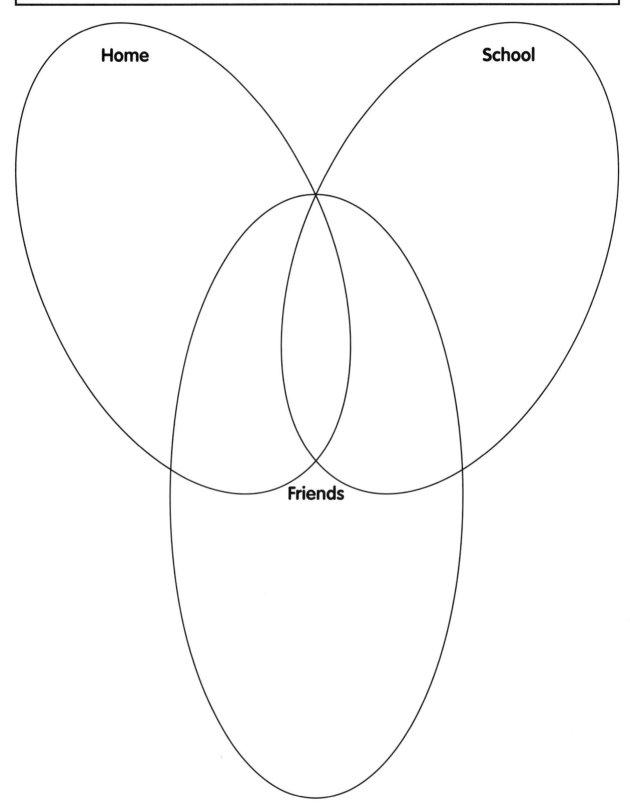

Home

School

Friends

Belly Breathing

Belly Breathing Instructions:

1. Take a deep breath in through your nose and fill your lungs. (If you are lying down on your bed or floor, you can see your belly rise.)

2. Slowly breathe out of your mouth. (If you are lying down, you will notice that your stomach starts to fall back down as you blow out.)

3. Complete Steps 1 and 2 at least three times in a row. (This completes **one set** of breathing.)

4. Try to do **one or two sets** of breathing at a time. You can do more if you want.

   Practice this activity at least three times (on three different days) before our next session.

Breathing Log

Child	Parents

Date: _____   _____

Date: _____   _____

Date: _____   _____

Family Project: Fix-It List (Sample)

Child Fix-It List

1. I'll play fairly with my brother.

2. If my brother is mean, I will quit playing with him.

3. I'll invite someone to play with me and plan to do what my friend wants to do.

Parent Fix-It List

1. I will stop yelling.

2. I will take 15 minutes/day for myself (e.g, walk around the neighborhood).

3. I will make sure that my spouse agrees before I give my child a major consequence.

Family Fix-It List

1. Every family member gets 15 minutes of "me" time.

2. Children will stop playing when they are treating each other unfairly.

3. Everyone in the family will use "inside" voices and not yell.

Family Project: Fix-It List

Child Fix-It List

1.

2.

3.

Parent Fix-It List

1.

2.

3.

Family Fix-It List

1.

2.

3.

PEP Parent Session Topics

1. Learn about mood symptoms and disorders.

2. Learn about medication.

3. Learn about "systems"—the school and treatment teams.

4. Learn about the negative family cycle and ways to change it.

5. Learn problem-solving skills and basic coping skills.

6. Learn further coping skills—improve communication.

7. Learn further coping skills—family issues, symptom/crisis management.

8. Wrap up—review and final Q & A.

PEP Child Session Topics

1. Learn about symptoms and disorders.

2. Learn about medication.

3. Learn about healthy habits.

4. Develop emotion regulation strategies (the "Tool Kit").

5. Learn the connections among thoughts, feelings, and actions (responsibility/choices).

6. Learn problem-solving strategies.

7. Improve nonverbal communication skills.

8. Improve verbal communication skills.

9. Final review (with parents).

Brain Differences in Mood Disorders

Note: More research has been completed with adolescents diagnosed with bipolar disorder (BD) than for children with BD or for youth with depression.

Bipolar Disorder (BD)

DIFFERENCES IN THE PREFRONTAL CORTEX

The prefrontal cortex is responsible for "executive functioning," which includes planning, decision making, managing reactions, modulating emotion, inhibiting impulses, shifting attention, initiating tasks, using working memory, maintaining effort, and perspective taking. It helps regulate the limbic system, which is highly involved in emotion.

- The amygdala (part of the limbic system) is more active in BD, while the prefrontal cortex is less active. In other words, emotional responses are stronger than rational/thinking responses.
- The part of the prefrontal cortex that controls how the body reacts to stimuli is less activated in BD during emotional situations. As a result, reactions to stress are more intense, making ordinary situations feel more like emergencies.
- The area of the prefrontal cortex that helps with understanding of past rewards and consequences is less activated, making it more difficult for people with BD to focus on the facts of a situation and make informed choices about behavior.
- The middle section of the prefrontal cortex, which helps understanding of others' perspectives and interprets emotional responses to events, shows decreased activation in BD. This makes it more difficult to take into account others' point of view when choosing what to do, as well as when inhibiting immediate responses.
- Lithium treatment increases the concentration of *N*-acetylaspartate, an indicator of health, in the prefrontal cortex in adolescents and adults. Improving functioning in the prefrontal cortex may be one mechanism by which lithium improves symptoms in people with BD.

DIFFERENCES IN THE LIMBIC SYSTEM

The limbic system perceives and processes emotional stimuli, and regulates responses to those stimuli. Dysfunction here contributes to problems with "theory of mind" (i.e., the ability to infer what others are thinking and feeling from their nonverbal and verbal communication) in people with BD.

- The connection between the amygdala (in the limbic system) and the temporal lobe helps to process certain types of stimuli (e.g., fear-provoking). Having fewer connections between these areas makes it harder for people with BD to perceive and process emotional stimuli.
- Emotion-focused parts of the network are more active in BD, while thinking-focused parts of the network are less active. This dysfunction appears to worsen across time with repeated episodes.

(cont.)

Depression

DIFFERENCES IN THE AMYGDALA

The amygdala is part of the limbic system that produces emotional reactions in response to environmental stimuli and stores emotional memory.

- Lower amygdala volumes may be associated with poor responses to social and emotional situations and with less intense emotional reactions (e.g., flat affect) in depression.

DIFFERENCES IN THE ANTERIOR CINGULATE CORTEX

The anterior cingulate cortex is involved in emotional and cognitive processing of information.

- Lower activity in this area leads to increased emotional reactivity and reduced thinking about a situation.

DIFFERENCES IN THE PREFRONTAL CORTEX

- Depressed youth with a family history of depression have less volume in this area than healthy controls do. Depressed youth without a family history have a greater volume than controls do. Volume differences may indicate dysfunction for depressed youth, with or without a family history.

BD and Depression: Cognitive Ability Deficits

- Learning disorders: Problems with reading, writing, and math are more common in youth with depression or BD than in typically developing peers.

Tracking Mood Changes:
Depressive Spectrum Disorders

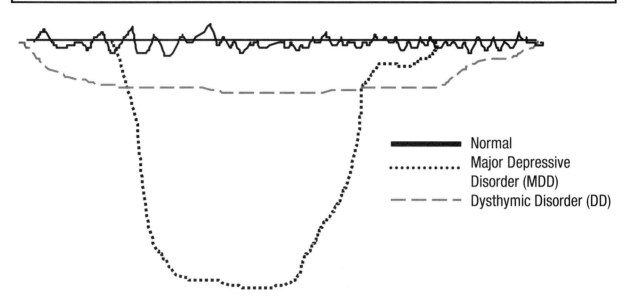

Major Depressive Disorder (MDD)

Need one or both of these:
Impaired mood
    Sad/anxious
    Irritable/angry
Loss of interest
    Complaints of boredom
    Previously fun activities aren't fun any more
Need three or four of these (five total):
    Impaired sleep
    Impaired appetite
    Poor concentration
    Fatigue
    Restlessness/lethargy
    Worthlessness/guilt
    Suicidal/morbid ideation
Symptoms last ≥ 2 weeks

The MDD Picture
Single-episode length: 7–9 months
90% get well by 1.5–2 years
6–10% stay impaired
Recurrence:
    40% after 2 years
    70% after 5 years

Dysthymic Disorder (DD)

Mood (lasting 1 year)
    Sad
    Irritable
Two or more of these:
    Impaired appetite
    Impaired sleep
    Fatigue
    Low self-esteem
    Impaired concentration/thinking
    Hopeless feelings
The DD Picture
Single untreated episode: 4 years
MDD episode usually comes 2–3 years after DD onset
Can lead to:
    Bipolar disorder: 13%
    Substance abuse: 15%

Seasonal Affective Disorder (SAD)

Most common:
Fall/winter: "Hibernating" depression—increased sleep and appetite, carbohydrate craving, decreased activity
Spring/summer: nondepressed or manic

Tracking Mood Changes:
Bipolar Spectrum Disorders

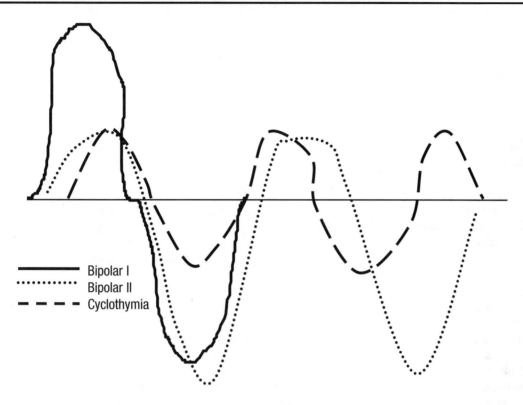

— Bipolar I
········· Bipolar II
– – – Cyclothymia

Manic Episode

Mood (1 week):
    Elevated
    Expansive
    Irritable

Three (four if just irritable mood) of these:
    Grandiosity
    Little need for sleep
    Increased talking
    Racing thoughts
    Distractible
    Increased activity/agitation
    Foolish/reckless behavior

Hypomanic Episode

Mood changes (4–7 days)
Associated symptoms (same as mania)
Functioning clearly "out of character"
Altered mood and behavior noted by others
Symptoms not severe enough to be called mania

Mixed State

Depressive and manic symptoms co-occur
This is relatively common

Who Is at Risk for Bipolar Spectrum Disorders?

About 25–50% of depressed children develop bipolar disorder within 2–5 years

Risk factors include these:
    Symptoms of psychomotor retardation or psychosis
    Bipolar spectrum disorder on one side of the family
    Mood disorder on both sides of the family
    Medication-induced hypomania

Additional Concerns

Suicidal Concerns

Time
> During/right after inpatient treatment
> During a crisis
> Following suicide of a close friend/relative
> Positive or negative life events

Warning signs
> Talking about death/suicide
> Saying goodbyes, making wills, giving away
>> belongings

Other factors
> Depressed/hopeless
> Drug/alcohol use
> Impulsivity/anger
> Physical/sexual abuse
> Running away
> Past attempt
> Self-destructiveness
> Perfectionism

Access to guns!

Psychotic Symptoms

Some children with mood disorders experience:

Hallucinations
> Hearing voices
> Seeing things
> Sometimes smelling or feeling things

Delusions
> Special messages
> Special powers
> Other unusual thoughts/ideas

These occur when mood symptoms are severe

They typically go away when the mood disorder is treated

Co-Occurring Disorders

Can be anything.

Behavior Disorders
> Attention-deficit/hyperactivity disorder (ADHD),
>> oppositional defiant disorder, conduct disorder

Anxiety Disorders
> Separation anxiety disorder, generalized anxiety
>> disorder, phobias, post traumatic stress disorder,
>> acute stress disorder, obsessive–compulsive
>> disorder, social phobia, panic disorder

Eating Disorders
> Anorexia nervosa, bulimia nervosa, obesity

Learning Disorders
> Reading, writing, math, language disabilities

Pervasive Developmental Disorders
> (aka autism spectrum disorders)

Some co-occurring disorders will be successfully treated *in part* by mood disorder treatments:
> Many anxiety disorders
> Some behavior disorders
> Some eating disorders

Most will require some other specialized intervention:
> Other medications/psychotherapy
> School intervention
> Learning to cope with symptoms of those disorders

Mood Record: Tracking Three Moods, Three Times per Day

Month: _____   Treatment providers/programs: _____

Medication, if any (type, dose, side effects): _____

Day	Date	Sad			Angry			Euphoric			Meds taken?	Comments (e.g., life event, med changes, med side effects, sleep/appetite changes, other)
		A.M.	P.M. 1	P.M. 2	A.M.	P.M. 1	P.M. 2	A.M.	P.M. 1	P.M. 2		
	1											
	2											
	3											
	4											
	5											
	6											
	7											
	8											
	9											
	10											
	11											
	12											
	13											
	14											
	15											
	16											
	17											
	18											
	19											
	20											
	21											
	22											
	23											
	24											
	25											
	26											
	27											
	28											
	29											
	30											
	31											

Directions: Rate each mood state at each time period, on a scale where 1 = normal/healthy and 10 = worst/most inappropriate to situation.

How Is _____ **Feeling Today?**

-5   -4   -3   -2   -1   0   1   2   3   4   5

M _____

_____

T _____

_____

W _____

_____

Th _____

_____

F _____

_____

S _____

_____

S _____

_____

Naming the Enemy

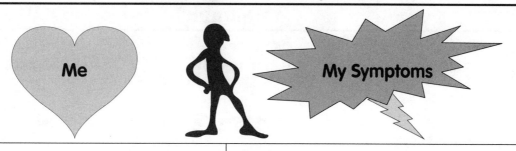

Get Help to Put the Enemy Behind You
(Sample)

School 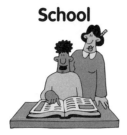   **Therapy** 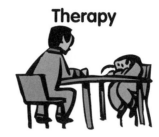   **Medication**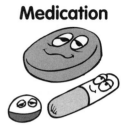

1. How do you know if it's **working**?

   My symptoms get better.

   I learn new ways to do things.

   I get the grades that I know I can achieve.

   _____

2. How do you know if it's **not working**?

   My symptoms don't change.

   My symptoms get worse.

   New symptoms appear.

   My grades are lower than what I know I can earn.

3. How can you be a team player to fight the **Enemy** and reveal more of **Me?**

   Gather clues. Keep a log of symptom changes and side effects. Tell my doctor.

   Communicate with my teacher and let him/her know when I am having a bad day.

   Let my school counselor know if I need more help at school. (Let my parents know

   if the school counselor doesn't help).

   Work in therapy to learn how to manage my thoughts, feelings, and actions.

Get Help to Put the Enemy Behind You

School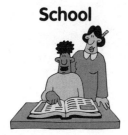

Therapy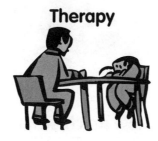

Medication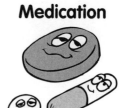

1. How do you know if it's **working**?

_____

_____

_____

_____

2. How do you know if it's **not working**?

_____

_____

_____

_____

3. How can you be a team player to fight the Enemy and reveal more of Me?

_____

_____

_____

_____

_____

My Medicine

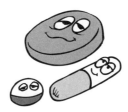

Name of medicine	How much/when	Reason for taking it
1.		
2.		
3.		
4.		
5.		

Summary of Medications
and the Enemies They Target

Antidepressants/antianxiety medications (mainly used for sleep; Prozac, Zoloft, Celexa, Lexapro, Luvox, Paxil, Wellbutrin)

Depressive symptoms (feeling sad, grouchy, irritable)

Anxiety symptoms (feeling worried or scared)

Mood stabilizers (Eskalith, Lithium Carbonate, Depakote, Lamictal, Tegretol)

Manic symptoms (feeling too "happy" or "too angry," thoughts racing, not needing sleep)

Antipsychotics (Risperdal, Abilify, Geodon, Seroquel, Zyprexa, Invega, Clozaril)

Manic symptoms and other problems (Hearing or seeing things that others don't hear or see; agitation and aggression)

Stimulants (Ritalin, Concerta, Metadate, Vyvanse, Focalin, Adderall, Dexedrine, Daytrana)

Nonstimulants (Strattera)

ADHD symptoms (feeling "hyper," trouble paying attention, being impulsive)

Antihypertensives (Catapres, Tenex, Intuniv)

(trouble sleeping, tics, too impulsive or restless)

Common Side Effects
and What to Do about Them

Side effects	Ways to feel better
Dizziness:	• Stand up slowly.
Dry mouth:	• Drink water. • Chew sugarless gum.
Constipation:	• Eat cereal, whole wheat bread, fruit, and raw vegetables. • Drink plenty of water.
Upset stomach:	• Take medication with food.
Increased thirst:	• Drink water.
Increased urination:	• Arrange bathroom breaks.
Weight gain:	• Increase exercise. • Eat a low-fat diet. • Drink plenty of water (not high-calorie juice/soda). • Eat lots of fiber to help fill you up. • Avoid junk food.

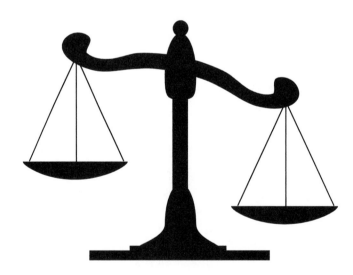

Bubble Breathing

Bubble Breathing Instructions

1. Take a deep breath in through your nose and fill your lungs.

2. Using a slow and steady breath, breathe out through your mouth. **Do this with the same kind of slow, steady breath you use when blowing bubbles.**

3. Complete Steps 1 and 2 at least three times in a row. (This completes **one set** of breathing.)

4. Try to do **one or two sets** of breathing at a time. You can do more if you want.

   Practice this activity at least three times (on three different days) before our next session.

Breathing Log

	Child	Parents
Date:	_____	_____
Date:	_____	_____
Date:	_____	_____

Family Project: Naming the Enemy (Sample)

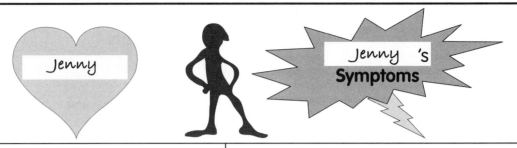

Jenny	Jenny's Symptoms
Caring	Depression
	Low energy
Good helper	Irritable, disrespectful
	Cries
Good swimmer	Hates herself
Very loving	
	Mania
Good student	Talks too fast
	Sleeps much less
Likes computers	Aggressive
	Acts wild, silly, inappropriately
Good at basketball	
	ADHD
Smart	Unorganized
	Homework struggles
Shares well with siblings and friends	Can't concentrate
	Other
	Hears voices

Family Project: Naming the Enemy

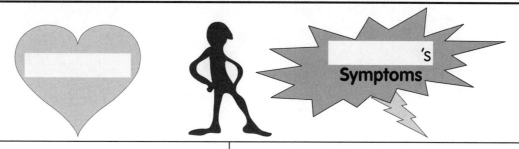

Mood–Medication Log (Sample)

Child's name: _Jasmine_   Month: _Nov._   Treatment providers/program: _PEP_

Medications (type, dose, side effects): _Risperdal 0.5mg 2x per day until 11/16 added 0.5mg at noon_

Day	Date	Overall rating 1 = great, 5 = so-so, 10 = terrible	Comments (e.g., life event, med changes, med side effects, sleep/appetite changes, other)
S	1	8	Sleepover Friday – tired & extremely irritable
M	2	7	
T	3	5	
W	4	5	Carb craving after school
Th	5	4	
F	6	4	
S	7	7	
S	8	7	Dad on business trip
M	9	7	Major meltdown after school
T	10	6	
W	11	5	
Th	12	5	Dad home
F	13	4	
S	14	6	
S	15	7	1st day with Risperdal 0.5mg 3x per day 60lbs at psychiatrist appt (has
M	16	6	gained 5 lbs in past month)
T	17	4	
W	18	4	
Th	19	3	
F	20	3	
S	21	4	
S	22	5	
M	23	4	
T	24	4	
W	25	4	
Th	26	3	
F	27	3	
S	28	3	
S	29	5	
M	30	4	
T	31	4	

From *Psychotherapy for Children with Bipolar and Depressive Disorders* by Mary A. Fristad, Jill S. Goldberg Arnold, and Jarrod M. Leffler. Copyright 2011 by The Guilford Press. Permission to photocopy this handout is granted to purchasers of this book for personal use only (see copyright page for details).

Mood–Medication Log

Child's name: _____   Month: _____   Treatment providers/program: _____

Medications (type, dose, side effects): _____

Day	Date	Overall rating 1 = great, 5 = so-so, 10 = terrible	Comments (e.g., life event, med changes, med side effects, sleep/appetite changes, other)
	1		
	2		
	3		
	4		
	5		
	6		
	7		
	8		
	9		
	10		
	11		
	12		
	13		
	14		
	15		
	16		
	17		
	18		
	19		
	20		
	21		
	22		
	23		
	24		
	25		
	26		
	27		
	28		
	29		
	30		
	31		

Medication Summary
for Depression and Anxiety Disorders

Selective Serotonin Reuptake Inhibitors (SSRIs)

Trade name	Generic name
Prozac	fluoxetine
Zoloft	sertraline
Luvox	fluvoxamine
Celexa	citalopram
Lexapro	escitalopram
Paxil	paroxetine

Atypical Antidepressants

Trade name	Generic name
Wellbutrin	bupropion
Effexor	venlafaxine
Cymbalta	duloxetine
Serzone	nefazodone
Desyrel	trazodone

Side Effect Management

Note: The U.S. FDA has issued "black-box warnings" for antidepressants in youth. Clinical guidelines suggest careful monitoring for increased suicidal thoughts and actions, particularly in the first 8 weeks of use. Monitoring is also advisable at any dosage increase.

Side effect	Management strategies
Increased thirst/urination:	• Drink six to eight glasses of liquid/day. • Avoid high-calorie beverages. • Make school plan to use bathroom often.
Tremor:	• Take medication with meals or in divided doses. • Avoid caffeine.
Increased appetite/weight gain:	• Develop and maintain balanced diet and regular, developmentally appropriate exercise. Avoid drastic diets and/or diet pills.
Skin sensitivity:	• Use sunscreen. • Wear protective clothing. • Avoid sunlight/sunlamps.
Impaired sleep:	• Have routine sleep habits. • Don't let the weekend disrupt these by more than 1 hour. • No exercise/caffeine in the evening. • Wake at regular times, even if tired. • Do not nap during the day.
Dizziness:	• Stand up slowly.
Dry mouth:	• Drink water. • Use sugarless gum/candy.
Constipation:	• Eat high-fiber diet. • Drink six to eight glasses of water/day.
Persistent nausea:	• Take medicine with meals or in divided doses.

Medication Summary
for Bipolar Disorder and ADHD

Mood Stabilizers

Target symptom: Mood.

Side effects: Multiple; need to monitor carefully, especially weight gain; get fact sheet for each medication.

Trade name	Generic name
Eskalith, Lithobid	lithium
Depakote, Depakene	valproic acid
Tegretol	carbamazepine
Lamictal	lamotrigine

Atypical Antipsychotics

Target symptoms: Mood, aggression, psychosis.

Side effects: Multiple; need to monitor carefully, especially weight gain; get fact sheet for each medication.

Trade name	Generic name
Risperdal	risperidone
Seroquel	quetiapine
Zyprexa	olanzapine
Clozaril	clozapine
Geodon	ziprasidone
Abilify	aripiprazole
Invega	paliperidone

Antihypertensives

Target symptoms: Agitation, sleep disruption, impulsivity, tics.

Side effects: Drowsiness, dizziness.

Trade name	Generic name
Catapres	clonidine
Tenex, Intuniv	guanfacine

(cont.)

Stimulants and Nonstimulants

Target symptoms: Attention, impulsivity, hyperactivity.

Side effects: Decreased appetite/weight, stomach pain, restlessness, dizziness, palpitations, insomnia, headache.

Note. Strattera is a nonstimulant. Also, the abbreviations in brackets [LA, etc.] indicate drugs that are available in various long-acting/extended-release forms, as well as in their standard forms.

Trade name	Generic name
Ritalin [LA], Metadate [ER, CD], Concerta	methylphenidate
Focalin	dexmethylphenidate
Dexedrine	dextroamphetamine
Adderall [XR]	amphetamine–dextroamphetamine
Daytrana	methylphenidate transdermal system
Vyvanse	lisdexamfetamine
Strattera	atomoxetine

Side Effect Management

Many side effects can be minimized by altering the dose, changing the number of administrations per day (e.g., splitting the dose into three instead of two administrations), or changing the timing of administration. The side effects of some medications may be of equal (or greater) concern than the symptoms the medications are treating; careful monitoring, and discussing the cost–benefit analysis with the prescriber, are important.

See Handout 33 (Medication Summary for Depression and Anxiety Disorders) for specific side effect management tips.

Understanding My Child's Medication

Medication and Dose	Target Symptom	Side Effects	How to Manage Side Effects	Important Things to Remember
1.				
2.				
3.				
4.				
5.				
6.				

The Important Healthy Habits

1. Sleep

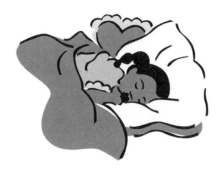

2. Eating

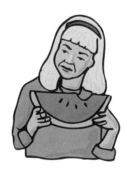

3. Exercise

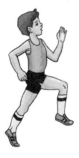

Enough sleep on a consistent schedule + healthy eating
+ regular exercise = healthier body + better mood.

Healthy Habits Worksheet

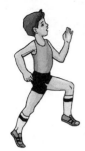 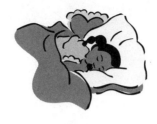 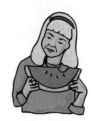

What daily activities help you stay healthy?

1. _____

2. _____

3. _____

4. _____

What are some of your and your family's unhealthy habits?

1. _____

2. _____

3. _____

4. _____

Why are healthy habits important? They help you:

- Feel good about yourself
- Improve mood
- Deal with stress
- Avoid illness
- Improve your schoolwork
- Stay at a healthy weight
- Reduce side effects of medication

Sleep

➡ The importance of sleep:
What happens when I don't get enough sleep?

_____

_____

_____

_____

_____

What happens when I get too much sleep?

_____

_____

_____

_____

_____

➡ How much sleep do I get?

Bedtime =

Fall-asleep time =

Wake-up time =

Total sleep =

➡ Am I getting enough sleep?   Yes   /   No

➡ If "No," use Handout 40 (Sleep Chart) to make and keep track of goals.

Sleep Chart (Sample)

	Bedtime	Fall-Asleep Time	Wake-Up Time	Total Sleep Time	Total Nap Time
Goals	Weekdays = 8:45 Weekends = 9:45	Weekdays = 9:00 Weekends = 10:00	Weekdays = 6:30 Weekends = 9:00	Weekdays = 9 hr 30 min Weekends = 11 hr	0 min
Mon. ↓ Tues.	8:50	9:00	6:30	10 hr	30 min
Tues. ↓ Wed.	8:45	9:00	6:40	9 hr, 40 min	0 min
Wed. ↓ Thurs.	9:00	9:30	6:00	8 hr, 50 min	20 min
Thurs. ↓ Fri.	8:45	9:00	6:30	10 hr	30 min
Fri. ↓ Sat.	10:00	10:30	10:00	11 hr, 30 min	0 min
Sat. ↓ Sun.	9:45	10:00	9:15	11 hr, 45 min	30 min
Sun. ↓ Mon.	8:45	9:00	6:30	10 hr	30 min

Sleep Chart

	Bedtime	Fall-Asleep Time	Wake-Up Time	Total Sleep Time	Total Nap Time
Goals	Weekdays = Weekends =	Weekdays = Weekends =	Weekdays = Weekends =	Weekdays = Weekends =	
Mon. ↓ Tues.					
Tues. ↓ Wed.					
Wed. ↓ Thurs.					
Thurs. ↓ Fri.					
Fri. ↓ Sat.					
Sat. ↓ Sun.					
Sun. ↓ Mon.					

Healthy Eating

➡ The importance of healthy eating:
What happens when I don't eat healthy foods?

_____

_____

_____

_____

_____

What happens when I eat healthy foods?

_____

_____

_____

_____

_____

➡ Healthy and unhealthy foods (see Handout 42, The Food Pyramid)

➡ Healthy foods I eat:

➡ Unhealthy foods I eat:

➡ Am I getting enough healthy foods? Yes / No

➡ If "No," use Handout 42 (The Food Pyramid) and Handout 44
(Healthy Food Chart) to make and keep track of goals.

The Food Pyramid

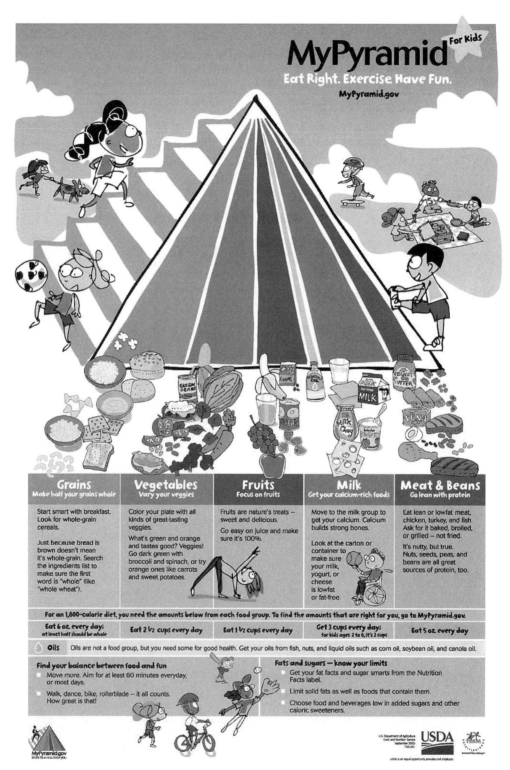

Healthy Food Chart (Sample)

	Bread Cereal Rice Pasta	Veggies	Fruits	Milk Yogurt Cheese	Meat Fish Eggs	Fats Oils Sweets
Goals	6–11	3–5	2–4	2–3	2–3	2
Mon.	9	4	3	2	2	2
Tues.	7	5	3	2	2	2
Wed.	9	3	4	3	3	1
Thur.	8	3	2	3	2	2
Fri.	10	5	4	2	3	1
Sat.	6	4	2	2	3	1
Sun.	9	5	3	3	2	2

Healthy Food Chart

	Bread Cereal Rice Pasta	Veggies	Fruits	Milk Yogurt Cheese	Meat Fish Eggs	Fats Oils Sweets
Goals	6–11	3–5	2–4	2–3	2–3	2
Mon.						
Tues.						
Wed.						
Thur.						
Fri.						
Sat.						
Sun.						

Exercise

➡ The importance of exercise:
What happens when I don't get enough exercise?

_____

_____

_____

What happens when I get too much exercise?

_____

_____

_____

➡ Three main types of exercise:
1. Stretching
2. Aerobic
3. Strengthening

➡ How many times do I exercise per week?
1. Stretching   _____
2. Aerobic   _____
3. Strengthening   _____

➡ Am I getting enough exercise?   Yes   /   No

➡ If "No," use Handout 47 (Exercise Chart) to make and keep track of goals.

Exercise Chart (Sample)

	Stretching	Cardiovascular	Strengthening
Ideas	Yoga, my own stretching routine	Playing tennis, running, soccer, walking, skateboarding	Push-ups, lifting weights, sit-ups
Goals	10—15 min daily	10—15 min daily	2—3 times a week for 5—10 min each
Mon.	10 min	15 min	1 time today
Tues.	0 min	30 min	
Wed.	15 min	10 min	
Thurs.	10 min	0 min	1 time today
Fri.	5 min	15 min	
Sat.	10 min	10 min	1 time today
Sun.	15 min	10 min	

Exercise Chart

	Stretching	**Cardiovascular**	**Strengthening**
Ideas			
Goals	_____ min daily	_____ min daily	_____ times a week for _____ min each
Mon.			
Tues.			
Wed.			
Thurs.			
Fri.			
Sat.			
Sun.			

Balloon Breathing

Balloon Breathing Instructions

1. Take a deep breath in through your nose and fill your lungs.

2. Keep your lips together tightly.

3. Allow one small "pinhole" between your upper and lower lips.

4. Blow out slowly through this small "pinhole" in your lips. **Do this the way air comes out of a balloon that has been poked with a pin.**

5. Complete Steps 1 through 4 at least three times in a row. (This completes **one set** of breathing.)

6. Try to do **one or two sets** of breathing at a time. You can do more if you want.

   Practice this activity at least three times (on three different days) before our next session.

Breathing Log

	Child	Parents
Date:	_____	_____
Date:	_____	_____
Date:	_____	_____

Who's Who and What's What
in the Mental Health System

Title	Degree/credentials	Role
		Who's Who
Psychiatrist	MD or DO	Completes evaluations; makes medication recommendations; monitors medication; sometimes provides therapy.
Psychologist	PhD, PsyD, or EdD	Completes evaluations; may do cognitive testing; provides individual/family/group therapy and/or parent guidance; collaborates with prescriber; may collaborate with educational team.
Social worker	LSW, LISW, LICSW, or MSW	May complete evaluations; may serve as a "gatekeeper" for psychiatric services; provides individual/family/group therapy and/or parent guidance; collaborates with prescribing physician; may collaborate with educational team.
Therapist (various degrees)	PC, PCC, PCC-S, MFT, IMFT	Usually plays a role comparable to a social worker's; these are professional counselors or marriage and family therapists.
Nurse with advanced training or physician assistant	APRN, RNCS, CRNP, MSN, PA	Completes evaluations; makes medication recommendations; monitors medication; sometimes provides therapy.
Case manager	MA, BA, or BS (may also have titles listed for "Therapist")	Helps coordinate services; makes home visits; works with child individually at school or home; may work with parents on strategies to manage problems at home; may work with educational team to coordinate services.
Others (e.g., Big Brother/Big Sister, neighbor, religious youth leader, family friend)	Varies	Respite; community mentoring.
		What's What: Levels of Care
Wrap-around care	Varies	Provides support to child/family to improve communication and behavior; provides crisis management services; can provide home-based services; in some cases, provides one-on-one behavioral support at home and (when not provided by the school district) at school.
Inpatient care	MD, APN, RN, MSW/LISW, PhD/PsyD, educators, various others	Provides safety when symptoms are severe and child is dangerous to self or others. Focus is on stabilization; child is usually discharged to less intensive care within 1 week; sometimes a few family therapy sessions occur; medications are probably adjusted; medical tests (e.g., drug screen, EEG, MRI) may be conducted; may coordinate return to school plan and evaluate academic needs.

(cont.)

Title	Degree/credentials	Role
Partial hospitalization programs	MD, APN, RN, MSW/LISW, PhD/PsyD, educators, various others	"Step down" from inpatient care: Child attends program during the day, goes home at night. Focus is on stabilization; child is usually discharged to less intensive care within 1–2 weeks. Some family therapy is possible; medication adjustment may continue.
Residential treatment programs	Similar to partial hospitalization program	Longer-term out-of-home treatment. Length of stay varies depending on severity of symptoms (can be a year or more). School on site. Focus is on changing behavior to allow return to less restrictive setting.

Important School Terms and Abbreviations

Acronym (if applicable)	Term	Definition
—	Due process	Parental right to approve or disapprove of plans proposed by the school/district special services team, and to call for a review process if the parents do not approve of a plan.
FAPE	Free and appropriate public education	School districts must provide all eligible students with special education and related services, allowing personalized instruction and sufficient support services to permit the child to benefit educationally, at the public's expense.
FBA	Functional behavioral assessment	An evaluation, usually conducted by one or more school staff members, to identify triggers that precede losses of control or other significant behavioral problems.
IDEA or IDEIA	Individuals with Disabilities Education Improvement Act of 2004	One of two federal laws mandating educational services to children with disabilities. The child's disorder must fall into one of the qualifying disability categories; the condition must adversely affect performance; child must need special education and related services. Requires a written IEP based on an MFE.
IEE	Independent educational evaluation	All parents have a right to obtain an IEE at the expense of the school if they are dissatisfied with the MFE and they have followed specific procedural requirements of the law.
IEP	Individualized education program	Specific plan devised by school personnel, with parental participation and approval. Establishes child's educational goals and specifies how they will be met.
—	Inclusion[a]	All special education services are provided within the context of the regular classroom with typical peers. A special education teacher coordinates services, oversees implementation of the IEP, consults, and sometimes teaches with the classroom teacher.
LRE	Least restrictive environment	Placement that provides a child with needed educational services while maintaining his/her maximum participation in regular education services with typical peers.
—	Mainstreaming[a]	Children who have been placed in a self-contained classroom rejoin their regular class for particular subjects or time periods. Sometimes used as an incentive for children with behavioral challenges, or as a transition from a self-contained classroom back to a regular classroom.
MFE	Multifactored evaluation	An evaluation completed by the school (by a multidisciplinary team) to determine eligibility for special services. Ensures that no single procedure is the sole criterion for determining a child's eligibility for services.

(cont.)

Acronym (if applicable)	Term	Definition
OHI	Other health impairment	Classification for a child whose health problem adversely affects school performance and prevents the child's needs from being met entirely by regular education services. Some parents prefer this classification over SED for their children with mood disorders.
504 Plan	Rehabilitation Act, Section 504	One of two federal laws mandating educational services for children with disabilities. Child is eligible if physical or mental impairment is present and has a negative impact on a major life activity. Requires an agreed-upon 504 plan. Adherence is dependent on regular education teacher.
SBH	Severe behavioral handicap	Term (now dated, but still used in some districts) describing significant behavioral dysregulation.
SED	Severe emotional disturbance	Term used to describe significant emotional needs.
SLD	Specific learning disability	Term used to describe achievement in particular academic areas (e.g., reading, math) that is below expected level (often, but not always, based on tested ability level).

[a]Under IDEA 2004, which replaced the Individuals with Disabilities Education Act of 1997, the emphasis is on inclusion rather than mainstreaming

Who's Who in the School System

Team member	Role(s)
Teachers (regular and special education)	Classroom teacher, school plan coordinator, case manager.
School counselor	Individual work with child; consultation with teacher, school plan coordinator; sometimes in charge of coordinating 504 plans.
School psychologist	Responsible for evaluation report; does testing with child; may provide direct intervention, consultation with teacher.
School social worker	Only present in some school settings; may provide direct intervention with child; may help families find resources.
Principal/vice principal	Administrator; may work directly with child; supports classroom teacher; attends IEP/504 meetings; has input into eligibility for services.
Special education coordinator	Works for the district coordinating special education services; knowledgeable about services throughout the district; consultation; sometimes attends IEP meetings; may help make eligibility determinations.
Local education agency (LEA) representative (may also be special education coordinator or another IEP team member)	Qualified to provide, or supervise the provision of, specially designed instruction to meet the unique needs of children with disabilities; knowledgeable about the general education curriculum; and knowledgeable about the availability of the LEA's resources.
Instructional support teacher	Title may vary from district to district; in charge of coordinating a team that meets to discuss children who may need academic or behavioral support prior to an evaluation's being initiated; may be in charge of developing 504 plans.
Occupational therapist	Direct intervention with students or consultation with teachers re: developing fine motor abilities/handwriting or making accommodations for fine motor weaknesses. Also provides consultation and intervention for children with sensory integration issues.
Physical therapist	Direct intervention with students or consultation with teachers re: developing gross motor abilities or making accommodations for gross motor weaknesses.
Speech–language pathologist	Direct intervention with students or consultation with teachers re: developing language abilities, developing compensatory strategies for auditory processing deficits, etc.
Other school personnel	A creative, flexible team uses all resources. Any staff members (attendance coordinators, in-school discipline specialists, custodial staff, secretarial staff, etc.) may become helpful members of an educational team.

My Child's Treatment Team

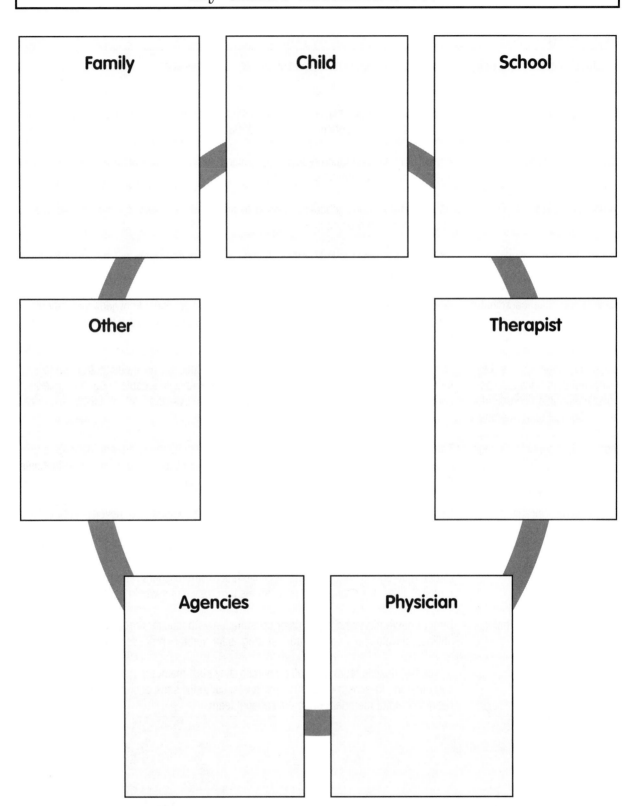

Family

Child

School

Other

Therapist

Agencies

Physician

My Child's Educational Team

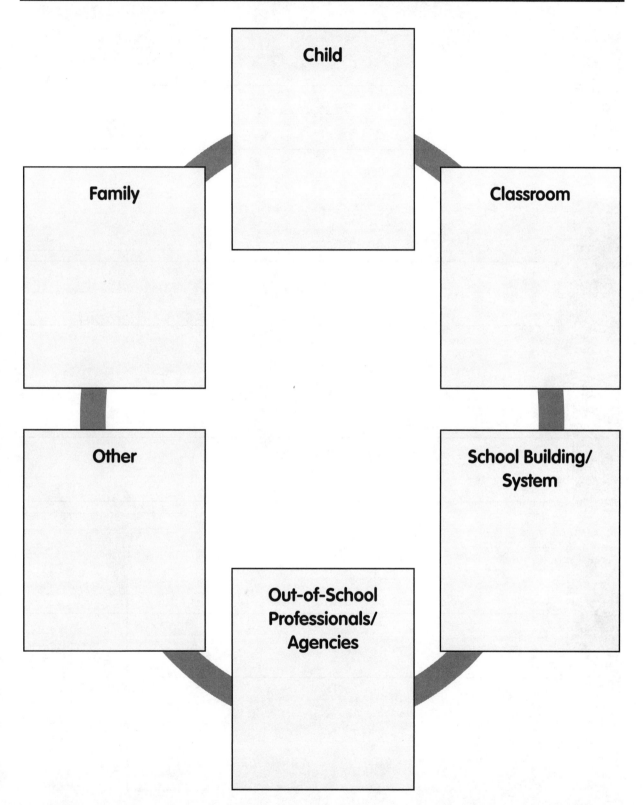

My Triggers for Mad, Sad, Bad Feelings

My Body Signals for Mad, Sad, Bad Feelings

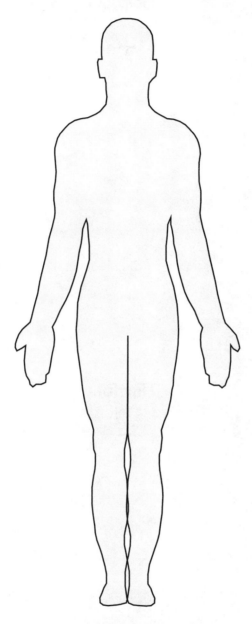

Red = Mad

Blue = Sad

Yellow = Bad

My Actions When I Feel Mad, Sad, Bad

Helpful

+

Hurtful

—

Building the Tool Kit (Sample)

Creative

Draw

Play music

Build with Legos

Write stories or a journal

Active

Take a walk

Ride bike

Play outside

Jump on trampoline

Dance

Social

Talk to parent or other adult

Talk to friends

Talk to pets

Play with a friend

R&R

Take a bath

Read a book

Get a drink/snack

Listen to music

Take a nap

Do 15 Bubble Breaths

Building the Tool Kit

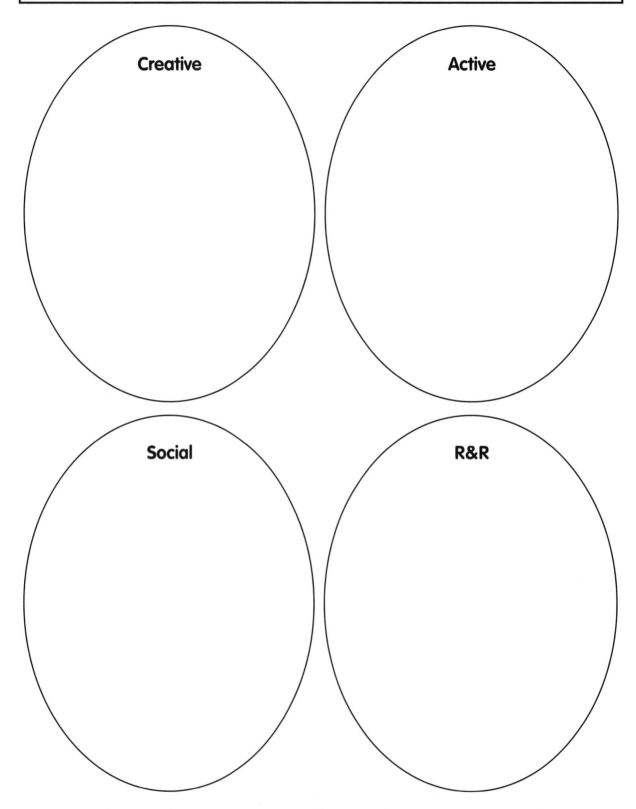

Creative

Active

Social

R&R

Taking Charge of Mad, Sad, Bad Feelings
(Sample)

My Tool Kit

Creative
Color.
Draw pictures.

Active
Play soccer.
Do jumping jacks.

R&R
Read a book
in my room.
Take a shower.

Social
Go outside
to play with
friends.
Talk to Mom.

I felt mad, sad, bad when ...
(Triggers)

When my sister took my game without asking.

My body felt ...
(Signals)

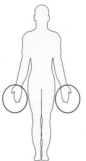

How I remembered to use my Tool Kit ...

Parent reminded me by ...
Telling me to think of my Tool Kit.

Or I remembered by ...
Putting it on my bedroom door.

From my tool kit, I used ...

I did 10 jumping jacks to calm myself down.

The outcome was ...
I calmed down and then asked my mom to help me get my game back.

| HANDOUT 60 | **Taking Charge of Mad, Sad, Bad Feelings** |

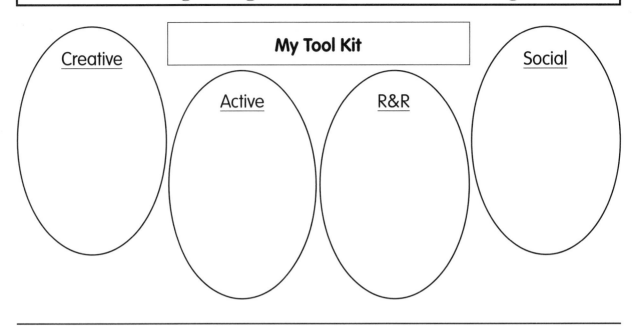

Creative   **My Tool Kit**   Social

Active   R&R

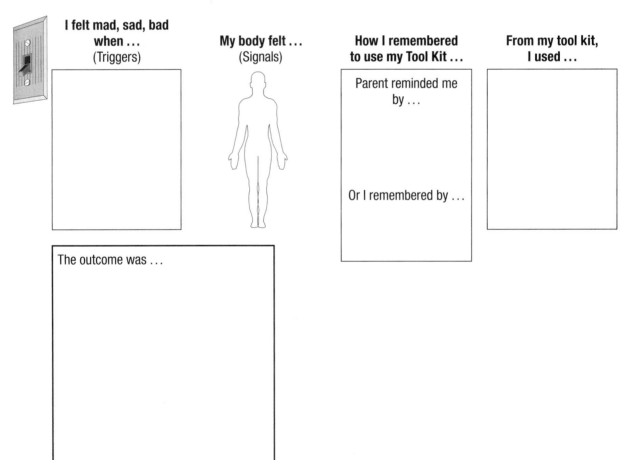

I felt mad, sad, bad when . . .
(Triggers)

My body felt . . .
(Signals)

How I remembered to use my Tool Kit . . .

Parent reminded me by . . .

Or I remembered by . . .

From my tool kit, I used . . .

The outcome was . . .

Thinking, Feeling, Doing (Sample for Parents)

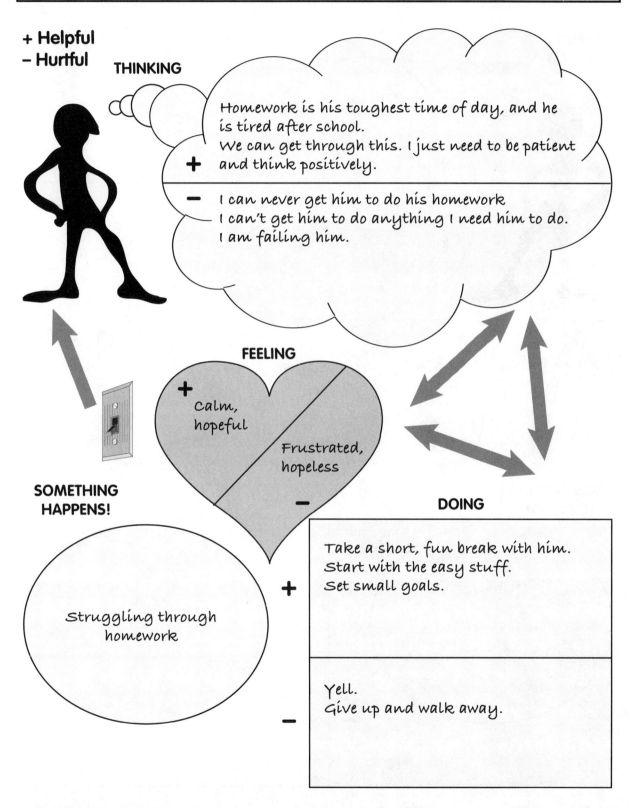

+ Helpful
– Hurtful

THINKING

+ Homework is his toughest time of day, and he is tired after school.
We can get through this. I just need to be patient and think positively.

– I can never get him to do his homework
I can't get him to do anything I need him to do.
I am failing him.

FEELING

+ Calm, hopeful

Frustrated, hopeless **–**

SOMETHING HAPPENS!

Struggling through homework

DOING

+ Take a short, fun break with him.
Start with the easy stuff.
Set small goals.

– Yell.
Give up and walk away.

Thinking, Feeling, Doing (Sample for Parents)

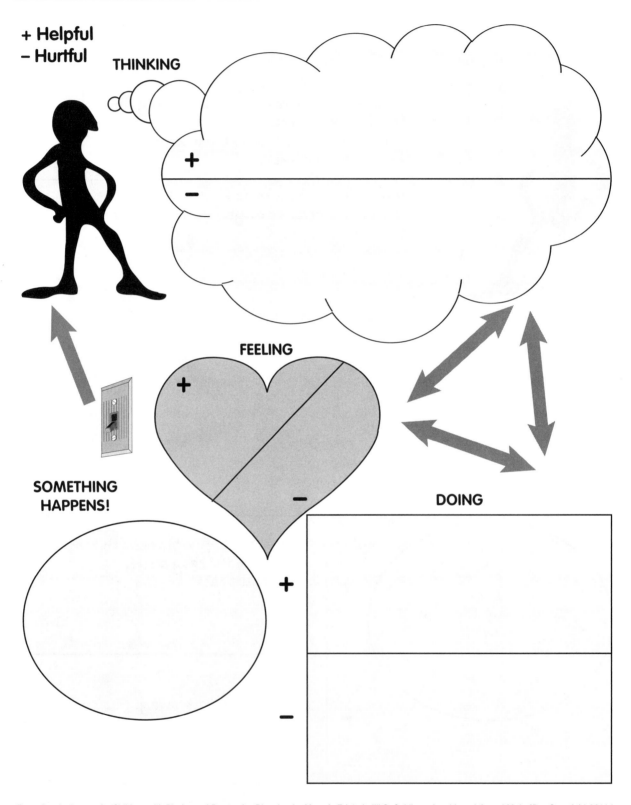

+ Helpful
– Hurtful

THINKING

+

–

FEELING

+

–

SOMETHING HAPPENS!

DOING

+

–

Thinking, Feeling, Doing (Sample 1 for Children)

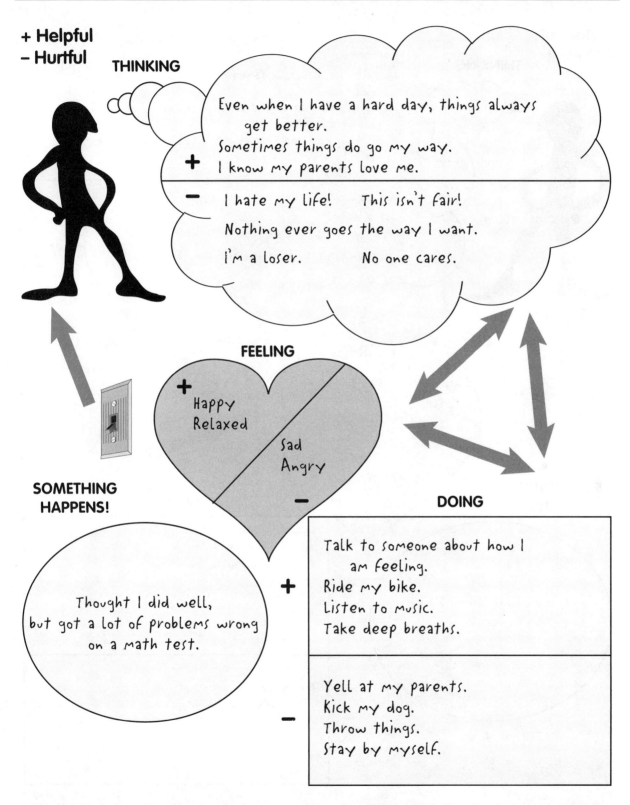

+ Helpful
– Hurtful

THINKING

+ Even when I have a hard day, things always get better.
Sometimes things do go my way.
I know my parents love me.

– I hate my life!   This isn't fair!
Nothing ever goes the way I want.
I'm a loser.   No one cares.

FEELING

+ Happy
Relaxed

Sad
Angry **–**

SOMETHING HAPPENS!

Thought I did well, but got a lot of problems wrong on a math test.

DOING

+ Talk to someone about how I am feeling.
Ride my bike.
Listen to music.
Take deep breaths.

– Yell at my parents.
Kick my dog.
Throw things.
Stay by myself.

Thinking, Feeling, Doing (Sample 2 for Children)

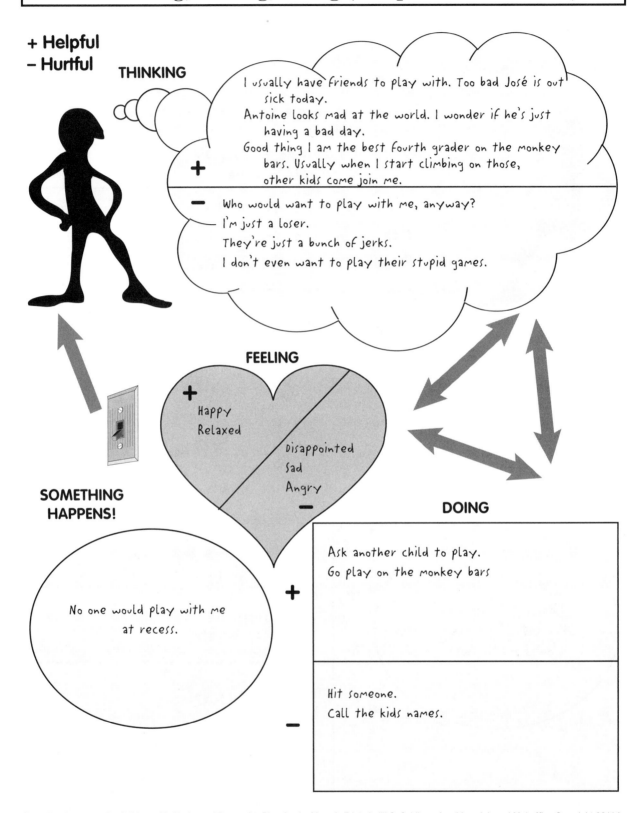

+ Helpful
– Hurtful

THINKING

+
I usually have friends to play with. Too bad José is out sick today.
Antoine looks mad at the world. I wonder if he's just having a bad day.
Good thing I am the best fourth grader on the monkey bars. Usually when I start climbing on those, other kids come join me.

–
Who would want to play with me, anyway?
I'm just a loser.
They're just a bunch of jerks.
I don't even want to play their stupid games.

FEELING

+
Happy
Relaxed

Disappointed
Sad
Angry
–

SOMETHING HAPPENS!

No one would play with me at recess.

DOING

+
Ask another child to play.
Go play on the monkey bars

–
Hit someone.
Call the kids names.

Problem Solving:
Symptoms and Family Conflicts

1. The problem is ...

2. I/We have talked to ...

3./4. We have thought of these possible solutions and weighed their pros and cons:

Solution?	Pros	Cons

5. We picked this one to try:

6. This is how it worked:

7. Next time we will:

Problem Solving (Sample)

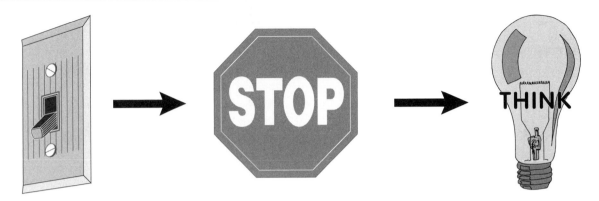

This is what happened:

I got angry because I don't understand my homework!

I used this tool to calm down:

I took deep breaths.

What is my problem?

I'm tired after school, and math is hard, so I get frustrated.

What can I do to solve my problem?

1. Copy my friend's homework!

2. Ask my mom for help.

3. Ask the teacher for help.

4. Do math in A.M. when I'm not tired.

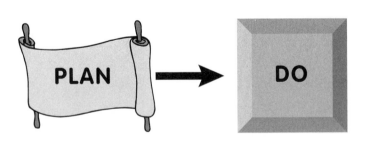

Which solution seems the best?   Do # ___3___

___3___

Did it work?   (Yes) No

Next time I will

Ask the teacher for help.

Problem Solving

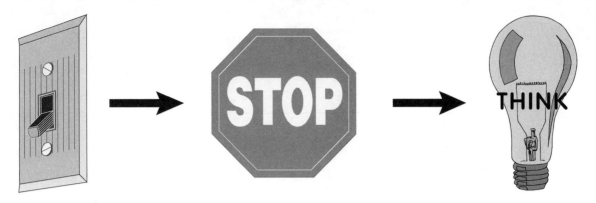

This is what happened:

I used this tool to calm down:

What is my problem?

What can I do to solve my problem?
1.

2.

3.

4.

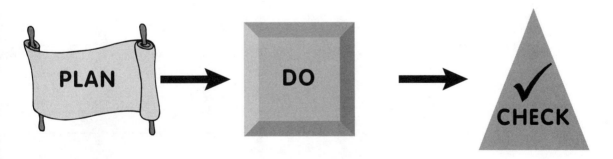

Which solution seems the best?   Do # _____
_____

Did it work?   Yes   No
Next time I will

_____

HANDOUT 68	**Communication**

What is communication? _____

_____

_____

_____

_____

Why is it important? _____

_____

_____

_____

_____

Two types of communication:

Nonverbal, which includes:

1. _____   4. _____

2. _____   5. _____

3. _____

Verbal, which includes: _____

_____

_____

_____

The Communication Cycle

All communication—verbal and nonverbal—involves both sending and getting a message.

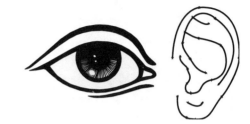

You send a message.

Person receives message.

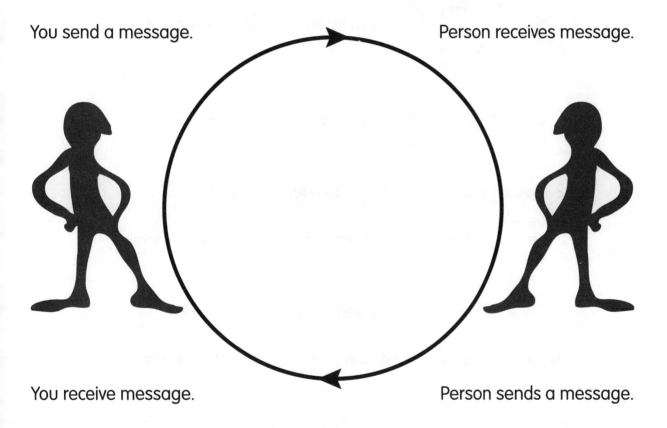

You receive message.

Person sends a message.

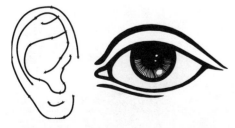

Nonverbal Communication

Look 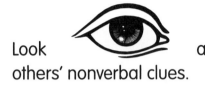 and listen  to your own and others' nonverbal clues.

1. **Facial Expressions**—happy, sad, scared, angry (see Handout 1, Feelings)

2. **Body Gestures**—hands, shoulders, head nods

3. **Body Posture**—relaxed, stressed, angry, bored, attentive, tired

4. **Tone of Voice**—happy, sad, angry, excited, bored

5. **Personal Space**—too close, too far, or arm's distance

Paying Attention to Feelings

Feeling	Child practices— Can adult guess? ✓ = Yes ? = Not sure	Adult practices— Can child guess? ✓ = Yes ? = Not sure
Sad		
Angry		
Scared		
Confused		
Stressed		
Bored		
Proud		
Other: _____		

Out with the Old Communication, In with the New (Sample)

Day	Old (hurtful) communication	When did I catch myself?*	New (helpful) communication
1	"Stop that now or else!"	When I saw my child's reaction	Use a calmer voice and don't threaten.
2	"You never listen to me."	The next day	Say, "Right now I feel that you aren't listening to me."
3	"Just snap out of it!"	As soon as I said it	Say, "I can tell you are feeling bad right now, and I'm also very frustrated," and then problem-solve later.
4	I don't remember—I just remember screaming at him.	Once I calmed down	Wait until I'm calmer to talk to him about what's making me feel unhappy.
5			
6			
7			

*Right away? When I saw my child's reaction? An hour/day later?

Out with the Old Communication, In with the New

Day	Old (hurtful) communication	When did I catch myself?*	New (helpful) communication
1			
2			
3			
4			
5			
6			
7			

*Right away? When I saw my child's reaction? An hour/day later?

Verbal Communication

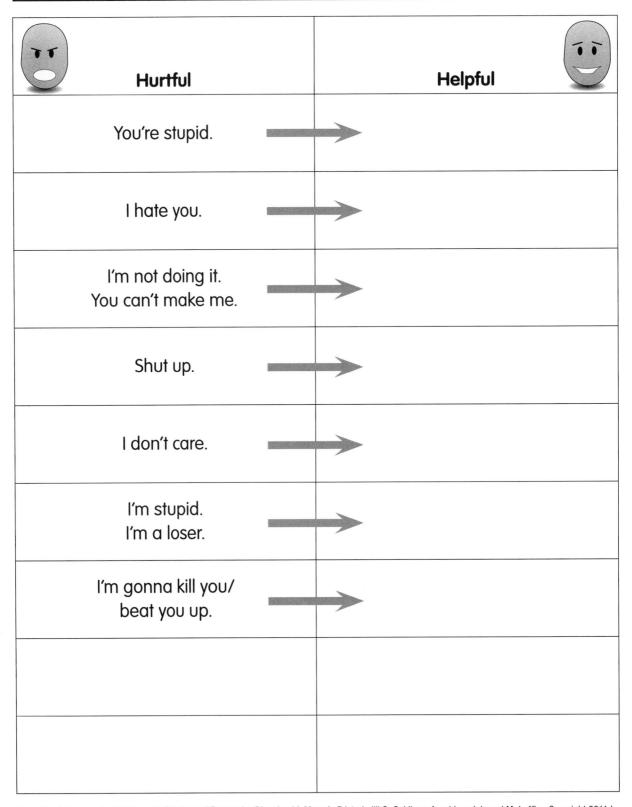

Hurtful	Helpful
You're stupid.	
I hate you.	
I'm not doing it. You can't make me.	
Shut up.	
I don't care.	
I'm stupid. I'm a loser.	
I'm gonna kill you/ beat you up.	

Let's Talk (Sample)

Kids did this:

1. Look at Mom and Dad when they're talking.

2. Wait until the other person is finished before talking.

3. Use a calm/inside voice.

We could all communicate better if . . .

Adults did this:

1. Use a calm, soft voice.

2. Let me talk too.

3. Use kind words.

Let's Talk

Kids did this:

1.

2.

3.

We could all communicate better if . . .

Adults did this:

1.

2.

3.

PEP Take-Home Messages for Parents

Topic	Take-home message	Follow-up actions
Symptoms and diagnoses	It's not your fault, but it is your challenge! Know the symptoms associated with mood episodes.	Track mood symptoms. Keep your team informed about symptoms.
Medications	Medications are often a part of treatment. They require a careful cost–benefit analysis.	Keep a medication log—work carefully with your child's prescriber.
Healthy habits	Good sleep hygiene, regular exercise, and healthy eating habits are "free medicines"	Work together on improving sleep, improving eating habits, and making regular exercise a family activity.
Psychosocial treatments—therapy and school-based intervention	It takes a village!	Build and then maintain mental health and school teams.
Negative family cycles	Mood symptoms tend to set off some negative family cycles.	Recognize negative cycles when they occur, and work together to change them.
Coping skills—problem solving	See symptoms and situations as problems that need solutions.	Use problem solving to address situations as they arise.
Coping skills—verbal communication	The way family members talk and listen to each other matters.	Have periodic check-ins about how family members are talking and listening.
Coping skills—nonverbal communication	Nonverbal communication is often misread or misunderstood.	Pay attention to nonverbal communication.
Symptom and crisis management	It pays to be prepared!	Have a plan for crisis management. Keep a mood/symptom log. Work with your treatment team to develop strategies that work.
Needs of other family members	A child's mood disorders affect the whole family.	Find creative ways to meet the needs of all family members.

When you have a problem that needs to be fixed:

1. Remember, it's okay to ask for help!

2. Where is your mood? _____

3. What are you feeling?

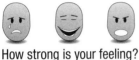 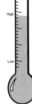

How strong is your feeling?

4. Keep healthy habits (sleeping, eating, exercise).

5. Get out your Tool Kit—what will be most helpful to "fix" the problem?

Creative   Active   R&R   Social

6. Can you change how you THINK? Or what you DO?

7. Use problem solving, and stay positive!

STOP   THINK   PLAN   DO   CHECK

8. Use helpful nonverbal and verbal communication

9. Remember: Practice, practice, practice your skills!

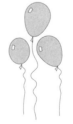 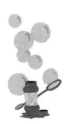 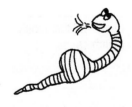

Medication Match Sample Cards

Depression

Bipolar Disorder

ADHD

Anxiety

Medication
Match

Medication
Match

Medication
Match

Medication
Match

Risperdal

Abilify

Lithium

Depakote

Medication
Match

Medication
Match

Medication
Match

Medication
Match

Prozac	**Ritalin**
Focalin	**Concerta**

Medication
Match

Medication
Match

Medication
Match

Medication
Match

Strattera

Clonidine

Seroquel

Sad

Medication
Match

Medication
Match

Medication
Match

Medication
Match

Really irritable

Grouchy

Angry

Nothing is fun

Medication Match

Medication Match

Medication Match

Medication Match

Worried

No energy

Scared

Too excited

Medication
Match

Medication
Match

Medication
Match

Medication
Match

From *Psychotherapy for Children with Bipolar and Depressive Disorders* by Mary A. Fristad, Jill S. Goldberg Arnold, and Jarrod M. Leffler. Copyright 2011 by The Guilford Press. Permission to photocopy this game is granted to purchasers of this book for personal use only (see copyright page for details).

Thinking too fast

Talking too fast

Can't pay attention

Can't concentrate

Medication Match

Medication Match

Medication Match

Medication Match

Hyperactive

Acting without thinking

Need less sleep than usual

Hard to fall asleep or stay asleep, but feel tired

Medication Match

Medication Match

Medication Match

Medication Match

Feeling guilty for things
that aren't your fault

Thinking about death or suicide

Hungry all the time
or not hungry at all

Feeling like you have
special powers

Medication Match

Medication Match

Medication Match

Medication Match

Medication
Match

Medication
Match

Medication
Match

Medication
Match

Thinking, Feeling, Doing
Activity Cards for Large and Small Spaces

Large Space	Small Space
Using a cone, whiffle ball, and bat, set up a batting-T and hit the whiffle ball into the large end of another cone.	Use a skinny marker to connect the dots in the PEP Connect the Dots game.
Ask someone to throw a pass with the football from one end of the room to the other, and do your best touchdown dance when you catch it.	Use a highlighter to find all of the words in one of the PEP Word Search games.
Holding a jump rope at knee level, jump over it side to side five times	Use a deck of playing cards to build a three-story card house.
Find a tennis ball and a sheet of paper. Balance the sheet of paper on your head, and bounce and catch the tennis ball from one end of the room to the other.	Use a small box of crayons to complete one of the Color by Number pictures.
Toss the ball from one hand to another while hopping across the room.	Use a pencil to complete one of the PEP Mazes leading from "My Symptoms" to "Me."

PEP Connect the Dots

PEP Word Search (Easy)

```
D  E  P  R  E  S  S  I  O  N  A  I  M  R  T
S  Q  D  E  X  C  I  T  E  D  C  N  A  F  R
V  C  U  O  H  A  P  P  Y  O  A  I  N  S  I
G  A  O  O  T  R  D  T  H  I  N  K  I  N  G
N  L  N  I  F  E  E  L  I  N  G  I  A  Z  G
F  M  K  S  A  D  L  L  M  G  R  O  Q  Y  E
K  E  K  E  U  F  A  M  I  L  Y  Y  D  O  R
C  H  A  L  L  E  N  G  E  N  R  S  R  S  Z
L  A  J  Y  T  O  O  L  K  I  T  P  J  I  E
```

Find the words listed below in the puzzle above. All of the words are either up-and-down or right-to-left. No words are diagonal.

ANGRY	DOING	FEELING	SCARED
CALM	EXCITED	HAPPY	THINKING
CHALLENGE	FAMILY	MANIA	TOOLKIT
DEPRESSION	FAULT	SAD	TRIGGER

PEP Word Search (Medium)

```
f r g a z k k b f d n z k r s p h s a v
d f z w i k a e d o o q m q y g f q s k
y p p a h a e q i f e i a h m p n a a q
w q a e g l w s j r b x n h p d i u d e
i w l r i u s y g m e z i g t e u m q a
h s k n z e u t w d f g a c o r m u n d
e t g d r c h a l l e n g e m o v g b i
p i h p u o g v p s e h j i s b r d c j
t g e i y o s j o u w t f j r y q l x q
y d s r n n r y y o i q i s q t w m a e
r c m a k k i p n l d m y h z o t l d q
r d l v c m i j l a d t y d t p v d v l
i v a b s d c n c e l s e d h a i t p z
j q c o a f t d g j m r z c a l i f i g
s t n l g t d f p b a m u h w k v m r e
i d d e t i c x e c f a m i l y h x w u
z g u f d r c q s x e e a o f y o s w h
b n o i t a c i n u m m o c q a k w x f
o q m t q h c h w g r t o s b f l d p n
l v v l u m z m i k z t e b s q j b z h
```

Find the words listed below in the puzzle above. Words can be up-and-down, sideways, or diagonal.

angry	depression	happy	scared
bored	doing	jealous	symptoms
calm	excited	mania	thinking
challenge	family	proud	toolkit
communication	feeling	sad	trigger

PEP Word Search (Hard)

```
K I T U T L R L J R N O N V E R B A L S
E O N N A H H E I Z T I K L O O T E F Y
Q C O M G D I M L A E S T N P C Q A E P
C Z I H A A E N B A G U J E R P M G M K
Y E S N Y N C T K L X N J P A I G D D X
J Z S O O P I O I I H A Z A L M R G V U
T A E I U E U A Q C N Z T Y K X C X S T
Z F R T R Z O H I G X G U I T K P W G C
G F P A C Y Q B B C G E M O O O Q R N A
C E E C H I G N I O D X P G Y N W R Y Q
N E D I A G N I V L O S M E L B O R P Y
W L S N L M X Y Y F Z N E C H P D X Z T
A I F U L W J I W W V E R B A L H Y P H
N N F M E Q K J Z U S C A R E D C H P V
G G Y M N B N A M I N G T H E E N E M Y
R O K O G B C S M O T P M Y S G S Z R R
Y D X C E S R T R I G G E R Q D W N N Q
```

Find the words listed below in the puzzle above. Words can be up-and-down, sideways, or diagonal.

ANGRY	MANIA	TEAM
COMMUNICATION	NAMINGTHEENEMY	THINKING
DEPRESSION	NONVERBAL	TOOLKIT
DOING	PROBLEMSOLVING	TRIGGER
EXCITED	RELAXATION	VERBAL
FAMILY	SCARED	YOURCHALLENGE
FEELING	SYMPTOMS	

Color by Number (Easy)

1 = Blue   2 = Red   3 = Yellow   4 = Green

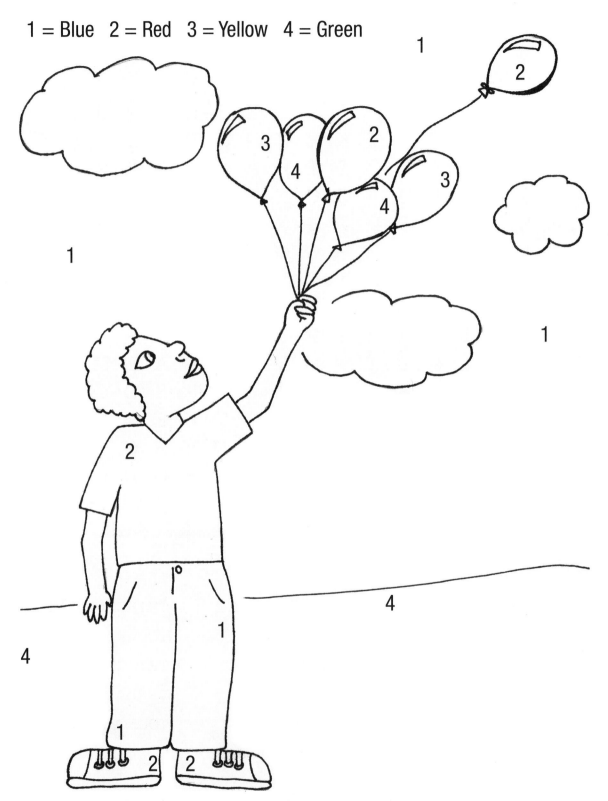

Color by Number (Hard)

1 = Green   2 = Blue   3 = Yellow   4 = Orange
5 = Purple   6 = Pink

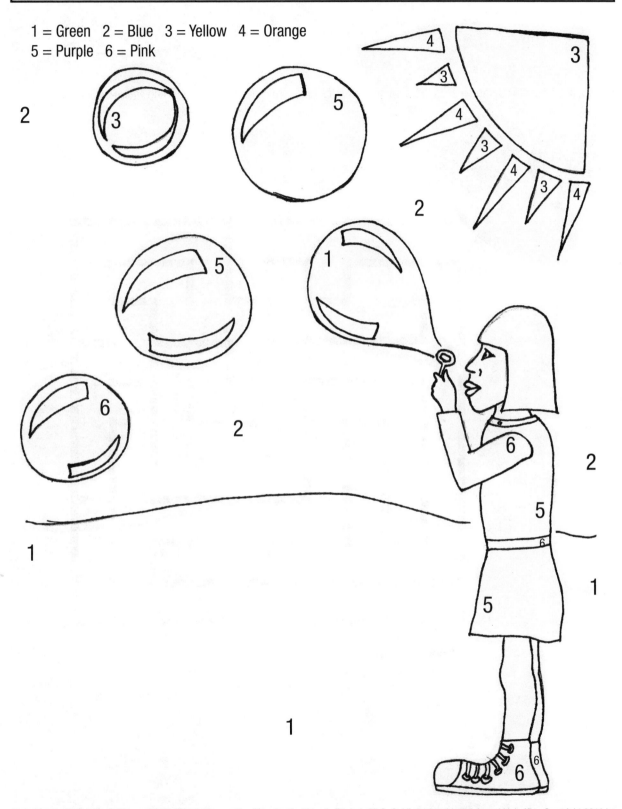

PEP Maze (Easy)

Draw a line from "My Symptoms" to "Me" without backtracking, crossing any walls, or lifting your pencil.

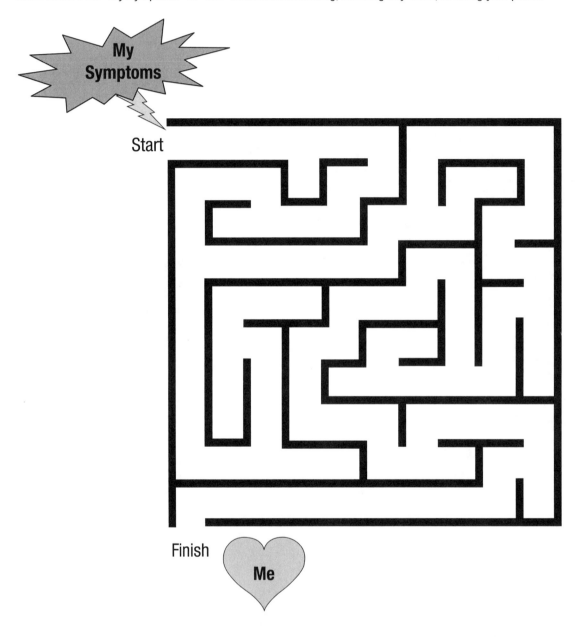

PEP Maze (Medium)

Draw a line from "My Symptoms" to "Me" without backtracking, crossing any walls, or lifting your pencil.

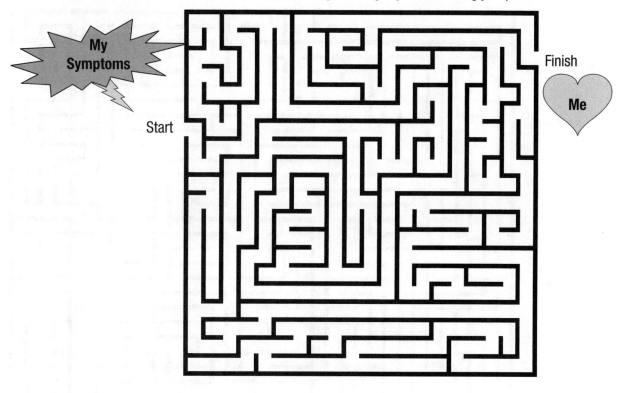

PEP Maze (Hard)

Draw a line from "My Symptoms" to "Me" without backtracking, crossing any walls, or lifting your pencil.

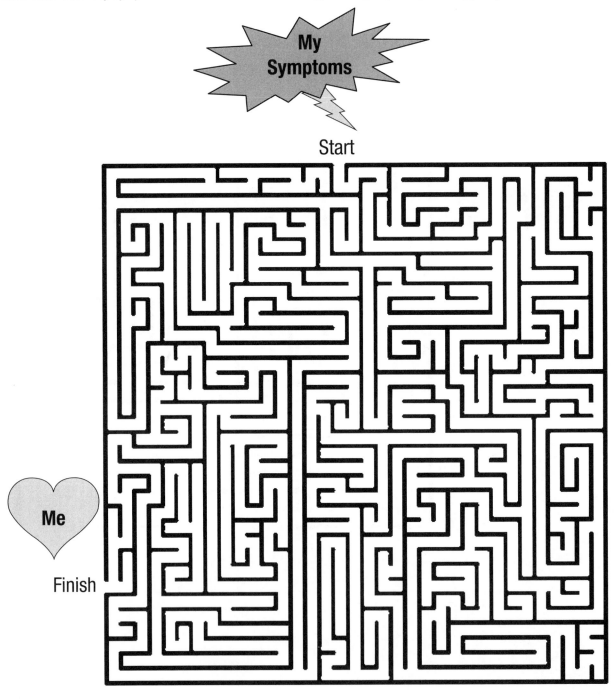

Key for PEP Connect the Dots

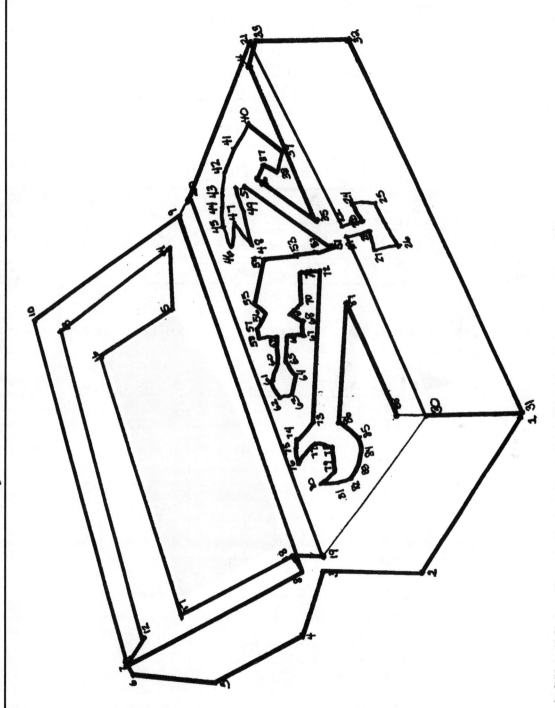

Key for PEP Word Search (Easy)

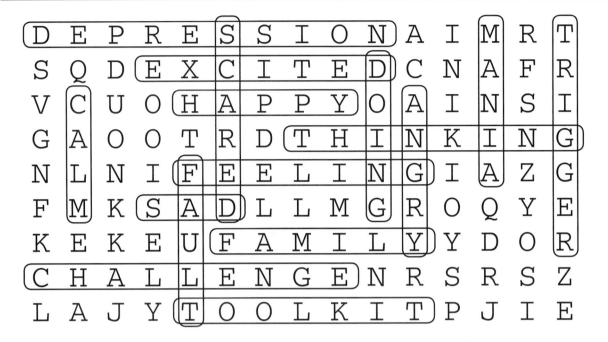

Find the words listed below in the puzzle above. All of the words are either up-and-down or right-to-left. No words are diagonal.

ANGRY	DOING	FEELING	SCARED
CALM	EXCITED	HAPPY	THINKING
CHALLENGE	FAMILY	MANIA	TOOLKIT
DEPRESSION	FAULT	SAD	TRIGGER

Key for PEP Word Search (Medium)

```
f r g a z k k b f d n z k r s p h s a v
d f z w i k a e d o o g m q y g f q s k
y p p a h a e g i f e i a h m p n a a q
w q a e g l w s j r b x n h p d i u d e
i w l r i u s y g m e z i g t e u m q a
h s k n z e u t w d f g a c o r m u n d
e t g d r c h a l l e n g e m o v g b i
p i h p u o g v p s e h j i s b r d c j
t g e i y o s j o u w t f j r y q l x q
y d s r n n r y o i q i s q t w m a e e
r c m a k k i p n l d m y h z o t l d q
r d l v c m i j l a d t y d t p v d v l
i v a b s d c n c e l s e d h a i t p z
j q c o a f t d g j m r z c a l i f i g
s t n l g t d f p b a m u h w k v m r e
i d d e t i c x e c f a m i l y h x w u
z g u f d r c q s x e e a o f y o s w h
b n o i t a c i n u m m o c q a k w x f
o q m t q h c h w g r t o s b f l d p n
l v v l u m z m i k z t e b s q j b z h
```

Find the words listed below in the puzzle above. Words can be up-and-down, sideways, or diagonal.

angry	depression	happy	scared
bored	doing	jealous	symptoms
calm	excited	mania	thinking
challenge	family	proud	toolkit
communication	feeling	sad	trigger

Key for PEP Word Search (Hard)

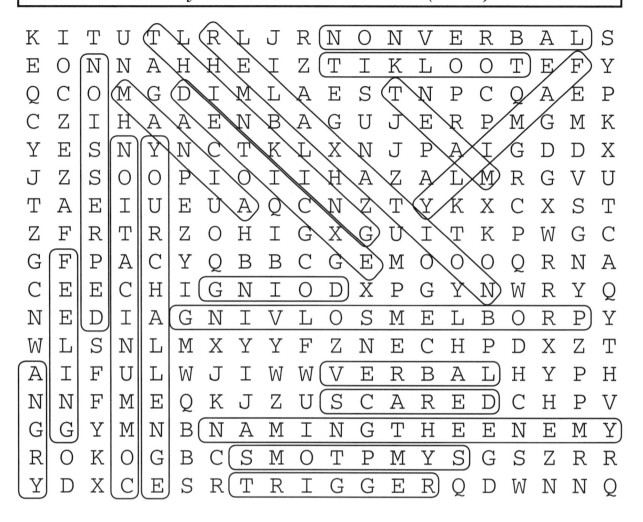

Find the words listed below in the puzzle above. Words can be up-and-down, sideways, or diagonal.

ANGRY	MANIA	TEAM
COMMUNICATION	NAMINGTHEENEMY	THINKING
DEPRESSION	NONVERBAL	TOOLKIT
DOING	PROBLEMSOLVING	TRIGGER
EXCITED	RELAXATION	VERBAL
FAMILY	SCARED	YOURCHALLENGE
FEELING	SYMPTOMS	

Key for PEP Maze (Easy)

Draw a line from "My Symptoms" to "Me" without backtracking, crossing any walls, or lifting your pencil.

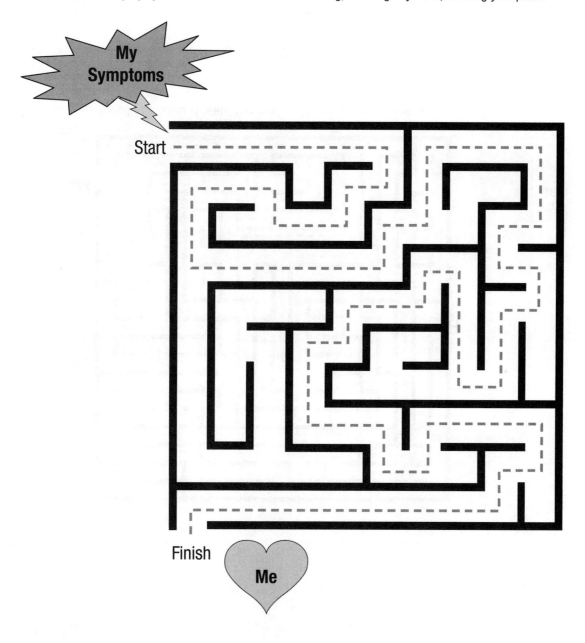

Key for PEP Maze (Medium)

Draw a line from "My Symptoms" to "Me" without backtracking, crossing any walls, or lifting your pencil.

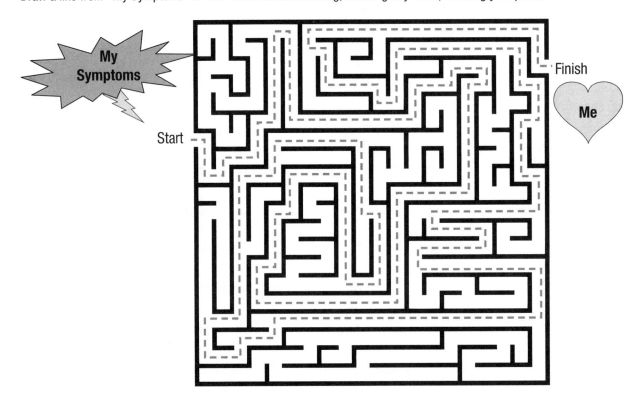

Key for PEP Maze (Hard)

Draw a line from "My Symptoms" to "Me" without backtracking, crossing any walls, or lifting your pencil.

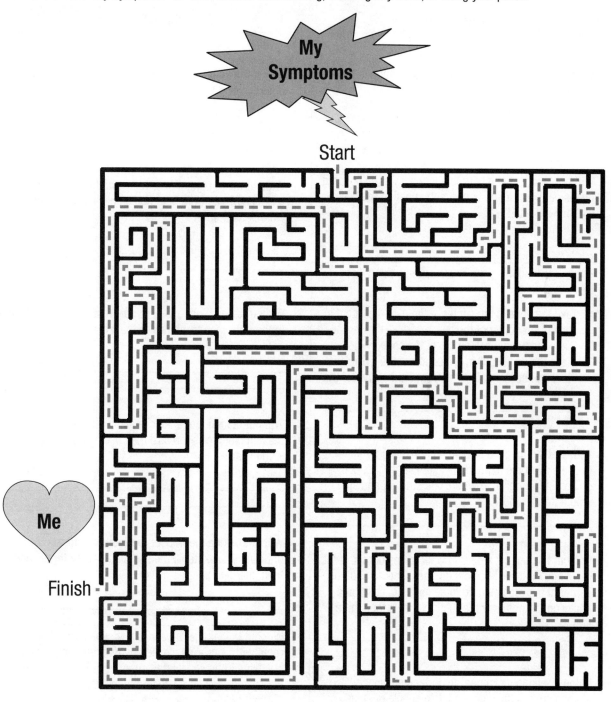

Follow-the-Leader Charades Cards
for Large and Small Spaces

Large Space

Without talking, get a peer to play underhand catch with you.

Without talking, get a peer to shoot a layup by hopping on his right foot to the basket and shooting the ball with his left hand.

Without talking, have the group arrange the gym in this order:

1. Take the cone in the center of the gym & place it in the far left corner of the gym.
2. Place the whiffle ball on top of the cone.
3. Place the basketball in the center of the gym.
4. Place the soccer ball in the front right corner of the gym.

Without talking, get a peer to hop on her right foot to one side of the room, do five jumping jacks, hop on her left foot back to where she started, and spin around three times.

Without talking, get a peer to walk to one corner of the room and do three knee bends; then walk to another corner of the room and do three jumping jacks; and finally go to another corner and touch his toes three times.

Without talking, get a peer to pretend she is ice-skating around the room and do a couple of spins, then skate backward for 10 feet, and then be a hockey player shooting a puck toward the net.

Small Space

Without talking, get a peer to pat his head with his right hand and rub his stomach with his left.

Without talking, get a peer to hop on her right foot to one side of the room, and hop on her left foot back to where she started.

Without talking, get a peer to spin in a circle five times to the right then five times to the left.

Without talking, get a peer to stand on one leg while making big circles forward then backward in the air with his arms.

Without talking, get a peer to pretend that he is dribbling a basketball, then shooting a free throw, and then guarding another player.

Without talking, get a peer to lead you across the room with your eyes closed and without bumping into anything. Then you lead the peer across the room with her eyes closed and without bumping into anything. Without talking, get a peer to stack two chairs, place a book on top of them, and walk around the stack four times. Then have the peer put the book and chairs back where they came from.

404

Letter Scramble Cards
for Large and Small Spaces

Large Space

Work with your teammate(s) to unscramble the six tasks. Then have your teammate(s) complete them in order.

1. Ckik the ccoser allb through the noces.
2. Toosh two absktes with a absktesallb.
3. Nur to the trheo dise of the myg and ckab.
4. Od ten umpjing cksaj.
5. Indf the rappe in oury etam's locor and utp it in the nectre of the myg.
6. Leyl, "Ew are infiedsh!"

Small Space

Work with your teammate(s) to unscramble the six tasks. Then have your teammate(s) complete them in order.

1. Terepdn to mjup peor for 20 sdeaocsn.
2. Klaw around the moro two mites. Yats scloe to the lwalas.
3. Muh the gnos "Pahyp Bdathiry."
4. Terepdn to hcaot a tofoallb and od a clbreeanoit cedna.
5. Tap oury deah and buroury mstahco.
6. Letl the dreales, "Ew are neod."

KEY: Work with your teammate to unscramble the six tasks. Then have your teammate complete them in order.

1. Kick the soccer ball through the cones.
2. Shoot two baskets with a basketball.
3. Run to the other side of the gym and back.
4. Do ten jumping jacks.
5. Find the paper in your team's color and put it in the center of the gym.
7. Yell, "We are finished!"

KEY: Work with your teammate(s) to unscramble the six tasks. Then have your teammate(s) complete them in order.

1. Pretend to jump rope for 20 seconds.
2. Walk around the room two times. Stay close to the walls.
3. Hum the song "Happy Birthday."
4. Pretend to catch a football and do a celebration dance.
5. Pat your head and rub your stomach.
6. Tell the leaders, "We are done."

PEP Review Game

Symptoms/Medications 100

Easy, Medium, Hard

True/False: Talking faster than usual is a symptom of mania.

(**Answer: True**)

Symptoms/Medications 200

Easy, Medium, Hard

True/False: Trouble sleeping is a symptom of depression.

(**Answer: True**)

Bonus: Where is your mood right now on the Strength of Feelings thermometer?

Symptoms/Medications 300

Easy, Medium

Name one side effect of one of the medications we talked about.

_____

Hard

Name one medication for depression.

Bonus: Name one symptom that this medication should affect.

Symptoms/Medications 400

Easy

Name two symptoms of depression.

_____

Medium

Name one medication for mania.

_____

Hard

Name one medication for mania and one for depression.

Bonus: Name two symptoms that these medications should affect.

Symptoms/Medications 500

Easy

Name one medication for depression or mania.

_____

Medium, Hard

Name three symptoms of depression.

Bonus: If your medication is working, what should happen to those symptoms?

(cont.)

Thinking, Feeling, Doing 100

Easy, Medium, Hard

True/False: Your thoughts can affect the way you feel.

(Answer: True)

Bonus: What does R&R stand for in the Tool Kit?

(Answer: Rest & relaxation)

Thinking, Feeling, Doing 200

Easy, Medium, Hard

True/False: One way to improve your mood is to change a hurtful thought or action into a helpful thought or action.

(Answer: True)

Bonus: You think somebody stole your binder. What's a more helpful thought? A more helpful action?

Thinking, Feeling, Doing 300

Easy, Medium, Hard

Jerome got shoved by a classmate in the hallway. Name one helpful action he might do.

Thinking, Feeling, Doing 400

Easy, Medium, Hard

Tiffani got a bad grade on a test. Name one helpful thought she might have.

Thinking, Feeling, Doing 500

Easy

Joe did not make the football team, and he really wanted to. Name one helpful thought he might have.

Medium

Antonio failed his math test. Name one helpful thought and one helpful action he could choose.

Hard

Latoya thinks, "My mother is *always* mean to me." Name 2 helpful thoughts to replace this.

(cont.)

Anger Management/Coping 100

Easy, Medium, Hard

Name one calming strategy you can try when you are really mad.

Anger Management/Coping 300

Easy

Out of your Tool Kit, name one physical coping strategy.

Medium

Out of your Tool Kit, name one creative coping strategy and one R&R strategy.

Hard

Name a Tool Kit coping skill that you can use anywhere.

Bonus: What Tool Kit category (Creative, Active, R&R, Social) is that skill from?

Anger Management/Coping 500

Easy

Out of your Tool Kit, name one social coping strategy.

Medium

Out of your Tool Kit, name one social and one active coping strategy.

Bonus: What does CARS stand for?

(Answer: Creative, Active, Rest & Relaxation [R&R] Social)

Hard

Out of your Tool Kit, name a coping strategy that you can use at school.

Bonus: Are triggers always external events, or can your mood change without an "outside" trigger?

(Answer: Your mood can change because of an internal trigger.)

Anger Management/Coping 200

Easy, Medium, Hard

Name one anger trigger for you.

Anger Management/Coping 400

Easy

Out of your Tool Kit, name one creative coping strategy.

Medium

Name one anger signal for you (something that lets you know you are mad).

Hard

Name one sadness trigger for you and one Tool Kit skill to cheer yourself up.

(cont.)

Problem Solving/Communication 100

Easy

Name one way to show someone you are listening.

Bonus: In order for communication to happen, you need a speaker and a _____ .

(**Answer: Receiver, Listener**)

Medium

Name one way in which you communicate to others that does not involve talking.

(**Answer: Tone of voice, facial expression, body posture, body gestures, or personal space**)

Hard

Name at least three of the five steps of problem solving.

(**Answer: Stop, Think, Plan, Do, Check**)

Problem Solving/Communication 200

Easy

Tell us one of the wishes you had for your parents for improving communication.

Medium

Name two helpful communication strategies.

Hard

Joey's big brother keeps mocking him in front of his friends. According to the five steps of problem solving, what's the *first* thing Joey should do?

(**Answer: Stop—do something to calm down.**)

Bonus: Brainstorm three plans to solve the problem.

Problem Solving/Communication 300

Easy, Medium

Maria is having trouble with her homework. Name two helpful actions that she could try to help solve her problem.

Hard

Name a more helpful communication than "I hate you!"

Problem Solving/Communication 500

Easy, Medium

Name all five steps of problem solving.

(**Answer: Stop, Think, Plan, Do, Check**)

Hard

Name all of the ways you communicate to others that do not involve talking.

(**Answer: Tone of voice, facial expression, body posture, body gestures, personal space**)

Problem Solving/Communication 400

Easy

Name two aspects of nonverbal communication that we practiced or talked about.

(**Answer: Tone of voice, facial expression, body posture, gestures, and/or personal space**)

Medium

At what stage/step of problem solving should you use your Tool Kit?

(**Answer: Stop**)

Bonus: What is one of the three ways to know if our talk or behavior is helpful or hurtful?

(**Answers: Does it hurt me?**

Does it hurt someone or something else?

Does it get anyone in trouble?)

Hard

Billy chose to ignore his little sister when she was bothering him, but she just kept bothering him. Using your five steps of problem solving, what should Billy do?

APPENDIX

Resources

Books

For Children

Anglada, T. (2004). *Brandon and the bipolar bear*. Victoria, BC, Canada: Trafford.—A storybook about a young boy newly diagnosed with BD.

Child and Adolescent Bipolar Foundation (CABF). (2003). *The storm in my brain*. Evanston, IL: Author.—An informational booklet that provides basic information about childhood BD (Also available at *www.bpkids.org*)

Dubuque, N., & Dubuque, S. (1996). *Kid power tactics for dealing with depression*. King of Prussia, PA: Center for Applied Psychology.—Written by an 11-year-old boy with depression and his mother; includes 15 strategies to deal with depression.

Hebert, B. (2001). *My bipolar, roller coaster, feelings book and workbook*. Murdock, FL: BPChildren.—A storybook about a young boy diagnosed with BD, and an accompanying workbook to help children better understand BD.

Hebert, B. (2005). *Anger mountain*. Murdock, FL: BPChildren.—A short story to help young children understand and deal with angry feelings.

McGee, C. (2002). *Matt, the moody hermit crab*. Nashville, TN: McGee & Woods.—A chapter book designed for 8- to 12-year-olds that portrays both the depressive and manic phases of BD.

For Adolescents

Calhoun, D. (2005). *The phoenix dance*. New York: Farrar, Straus & Giroux.—Fiction based on the Grimms' "The Twelve Dancing Princesses"; explores an adolescent girl's experience of BD.

Cobain, B. (2007). *When nothing matters anymore: A survival guide for depressed teen* (rev. ed.). Minneapolis, MN: Free Spirit.—A two-part book that describes depression and its treatment strategies.

Copeland M. E., & Copans, S. (2002). *Recovering from depression: A workbook for teens*. Baltimore, MD: Brookes.—A workbook to help adolescents understand depression and learn coping strategies.

Irwin, C. (1998). *Conquering the beast within: How I fought depression and won—and how you can, too*. New York: Random House.—Written and illustrated by a young adult, describes depression, its impact on loved ones, and steps to recovery.

Jamieson, P. E., & Rynn, M. A. (2006). *Mind race: A firsthand account of one teenager's experience with bipolar disorder*. New York: Oxford University Press.—Autobiography interwoven with facts about BD and its treatment.

For Parents

Anglada, T. (2006). *Intense minds.* Victoria, BC, Canada: Trafford.—A collection of personal reflections by adolescents and young adults describing the experience of mania and depression.

Anglada, T., & Hakala, S. M. (2008). *The childhood bipolar disorder answer book.* Naperville, IL: Sourcebooks.—Written in question-and-answer format by the parent of two children with BD and a psychiatrist who treats mood-disordered children.

Birmaher, B. (2000). *New hope for children and teens with bipolar disorder.* New York: Three Rivers Press.—Provides information about BD and its treatment.

Dubuque, S. (1996). *A parent's survival guide to childhood depression.* King of Prussia, PA: Center for Applied Psychology.—Describes depression in children and coping strategies.

Fristad, M. A., & Goldberg Arnold, J. S. (2004). *Raising a moody child: How to cope with depression and bipolar disorder.* New York: Guilford Press.—Describes the diagnosis, professional treatment, and relevant coping strategies for a mood disordered child and his or her family.

Koplewicz, H. (1997). *It's nobody's fault.* New York: Three Rivers Press.—Describes 13 common psychiatric disorders in children; outlines the diagnostic and treatment process in a non-blaming manner.

Miklowitz, D. J., & George, E. L. (2007). *The bipolar teen: What you can do to help your child and your family.* New York: Guilford Press.—Describes the diagnosis, professional treatment, and relevant coping strategies for adolescents with bipolar disorder and their families.

Papolos, D. & Papolos, J. (2006). *The bipolar child.* New York: Broadway Books.—Provides a compendium of information on BD and its treatment in youth.

Wilens, T. (2009). *Straight talk about psychiatric medications for kids* (3rd ed.). New York: Guilford Press.—An educational guide that outlines diagnosis, treatment and medication strategies for a variety of childhood disorders.

For Adults with Mood Disorders and Their Families

Beardslee, W. (2002). *Out of the darkened room: Protecting the children and strengthening the family when a parent is depressed.* Boston: Little, Brown.—Describes depression and its treatment in adults, and discusses how to prevent secondary damage in children.

Copeland, M. E. (1994). *Living without depression and manic depression.* Oakland, CA: New Harbinger.—A workbook that provides coping strategies to minimize the impact of mood disorders on life.

Jamison, K. R. (1995). *An unquiet mind.* New York: Knopf—An autobiography that discusses stigma, experiences of depression and mania, and the critical roles of medication and psychotherapy in managing BD.

Last, C. G. (2009). *When someone you love is bipolar: Help and support for you and your partner.* New York: Guilford Press.—A psychologist with BD uses both personal and professional experience to provide guidance on maintaining relationships through the challenges of bipolar disorder.

McKay, M., Davis, M., & Fannin, P. (1998). *Thoughts and feelings: Taking control of your moods and your life.* Oakland, CA: New Harbinger.—A handbook of cognitive-behavioral strategies to improve mood and functioning.

McManamy, J. (2006). *Living well with depression and bipolar disorder.* New York: HarperCollins.—Describes differential diagnosis, impact of mood disorders on relationships, and treatment/coping strategies.

Miklowitz, D. J. (2011). *The bipolar disorder survival guide: What you and your family need to know* (2nd ed.). New York: Guilford Press.—A guide to understanding BD and its treatment.

Rosenthal, N. E. (2006). *Winter Blues: Everything you need to know about seasonal affective disorder* (rev. ed.). New York: Guilford Press.—Describes SAD and its treatment, including light therapy and medication.

General Parenting

Faber, A., & Mazlish, E. (1999). *How to talk so kids will listen and listen so kids will talk.* New York: Avon Books.—Cartoons, illustrations, and exercises are used to provide guidance on communication strategies.

Greene, R. (2005). *The explosive child.* New York: Harper.—Describes a strategy to lessen hostility and noncompliance in parent–child interactions.

Seligman, M. (1996). *The optimistic child.* New York: Harper Perennial.—Provides strategies to promote self-esteem in children, and discusses the importance of optimism in reducing the threat of depression.

Sibling Issues

Faber, A., & Mazlish, E. (1998). *Siblings without rivalry.* New York: Avon Books.—Stories and illustrations are used to exemplify ways to improve sibling relationships.

Anglada, T. (2001). *Turbo Max: A story for siblings of bipolar children.* Murdock, FL: BPChildren.—Story for 8- to 12-year-olds, written as a boy's summer diary about coming to accept his sibling with BD.

Miscellaneous

Amador, X., & Johanson, A. L. (2000). *I am not sick, I don't need help!* Peconic, NY: Vida Press.—Guides family members in assisting a loved one to accept the need for treatment of a mood disorder or other mental health problem.

Rosenthal, M. S. (2000). *The thyroid sourcebook.* Los Angeles: Lowell House.—Describes thyroid disorders and their nutritional and pharmacological treatments.

Educational Resources

Anglada, T. (2009). *SWIVEL to success—Bipolar disorder in the classroom: A teacher's guide to helping students succeed.* Murdock, FL: BPChildren.—Describes the impact of BD on a student in the classroom, and suggests school-based interventions.

The following websites contain useful information regarding planning for children with mood disorders in the school setting.

www.bpchildren.org—BPChildren

www.schoolbehavior.com

www.bpkids.org—Child and Adolescent Bipolar Foundation (CABF)

www.josselyn.org/store.htm—The Josselyn Center

www.wrightslaw.com—Wrightslaw

www.natsap.org—National Association of Therapeutic Schools and Programs

www.iser.com/index.shtml—Internet Special Education Resources (ISER)

National Organizations and Support Groups

National Alliance on Mental Illness (NAMI), 1-800-950-6264, *www.nami.org*
Mental Health America (MHA), 1-703-684-7722, *www.nmha.org*
Depressive and Bipolar Support Alliance (DBSA), 1-800-826-3632, *www.dbsalliance.org*
Child and Adolescent Bipolar Foundation (CABF), 1-847-492-8519, *www.bpkids.org*
Juvenile Bipolar Research Foundation (JBRF), 1-866-333-JBRF, *www.jbrf.org*
BP Children, 1-732-909-9050 (fax), *www.bpchildren.org*
Families for Depression Awareness, 1-781-890-0220, *www.familyaware.org*

Phototherapy

Center for Environmental Therapeutics. *www.cet.org*

Nutritional Interventions

Truehope, 1-888-878-3467, *www.truehope.com*—EMPowerplus.
OmegaBrite, 1-800-383-2030, *www.omegabrite.com*—Omega 3 fatty acids.

PEP Workbooks

Child, parent, and child therapist MF-PEP workbooks, and child and parent IF-PEP workbooks, can be purchased at *www.moodychildtherapy.com*

References

Abela, J. R. Z., & Hankin, B. L. (2008). Cognitive vulnerability to depression in children and adolescents: A developmental psychopathology perspective. In J. R. Z. Abela & B. L. Hankin (Eds.), *Handbook of depression in children and adolescents* (pp. 35–78). New York: Guilford.

Abu-Omar, K., Rütten, A., & Lehtinen, V. (2004). Mental health and physical activity in the European Union. *Sozial-Präventivmedizin, 49*, 301–309.

Adler, C. M., DelBello, M. P., & Strakowski, S. M. (2006). Brain network dysfunction in bipolar disorder. *CNS Spectrums, 11*, 312–320.

American Psychiatric Association. (1994). *Diagnostic and statistical manual of mental disorders* (4th ed.). Washington, DC: Author.

Asarnow, J. R., Goldstein, M. J., Tompson, M., & Guthrie, D. (1993). One-year outcomes of depressive disorders in child psychiatric in-patients: Evaluation of the prognostic power of a brief measure of expressed emotion. *Journal of Child Psychology and Psychiatry, 34*(2), 129–137.

Asarnow, J. R., Scott, C. V., & Mintz, J. (2002). A combined cognitive-behavioral family education intervention for depression in children: A treatment development study. *Cognitive Therapy and Research, 26*(2), 221–229.

Barbini, B., Benedetti, F., Colombo, C., Dotoli, D., Bernasconi, A., Cigala-Fulgosi, M., et al. (2005). Dark therapy for mania: A pilot study. *Bipolar Disorders, 7*, 98–101.

Barbini, B., Bertelli, S., Colombo, C., & Smeraldi, E. (1996). Sleep loss, a possible factor in augmenting manic episode. *Psychiatry Research, 65*(2), 121–125.

Bersani, G., & Gravini, A. (2000). Melatonin add-on in manic patients with treatment resistant insomnia. *Progress in Neuro-Psychopharmacology and Biological Psychiatry, 24*, 185–191.

Birmaher, B., Axelson, D., Goldstein B., Strober M., Gill M. K., Hunt J., et al. (2009). Four-year longitudinal course of children and adolescents with bipolar spectrum disorders: The Course and Outcome of Bipolar Youth (COBY) study. *American Journal of Psychiatry, 166*(7), 795–804.

Birmaher, B., Brent, D., & the AACAP Work Group on Quality Issues. (2007). Practice parameter for the assessment and treatment of children and adolescents with depressive disorders. *Journal of the American Academy of Child and Adolescent Psychiatry, 46*, 1503–1526.

Birmaher, B., Axelson, D., Strober, M., Gill, M. K., Valeri, S., Chiappetta, L., et al. (2006). Clinical course of children and adolescents with bipolar spectrum disorders. *Archives of General Psychiatry, 63*(2), 175–183.

Bridge, J. A., Iyengar, S., Salary, C. B., Barbe, R. P., Birmaher, B., Pincus, H. A., et al. (2007). Clinical response and risk for reported suicidal ideation and attempts in pediatric antidepressant treatment: A meta-analysis of randomized controlled trials. *Journal of the American Medical Association, 297*, 1683–1696.

Butzlaff, R. L., & Hooley, J. M. (1998). Expressed emotion and psychiatric relapse. *Archives of General Psychiatry, 55,* (6), 547–552.

Campbell, M., & Cueva, J. E. (1995). Psychopharmacology in child and adolescent psychiatry: A review of the past seven years. Part II. *Journal of the American Academy of Child and Adolescent Psychiatry, 34*(10), 1262–1272.

Carlson, G. A. (2009). Treating the childhood bipolar controversy: A tale of two children. *American Journal of Psychiatry, 166,* 18–24.

Caspi, A., Sugden, K., Moffitt, T. E., Taylor, A., Craig, I. W., Harrington, H., et al. (2003). Influence of life stress on depression: Moderation by a polymorphism in the 5-HTT gene. *Science, 301*(5631), 386–389.

Centers for Disease Control and Prevention. (2008). Physical activity and health. Retrieved February 11, 2009, from *www.cdc.gov/physicalactivity/everyone/health/index.html.*

Centers for Disease Control. (2010). *Morbidity and Mortality Weekly Report, 59*(38), 1–7.

Chang, K., Saxena, K., Howe, M. (2006). An open-label study of lamotrigine adjunct or monotherapy for the treatment of adolescents with bipolar depression. *Journal of the American Academy of Child and Adolescent Psychiatry, 45,* 298–304.

Correll, C. U., & Carlson, E. (2006). Endocrine and metabolic adverse effects of psychotropic medications in children and adolescents. *Journal of the American Academy of Child and Adolescent Psychiatry, 45*(7), 771–791.

Craddock, N., & Jones, I. (1999). Genetics of bipolar disorder. *Journal of Medical Genetics, 36,* 585–594.

David-Ferdon, C., & Kaslow, N. J. (2008). Evidence-based treatments for child and adolescent depression. *Journal of Clinical Child and Adolescent Psychology, 37,* 62–104.

Davidson, K. H., & Fristad, M. A. (2008). Psychoeducational psychotherapy. In B. Geller & M. P. DelBello (Eds.), *Treatment of bipolar disorder in children and adolescents* (pp. 184–204). New York: Guilford Press.

Davies, P. T., & Cummings, E. M. (1994). Marital conflict and child adjustment: An emotional security hypothesis. *Psychological Bulletin, 116,* 387–411.

DelBello, M. P., Soutollo, C. A., Hendricks, W., Neimeier, T., McElray, S. L., & Strakowski, S. M. (2001). Prior stimulant treatment in adolescents with bipolar disorder: An association with age at onset. *Bipolar Disorders, 3,* 53–57.

Emslie, G. J., Rush, A. J., Weinberg, W. A., Rintelmann, J. W., & Roffwarg, H. P. (1990). Children with major depression show reduced rapid eye movement latencies. *Archives of General Psychiatry, 47*(2), 119–124.

Findling, R. L., Youngstrom, E. A., Fristad, M. A., Birmaher, B., Kowatch, R. A., Arnold, L. E., et al. (2010). Characteristics of children with elevated symptoms of mania: The Longitudinal Assessment of Manic Symptoms (LAMS) Study. *Journal of Clinical Psychiatry, 71*(12), 1664–1672.

Frazier, E. A., Fristad, M. A., & Arnold, L.E. (2009). Multinutrient supplement as treatment: Literature review and case report of a 12-year-old boy with bipolar disorder. *Journal of Child and Adolescent Psychopharmacology, 19*(4), 453–460.

Frazier, E. A., Fristad, M. A., & Arnold, L. E. (2010, August). Multi-nutrients in the treatment of childhood mood dysregulation. In M. Fristad (Chair), *The role of pharmacotherapy and nutrition in the treatment of childhood psychiatric disorders.* Symposium conducted at the 118th annual meeting of the American Psychological Association, San Diego, CA.

Fristad, M. A. (2006). Psychoeducational treatment for school-aged children with bipolar disorder. *Development and Psychopathology, 18,* 1289–1306.

Fristad, M. A. (2010). Development of emotion regulation in children of bipolar parents: Treatment implications. *Clinical Psychology: Science and Practice, 17*(3), 187–190.

Fristad, M. A., Davidson, K. H., & Leffler, J. (2007). Thinking–Feeling–Doing: A therapeutic technique for children with bipolar disorder and their parents. *Journal of Family Psychotherapy, 18*(4), 81–104.

Fristad, M. A., Gavazzi, S. M., & Soldano, K. W. (1998). Multi-family psychoeducation groups for childhood mood disorders: Program description and preliminary efficacy data. *Contemporary Family Therapy, 20*(3), 385–402.

Fristad, M. A., Gavazzi, S. M., Soldano, K. W. (1999). Naming the enemy: Learning to differentiate mood disorder "symptoms" from the "self" that experiences them. *Journal of Family Psychotherapy, 10*(1), 81–88.

Fristad, M. A., & Goldberg Arnold, J. S. (2004). *Raising a moody child: How to cope with depression and bipolar disorder.* New York: Guilford Press.

Fristad, M. A., Goldberg Arnold, J. S., & Gavazzi, S. M. (2002). Multifamily psychoeducation groups (MFPG) for families of children with bipolar disorder. *Bipolar Disorders, 4*, 254–262.

Fristad, M. A., Goldberg Arnold, J. S., & Gavazzi, S. M. (2003). Multi-family psychoeducation groups in the treatment of children with mood disorders. *Journal of Marital and Family Therapy, 29*(4), 491–504.

Fristad, M. A., Topolosky, S., Weller, E. B., & Weller, R. A. (1992). Depression and learning disabilities in children. *Journal of Affective Disorders, 26*, 53–58.

Fristad, M. A., Verducci, J. S., Walters, K., & Young, M. E. (2009). Impact of multifamily psychoeducational psychotherapy in treating children aged 8–12 with mood disorders. *Archives of General Psychiatry, 66*(9), 1013–1021.

Geller, B., Craney, J. L., Bolhofner, K., Nickelsburg, M. J., Williams, M., & Zimerman, B. (2002). Two-year prospective follow-up of children with a prepubertal and early adolescent bipolar disorder phenotype. *American Journal of Psychiatry, 59*(6), 927–933.

Geller, B., Fox, L. W., & Clark, K. A. (1994). Rate and predictors of prepubertal bipolarity during follow-up of 6- to 12-year-old depressed children. *Journal of the American Academy of Child and Adolescent Psychiatry, 33*, 461–469.

Geller, B., Zimerman, B., Williams, M., Bolhofner, K., & Craney, J. L. (2001). Bipolar disorder at prospective follow-up of adults who had prepubertal major depressive disorder. *American Journal of Psychiatry, 158*(1), 125–127.

Geller, B., Zimerman, B., Williams, M., DelBello, M. P., Bolhofner, K., Craney, J. L., et al. (2000). Diagnostic characteristics of 93 cases of a prepubertal and early adolescent bipolar disorder phenotype by gender, puberty and comorbid attention deficit hyperactivity disorder. *Journal of Child and Adolescent Psychopharmacology, 10*(3), 157–164.

Getz, G. E., Shear, P. K., & Strakowski. S. M. (2003). Facial affect recognition deficits in bipolar disorder. *Journal of the International Neuropsychological Society, 9*, 623–632.

Gillham, J. E., Hamilton, J., Freres, D. R., Patton, K., & Gallop, R. (2006). Preventing depression among early adolescents in the primary care setting: A randomized controlled study of the Penn Resiliency Program. *Journal of Abnormal Child Psychology, 34*(2), 203–219.

Gillham, J. E., Reivich, K. J., Freres, D. R., Chaplin, T. M., Shatté, A. J., Samuels, B., et al. (2007). School-based prevention of depressive symptoms: A randomized controlled study of the effectiveness and specificity of the Penn Resiliency Program. *Journal of Consulting and Clinical Psychology, 75*(1), 9–19.

Gillham, J. E., Reivich, K. J., Freres, D. R., Lascher, M., Litzinger, S., Shatté, A., et al. (2006). School-based prevention of depression and anxiety symptoms in early adolescence: A pilot of the parent intervention component. *School Psychology Quarterly, 21*(3), 323–348.

Goldberg Arnold, J. S., Fristad, M. A., & Gavazzi, S. M. (1999). Family psychoeducation: Giving caregivers what they want and need. *Family Relations, 48*(4), 411–417.

Goldstein, T. R., Axelson, D. A., Birmaher, B., & Brent, D. A. (2007). Dialectical behavior therapy for adolescents with bipolar disorder: A 1-year open trial. *Journal of the American Academy of Child and Adolescent Psychiatry, 46*(7), 820–830.

Gould, M. S., Marrocco, F. A., Kleinman, M., Thomas, J. G., Mostkoff, K., Cote, J., et al. (2005). Evaluating iatrogenic risk of youth suicide screening programs: A randomized controlled trial. *Journal of the American Medical Association, 293*, 1635–1643.

Grave, J., & Blissett, J. (2004). Is cognitive behavior therapy developmentally appropriate for young children?: A critical review of the evidence. *Clinical Psychology Review, 24*(4), 399–420.

Green, M. J., Cahill, C. M., & Malhi, G. S. (2007). The cognitive and neurophysiological basis of emotion dysregulation in bipolar disorder. *Journal of Affective Disorders, 103*, 29–42.

Harris, A. H. S., Cronkite, R., & Moos, R. (2006). Physical activity, exercise coping, and depression in a 10-year cohort study of depressed patients. *Journal of Affective Disorders, 93*(1–3), 79–85.

Hellander, M., Sisson, D. P., & Fristad, M. A. (2003). Internet support for parents of children with early-onset bipolar disorder. In B. Geller & M. P. DelBello (Eds.), *Bipolar disorder in childhood and early adolescence* (pp. 314–329). New York: Guilford Press.

Herjanic, B., Hudson, R., & Kotloff, K. (1976). Does interviewing harm children? *Research Communications in Psychology, Psychiatry, and Behavior, 1*(4), 523–531.

Hibbeln, J. R. (1998). Fish consumption and major depression [Comment]. *Lancet, 351*, 1213.

Hibbeln, J. R., Ferguson, T. A., & Blasbalg, T. L. (2006). Omega-3 fatty acid deficiencies in neurodevelopment, aggression and autonomic dysregulation: Opportunities for intervention. *International Review of Psychiatry, 18*, 107–118.

Horrigan, J. P., & Barnhill, L. J. (1999). Guanfacine and secondary mania in children. *Journal of Affective Disorders, 54*, 309–314.

Kaplan, B. J., Crawford, S. G., Gardner, B., & Farrelly, G. (2002). Treatment of mood lability and explosive rage with minerals and vitamins: Two case studies in children. *Journal of Child and Adolescent Psychopharmacology, 12*(3), 205–219.

Kaplan, B. J., Fisher, J. E., Crawford, S. G., Field, C. J., & *Kolb, B.* (2004). Case report. Improved mood and behavior during treatment with a mineral–vitamin supplement: An open-label case series of children. *Journal of Child and Adolescent Psychopharmacology, 14*(1), 115–122.

Kaplan, B. J., Simpson, S. A., Ferre, R., C., Gorman, C. P., McMullen, D. M., & Crawford, S. G. (2001). Effective mood stabilization with a chelated mineral supplement: An open-label trial in bipolar disorder. *Journal of Clinical Psychiatry, 62*(12), 936–944.

Kaufman, J., Yang, B. Z., Douglas-Palumberi, H., Grasso, D., Lipschitz, D., Houshyar, S., et al. (2006). Brain-derived neurotrophic factor–5-HTTLPR gene interactions and environmental modifiers of depression in children. *Biological Psychiatry, 59*, 673–680.

Kendall, P. C., & Beidas, R. S. (2007). Smoothing the trail for dissemination of evidence-based practices for youth: Flexibility within fidelity. *Professional Psychology: Research and Practice. 38*, 13–20.

Kovacs, M., Sherrill, J., George, C. J., Pollock, M., Tumuluru, R. V., & Ho, V. (2006). Contextual emotion-regulation therapy for childhood depression: Description and pilot testing of a new intervention. *Journal of the American Academy of Child and Adolescent Psychiatry, 45*(8), 892–903.

Kowatch, R. A. (2009a). Pharmacotherapy 1: Mood stabilizers. In R. A. Kowatch, M. A. Fristad, R. L. Findling, & R. M. Post (Eds.), *Clinical manual for management of bipolar disorder in children and adolescents* (pp. 133–156). Arlington, VA: American Psychiatric Publishing.

Kowatch, R. A. (2009b). Pharmacotherapy 2: Atypical antipsychotics. In R. A. Kowatch, M. A. Fristad, R. L. Findling, & R. M. Post (Eds.), *Clinical manual for management of bipolar disorder in children and adolescents* (pp. 157–172). Arlington, VA: American Psychiatric Publishing.

Kowatch, R. A., Fristad, M., Birmaher, B., Wagner, K. D., Findling, R. L., Hellander, M., et al. (2005). Treatment guidelines for children and adolescents with bipolar disorder: Child psychiatric workgroup on bipolar disorder. *Journal of the American Academy of Child and Adolescent Psychiatry, 44*(3), 213–235.

Kowatch, R. A., Fristad, M. A., Findling, R. L., & Post, R. M. (Eds.). (2009). *Clinical manual for management of bipolar disorder in children and adolescents.* Arlington, VA: American Psychiatric Publishing.

Kowatch, R. A., Strawn, J. R., & DelBello, M. P. (2010). Developmental considerations in the pharmacological treatment of youth with bipolar disorder. In D. J. Miklowitz & D. Cicchetti (Eds.), *Understanding Bipolar Disorder: A Developmental Psychopathology Perspective.* New York: Guilford Press.

Kramer, T. (2004). Talking points about antidepressants and suicide. *Medscape General Medicine, 6*(2), 30.

Leffler, J. M., Fristad, M. A., & Klaus, N. (2010). Adaptation and extension of individual family psychoeducational psychotherapy (IF-PEP) for children with bipolar disorder. *Journal of Family Psychotherapy, 21*(4), 269–286.

Lofthouse, N., & Fristad, M. A. (2004). Psychosocial interventions for children with bipolar disorder. *Clinical Child and Family Psychology Review, 7*(2), 71–88.

Lofthouse, N., Fristad, M. A., Splaingard, M., Kelleher, K., Hayes, J., & Resko, S. (2008). Web survey of sleep problems associated with early-onset bipolar spectrum disorders. *Journal of Pediatric Psychology, 33*(4), 349–357.

Maag, J. W., & Reid, R. (2006). Depression among students with learning disabilities: Assessing the risk. *Journal of Learning Disabilities, 29*(1), 3–10.

Mackinaw-Koons, B., & Fristad, M. A. (2004). Children with bipolar disorder: How to break down barriers and work effectively together. *Professional Psychology: Research and Practice, 35*(5, 481–484.

Magistretti, P., Pellerin, L., Rothman, D., & Shulman, R. (1999). Energy on demand. *Science, 283*(5401), 496–497.

Marsh, R., Gerber, A. J., & Peterson, B. S. (2008). Neuroimaging studies of normal brain development and their relevance for understanding childhood neuropsychiatric disorders. *Journal of the American Academy of Child and Adolescent Psychiatry, 47*(11), 1233–1251.

Mayes, S. D., & Calhoun, L. (2007). Learning, attention, writing, and processing speed in typical children and children with ADHD, autism, anxiety, depression, and oppositional-defiant disorder. *Child Neuropsychology, 13*(6), 469–493.

Mendenhall, A. N., Fristad, M. A., & Early, T. (2009). Factors influencing service utilization and mood symptom severity in children with mood disorders: Effects of multifamily psychoeducation groups (MFPGs). *Journal of Consulting and Clinical Psychology, 77*(3), 463–473.

Miklowitz, D. J. (2008). *Bipolar disorder: A family-focused treatment approach* (2nd ed.). New York: Guilford Press.

Miklowitz, D. J., & Goldstein, T. R. (2010). Family-based approaches to treating bipolar disorder in adolescence: Family-Focused Therapy and Dialectical Behavior Therapy. In D. J. Miklowitz & D. Cicchetti (Eds.), *Understanding Bipolar Disorder: A Developmental Psychopathology Perspective.* New York: Guilford Press.

Miklowitz, D. J., Goldstein, M. J., Nuechterlein, K. H., Snyder, K. S., & Mintz, J. (1988). Family factors and the course of bipolar affective disorder. *Archives of General Psychiatry, 45*(3), 225–231.

Ming, X., Gordon, E., Kang, N., & Wagner, G. C. (2008). Use of clonidine in children with autism spectrum disorders. *Brain and Development, 30*(7), 454–460.

Muratori, F., Picchi, L., Bruni, G., Patarnello, M., & Romagnoli, G. (2003). A two-year follow-up of psychodynamic psychotherapy for internalizing disorders in children. *Journal of the American Academy of Child and Adolescent Psychiatry, 42*(3), 331–339.

National Institute of Mental Health. (2010a). Prevalence of depression among U.S. youth ages 12–15. (2005–2008). Retrieved December 28, 2010, *nimh.nih.gov/statistics/pdf/nsduh-data-depression_prev_youth.pdf.*

National Institute of Mental Health. (2010b). 12-month prevalence for children (8 to 15 years). Retrieved December 28, 2010, from *nimh.nih.gov/statistics/pdf/nhanes-overallprevalence.pdf.*

Nelson, E., Barnard, M., & Cain, S. (2003). Treating childhood depression over videoconferencing. *Telemedicine Journal and e-Health, 9*(1), 49–55.

Nemets, H., Nemets, B., Apter, A., Bracha, Z., & Belmaker, R. H. (2006). Omega-3 treatment of childhood depression: A controlled, double-blind pilot study. *American Journal of Psychiatry. 163*(6), 1098–1100.

Noaghiul, S., & Hibbeln, R. (2003). Cross-national comparisons of seafood consumption and rates of bipolar disorders. *American Journal of Psychiatry, 160*(12), 2222–2227.

Nolan, C. L., Moore, G. J., Madden, R., Farchione, T., Bartoi, M., Lorch, E., et al. (2002). Prefrontal cortical volume in childhood-onset major depression: Preliminary findings. *Archives of General Psychiatry, 59*, 173–179.

Ogden, C. L., Carroll, M. D., & Flegal, K. M. (2008). High body mass index for age among US children and adolescents, 2003–2006. *Journal of the American Medical Association, 299*, 2401–2405.

Owen, C., Rees, A.-M., & Parker, G. (2008). The role of fatty acids in the development and treatment of mood disorders. *Current Opinion in Psychiatry, 21*, 19–24.

Pagano, M. E., Demeter, C. A., Faber, J. E., Calabrese, J. R., & Findling, R. L. (2008). Initiation of stimulant and antidepressant medication and clinical presentation in juvenile bipolar disorder. *Bipolar Disorders, 10*, 334–341.

Parfitt, G., & Eston, R. G. (2005). The relationship between children's habitual activity level and psychological well-being. *Acta Psychiatrica Scandanavica, 94*, 1791–1797.

Parker, G., Gibson, N. A., Brotchie, H., Heruc, G., Rees, A. M., & Hadzi-Pavlovic, D. (2006). Omega-3 fatty acids and mood disorders. *American Journal of Psychiatry, 163*(6), 969–978.

Pavuluri, M. (2008). *What works for bipolar kids: Help and hope for parents.* New York: Guilford Press.

Pavuluri, M. N., Graczyk, P. A., Henry, D. B., Carbray, J. A., Heidenreich, J., & Miklowitz, D. J. (2004). Child- and family-focused cognitive-behavioral therapy for pediatric bipolar disorder: Development and preliminary results. *Journal of the American Academy of Child and Adolescent Psychiatry, 43*, 528–537.

Pavuluri, M. N., & Sweeney, A. (2008). Integrating functional brain neuroimaging and developmental cognitive neuroscience in child psychiatry research. *Journal of the American Academy of Child and Adolescent Psychiatry, 47*(11), 1273–1288.

Pfeffer, C. R., Jiang, H., Kakuma, T., Hwang, J., & Metsch, M. (2002). Group intervention for children bereaved by the suicide of a relative. *Journal of the American Academy of Child and Adolescent Psychiatry, 41*(5), 505–513.

Plante, D. T., & Winkelman, J. W. (2008). Sleep disturbance in bipolar disorder: Therapeutic implications. *American Journal of Psychiatry, 165*, 830–843.

Pliszka, S., & the AACAP Work Group on Quality Issues. (2007). Practice parameter for the assessment and treatment of children and adolescents with attention-deficit/hyperactivity disorder. *Journal of the American Academy of Child and Adolescent Psychiatry, 46*, 894–921.

Popper, C. W. (2001). Do vitamins or minerals (apart from lithium) have mood-stabilizing effects? *Journal of Clinical Psychiatry, 62*(12), 933–935.

Post, R. M. (2007a). Kindling and sensitization as models for affective episode recurrence, cyclicity, and tolerance phenomena. *Neuroscience and Biobehavioral Reviews, 31*, 858–873.

Post, R. M. (2007b). Role of BDNF in bipolar and unipolar disorder: Clinical and theoretical implications. *Journal of Psychiatry Research, 41*, 971–990.

Post, R. M. (2009). Etiology. In R. A. Kowatch, M. A. Fristad, R. L. Findling, & R. M. Post (Eds.), *Clinical manual for management of bipolar disorder in children and adolescents* (pp. 71–131). Arlington, VA: American Psychiatric Publishing.

Post, R. M., & Miklowitz, D. J. (2010). The role of stress in the onset, course, and progression of bipolar illness and its comorbidities. In D. J. Miklowitz & D. Cicchetti (Eds.), *Understanding bipolar disorder: A developmental psychopathology perspective* (pp. 370–413). New York: Guilford Press.

Reeves, G. M., Postolache, T. T., & Snitker, S. (2008). Childhood obesity and depression: Connection between these growing problems in growing children. *International Journal of Child Health and Human Development, 1*, 103–114.

Rich, B. A., Fromm, S. J., Berghorst, L. H., Dickstein, D. P., Brotman, M. A., Pine, D. S., et al.. (2008). Neural connectivity in children with bipolar disorder: Impairment in the face emotion processing circuit. *Journal of Child Psychology and Psychiatry, 49*, 88–96.

Riggs, N. R., Jahromi, L. B., Razza, R. P., Dillworth-Bart, J. E., & Mueller, U. (2006). Executive function and the promotion of social-emotional competence. *Journal of Applied Developmental Psychology, 27*(4), 300–309.

Rosenberg, D. R., MacMaster, F. P., Mirza, Y., Smith, J. M., Easter, P. C., Banerjee, S. P., et al. (2005). Reduced anterior cingulate glutamate in pediatric major depression: A magnetic resonance spectroscopy study. *Biological Psychiatry, 58*, 700–704.

Rosso, I. M., Cintron, C. M., Steingard, R. J., Renshaw, P. F., Young, A. D., & Yurgelun-Todd, D. A. (2005). Amygdala and hippocampus volumes in pediatric major depression. *Biological Psychiatry, 57*(1), 21–26.

Schachter, H., Kourad, K., Merali, Z., Lumb, A., Tran, K., Miguelez, M., et al. (2005). *Effects of omega-3 fatty acids on mental health* (Evidence Report/Technology Assessment No. 116, prepared by the University of Ottawa Evidence-Based Practice Center under Contract No. 290-02-0021, AHRQ Publication No. 05-E022-2). Rockville, MD: Agency for Healthcare Research and Quality.

Schenkel, L. S., Marlow-O'Connor, M., Moss, M., Sweeney, J. A., & Pavuluri, M. N. (2008). Theory of mind and social inference in children and adolescents with bipolar disorder. *Psychological Medicine, 38*(6), 791–800.

Schnoes, C. J., Kuhn, B. R., Workman, E. F., & Ellis, C. R. (2006). Pediatric prescribing practices for clonidine and other pharmacologic agents for children with sleep disturbance. *Clinical Pediatrics, 45*, 229–238.

Schwartz, C. E., Dorer, D. J., Beardslee, W. R., Lavori, P. W., & Keller, M. B. (1990). Maternal expressed emotion and paternal affective disorder: Risk for childhood depressive disorder, substance abuse or conduct disorder. *Journal of Psychiatric Research, 24*, 231–250.

Serene, J. A., Ashtari, M., Szeszko, P. R., & Kumra, S. (2007). Neuroimaging studies of children with serious emotional disturbances: A selective review. *Canadian Journal of Psychiatry, 52*, 135–145.

Simmons, M. (2003). Nutritional approach to bipolar disorder [Comment]. *Journal of Clinical Psychiatry, 64*(3), 338.

Stark, K. D., Hargrave, J., Janay, S., Custer, G., Schnoebelen, S., Simpson, J., et al.. (2006). Treatment of childhood depression: The ACTION Treatment Program. In P. Kendall (Ed.), *Child and adolescent therapy: Cognitive-behavioral procedures* (3rd ed., pp. 169–216). New York: Guilford Press.

Stark, K. D., Reynolds, W. M., & Kaslow, N. J. (1987). A comparison of the relative efficacy of self-control therapy and behavioral problem-solving therapy for depression in children. *Journal of Abnormal Child Psychology, 15*(1), 91–113.

Stathopoulou, G., Powers, M. B., Berry, A. C., & Smits, J. A. J., & Otto, M. W. (2006). Exercise interventions for mental health: A quantitative and qualitative review. *Clinical Psychology: Science and Practice, 13*, 179–193.

Staton, D. (2008). The impairment of pediatric bipolar sleep: Hypotheses regarding a core defect and phenotype-specific sleep disturbances. *Journal of Affective Disorders, 108*, 199–206.

Steingard, R., Renshaw, P., Yurgelun-Todd, D., Appelmans, K., Lyoo, I., Shorrock, K. et al. (1996). Structural abnormalities in brain magnetic resonance images of depressed children. *Journal of the American Academy of Child and Adolescent Psychiatry, 35*(3), 307–311.

Strober, M., & Carlson, G. (1982). Predictors of bipolar illness in adolescents with major depression: A follow-up investigation. *Adolescent Psychiatry, 10*, 299–319.

Ströhle, A., Höfler, M., Pfister, H., Müller, A., Hoyer, J., Wittchen, H., et al.. (2007). Physical activity an prevalence and incidence of mental disorders in adolescents and young adults. *Psychological Medicine, 37,* 1657–1666.

Tompson, M. C., Pierre, C. B., McNeil Haber, F., Fogler, J. M., Groff, A., & Asarnow, J. R. (2007). Family-focused treatment for childhood-onset depressive disorders: Results of an open trial. *Clinical Child Psychology and Psychiatry, 12,* 403–420.

Trowell, J., Joffe, I., Campbell, J., Clemente, C., Almqvist, F., Soininen, M., et al. (2007). Childhood depression: A place for psychotherapy. *European Child and Adolescent Psychiatry, 16,* 157–167.

Tsuang, M. T. & Faraone, S. V. (1990). *The genetics of mood disorders.* Baltimore: Johns Hopkins University Press.

U.S. Food and Drug Administration (FDA). (2004). Relationship between psychotropic drugs and pediatric suicidality: Review and evaluation of clinical data. Retrieved June 2, 2008, from *www.fda.gov/ohrms/dockets/ ac/04/briefing/2004-4065b1-10-TAB08-Hammads-Review.pdf*

Vygotsky, L. (1978). *Mind in society: The development of higher mental processes.* Cambridge, MA: Harvard University Press.

Wagner, K. D., Kowatch, R. A., Emslie, G. J., Findling, R. L., Wilens, T. E., McCague, K., S'Souza, J., Wamil, A., Lehman, R. B., Berv, D., & Linden, D. (2006). A double-blind, randomized, placebo-controlled trial of oxcarbazepine in the treatment of bipolar disorder in children and adolescents. *American Journal of Psychiatry, 163*(7), 1179–1186.

Wehr, T. A., Turner, E. H., Shimada, J. M., Lowe, C. H., Barker, C., & Leibenluft, E. (1998). Treatment of a rapidly cycling bipolar patient by using extended bed rest and darkness to stabilize the timing and duration of sleep. *Biological Psychiatry, 43*(11), 822–828.

Weisler, R. H., Cutler, A. J., Ballenger, J. C., Post, R. M., & Ketter, T. A. (2006). The use of antiepileptic drugs in bipolar disorders: a review based on evidence from controlled trials. *CNS Spectrums, 11,* 788–799.

Weisz, J. R., Thurber, C. A., Sweeney, L., Proffitt, V. D., & LeGagnoux, G. L. (1997). Brief treatment of mild-to-moderate child depression using primary and secondary control enhancement training. *Journal of Consulting and Clinical Psychology, 65*(4), 703–707.

White, M., & Epston, D. (1990). *Narrative means to therapeutic ends.* New York: Norton.

Wilens, T. (2009). *Straight talk about psychiatric medications for kids* (3rd ed.). New York: Guilford Press.

Wiles, N. J., Jones, G. T., Haase, A. M., Lawlor, D. A., Macfarlane, G. J., & Lewis, G. (2008). Physical activity and emotional problems amongst adolescents. *Social Psychiatry and Psychiatric Epidemiology, 43,* 765–772.

Yu, D. L., & Seligman, P. (2002). Preventing depressive symptoms in Chinese children. *Prevention and Treatment, 5*(1), no pagination specified.

Zuckerman, E. L. (2010). *Clinician's thesaurus: The guide to conducting interviews and writing psychological reports* (7th ed.). New York: Guilford Press.

Index